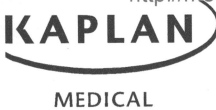

KAPLAN

MEDICAL

USMLE®
STEP 1 | Anatomy
Lecture Notes
2016

Editors

James White, Ph.D.
Assistant Professor of Cell Biology
School of Osteopathic Medicine
Rowan University
Stratford, NJ

Adjunct Assistant Professor of Cell and Developmental Biology
University of Pennsylvania School of Medicine
Philadelphia, PA

David Seiden, Ph.D.
Professor of Neuroscience and Cell Biology
Rutgers-Robert Wood Johnson Medical School
Piscataway, NJ

Contents

Preface

These volumes of Lecture Notes represent the most-likely-to-be-tested material on the current USMLE Step 1 exam.

We want to hear what you think. What do you like about the Notes? What could be improved? Please share your feedback by e-mailing us at **medfeedback@kaplan.com**.

Best of luck on your Step 1 exam!

Kaplan Medical

KAPLAN) MEDICAL vii

SECTION

I

Early Embryology and Histology: Epithelia

Gonad Development

1

Learning Objectives

❏ Explain information related to indifferent gonad

❏ Interpret scenarios on testis and ovary

❏ Answer questions about meiosis

❏ Interpret scenarios on spermatogenesis

❏ Solve problems concerning oogenesis

INDIFFERENT GONAD

Although sex is determined at fertilization, the gonads initially go through an **indifferent stage** between weeks 4 and 7 when there are no specific ovarian or testicular characteristics.

The indifferent gonads develop in a longitudinal elevation or ridge of **intermediate mesoderm** called the **urogenital ridge**.

Primordial Germ Cells

Primordial germ cells arise from the lining cells in the **wall of the yolk sac**.

At week 4, primordial germ cells migrate into the indifferent gonad.

Components of the Indifferent Gonad

- **Primordial germ cells** migrate into the gonad from the yolk sac and provide a critical inductive influence on gonad development.
- **Primary sex cords** are fingerlike extensions of the surface epithelium that grow into the gonad that are populated by the migrating primordial germ cells.
- **Mesonephric (Wolffian)** and the **paramesonephric (Mullerian)** ducts of the indifferent gonad contribute to the male and female genital tracts, respectively.

KAPLAN) MEDICAL   **3**

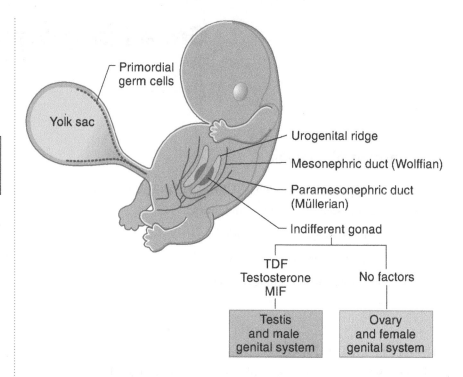

MIF: Müllerian-inhibiting factor

TDF: testis-determining factor

Figure I-1-1. Development of Testis and Ovary

TESTIS AND OVARY

The indifferent gonad will develop into either the testis or ovary (Figure I-1-1).

Testis

Development of the testis and male reproductive system is directed by:

- The **Sry gene** on the short arm of the **Y chromosome**, which encodes for **testis-determining factor** (TDF)
- **Testosterone**, which is secreted by the **Leydig cells**
- **Müllerian-inhibiting factor** (MIF), which is secreted by the **Sertoli cells**
- **Dihydrotestosterone (DHT):** external genitalia

Ovary

Development of the female reproductive system requires estrogen.

MEIOSIS

Meiosis occurs within the testis and ovary. This is a specialized process of cell division that produces the male gamete (**spermatogenesis**) and female gamete (**oogenesis**). There are notable differences between spermatogenesis and oogenesis, discussed below.

Meiosis consists of 2 cell divisions, meiosis I and meiosis II (Figure I-1-2).

Meiosis I

In meiosis I, the following events occur:

- **Synapsis**—the pairing of 46 homologous chromosomes
- **Crossing over**—the exchange of segments of DNA
- **Disjunction**—the separation of 46 homologous chromosome pairs (no centromere-splitting) into 2 daughter cells, each containing 23 chromosome pairs

Meiosis II

In meiosis II:

- Synapsis does not occur.
- Crossing over does not occur.
- Disjunction occurs **with** centromere-splitting.

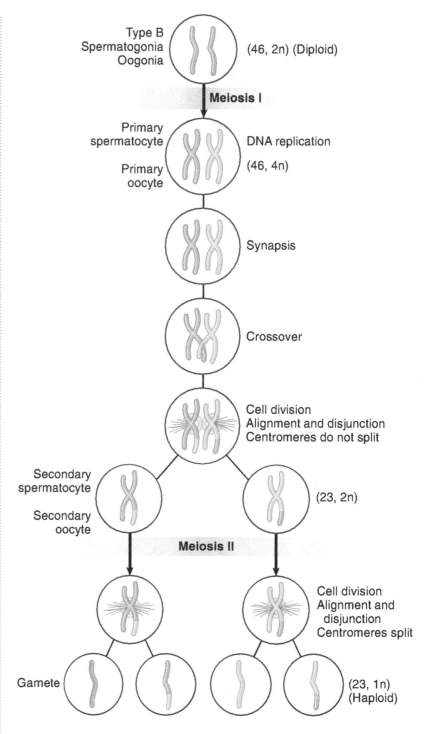

Figure I-1-2. Meiosis

SPERMATOGENESIS

- Primordial germ cells arrive in the indifferent gonad at week 4 and remain **dormant until puberty.**
- When a boy reaches puberty, primordial germ cells differentiate into **type A spermatogonia,** which serve as stem cells throughout adult life.
- Some type A spermatogonia differentiate into **type B spermatogonia.**
- Type B spermatogonia enter meiosis I to form **primary spermatocytes.**
- Primary spermatocytes form 2 **secondary spermatocytes.**
- Secondary spermatocytes enter meiosis II to form 2 **spermatids.**
- Spermatids undergo **spermiogenesis,** which is a series of morphological changes resulting in the mature **spermatozoa.**

OOGENESIS

- Primordial germ cells arrive in the indifferent gonad at week 4 and differentiate into oogonia.
- Oogonia enter meiosis I to form **primary oocytes.** All primary oocytes are formed by **month 5 of fetal life** and are **arrested the first time in prophase (diplotene) of meiosis I** and remain arrested until puberty.
- Primary oocyte arrested in meiosis I are present at birth.
- When a girl reaches puberty, during each monthly cycle a primary oocyte becomes unarrested and completes meiosis I to form a secondary oocyte and polar body.
- The secondary oocyte becomes **arrested the second time in metaphase of meiosis II** and is ovulated.
- At fertilization within the uterine tube, the secondary oocyte completes meiosis II to form a **mature oocyte** and **polar body.**

Chapter Summary

- The indifferent gonad begins development in a column of intermediate mesoderm called the urogenital ridge during week 4. Primordial germ cells arise in the wall of the yolk sac and migrate to the indifferent gonad.

  - In the male, a testis develops from the indifferent gonad due to the presence of testis-determining factor (TDF), which is produced on the short arm of the Y chromosome. Testosterone secreted by the Leydig cells and Müllerian-inhibiting factor (MIF) secreted by the Sertoli cells also contribute to the development of the genital system.

  - In the female, an ovary develops in the absence of any factors.

- Meiosis is a specialized type of cell division that produces the male and female gametes during spermatogenesis and oogenesis, respectively. Meiosis consists of 2 cell divisions: meiosis I and meiosis II.

  - In meiosis I, the events include synapsis, exchange of DNA, and disjunction, resulting in a reduction from 46 to 23 chromosomes.

  - In meiosis II, there is a reduction of DNA from 2n to 1n.

- Oogenesis begins in the female during the early weeks of development, and by month 5 of fetal life all of the primary oocytes are formed and become arrested in prophase of meiosis I until puberty. After puberty, during each monthly menstrual cycle, a secondary oocyte develops in the Graafian follicle and is then arrested a second time in metaphase of meiosis II, which is then ovulated. Meiosis II is completed only if there is fertilization.

- In the male, spermatogenesis begins after puberty in the seminiferous tubules and moves through meiosis I and II without any arrested phases to produce spermatids. Spermatids undergo spermiogenesis to develop into the adult spermatozoa.

Week 1: Beginning of Development

2

Learning Objectives

❑ Solve problems concerning beginning of development

BEGINNING OF DEVELOPMENT

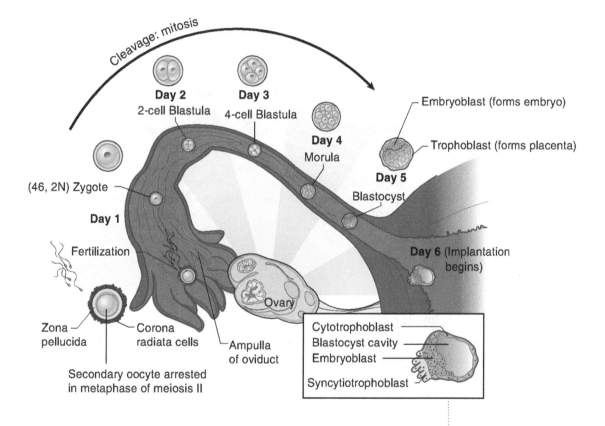

Figure I-2-1. Week 1

Fertilization occurs in the **ampulla of the uterine tube** when the male and female pronuclei fuse to form a **zygote**. At fertilization, the secondary oocyte rapidly completes meiosis II.

Prior to fertilization, spermatozoa undergo 2 changes in the female genital tract:

1. **Capacitation:** Occurs over about 7 hours in the female reproductive tract and consists of the removal of several proteins from the plasma membrane of the acrosome of the spermatozoa.

2. **Acrosome Reaction**: Release of hydrolytic enzymes from the acrosome used by the sperm to penetrate the zona pellucida. This results in a **cortical reaction** that prevents other spermatozoa penetrating the zona pellucida thus preventing polyspermy.

During the first 4 to 5 days of the first week, the zygote undergoes rapid mitotic division (**cleavage**) in the oviduct to form a **blastula**, consisting of increasingly smaller **blastomeres**. This becomes the **morula** (32-cell stage).

A **blastocyst** forms as fluid develops in the morula. The blastocyst consists of an inner cell mass known as the **embryoblast**, and the outer cell mass known as the **trophoblast**, which becomes the placenta.

At the end of the first week, the trophoblast differentiates into the **cytotrophoblast** and **syncytiotrophoblast** and then implantation begins (see below).

Clinical Correlate

Ectopic Pregnancy

Tubal

- The **most common form** of ectopic pregnancy; usually occurs when the blastocyst **implants within the ampulla** of the uterine tube because of delayed transport
- **Risk factors:** endometriosis, pelvic inflammatory disease (PID), tubular pelvic surgery, or exposure to diethylstilbestrol (DES)
- **Clinical signs:** abnormal or brisk uterine bleeding, sudden onset of abdominal pain that may be confused with appendicitis, missed menstrual period (e.g., LMP 60 days ago), positive human chorionic gonadotropin (hCG) test, culdocentesis showing intraperitoneal blood, positive sonogram

Abdominal

- Most commonly occurs in the **rectouterine pouch** (pouch of Douglas)

Implantation

The **zona pellucida** must degenerate for implantation to occur.

The blastocyst usually implants within the **posterior wall of the uterus.**

The embryonic pole of blastocyst implants first.

The blastocyst implants within the **functional layer** of the endometrium during the **progestational phase** of the menstrual cycle.

Chapter Summary

- Fertilization occurs in the ampulla of the uterine tube with the fusion of the male and female pronuclei to form a zygote. During the first 4–5 days of the first week, the zygote undergoes rapid mitotic division (cleavage) in the oviduct to form a morula before entering the cavity of the uterus.

- A blastocyst forms as fluid develops in the morula, resulting in a blastocyst that consists of an inner cell mass known as the embryoblast (becomes the embryo) and the outer cell mass known as the trophoblast (becomes the placenta). At the end of the first week, the trophoblast differentiates into the cytotrophoblast and syncytiotrophoblast and then implantation begins.

Week 2: 3
Formation of the Bilaminar Embryo

Learning Objectives

❑ Demonstrate understanding of the formation of the bilaminar embryo

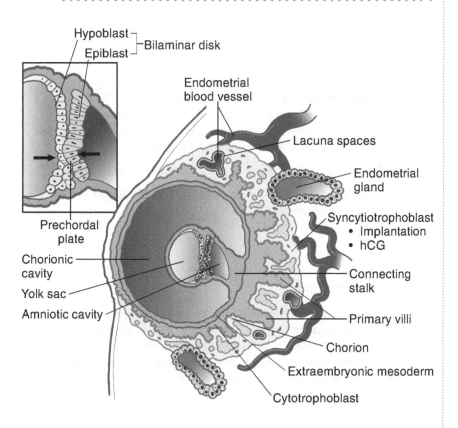

Figure I-3-1. Week 2

- The embryoblast differentiates into the **epiblast** and **hypoblast**, forming a **bilaminar embryonic disk**.
- The epiblast forms the **amniotic cavity** and hypoblast cells migrate to form the **primary yolk sac**.
- The **prechordal plate**, formed from fusion of epiblast and hypoblast cells, is the site of the future **mouth**.

Extraembryonic mesoderm is derived from the epiblast. **Extraembryonic somatic mesoderm** lines the cytotrophoblast, forms the connecting stalk, and covers the amnion. **Extraembryonic visceral mesoderm** covers the yolk sac.

The connecting stalk suspends the conceptus within the chorionic cavity. The wall of the chorionic cavity is called the **chorion**, consisting of extraembryonic somatic mesoderm, the cytotrophoblast, and the syncytiotrophoblast.

The **syncytiotrophoblast** continues its growth into the endometrium to make contact with endometrial blood vessels and glands. **No mitosis occurs in the syncytiotrophoblast.** The cytotrophoblast is mitotically active.

Hematopoiesis occurs initially in the mesoderm surrounding the yolk sac (up to 6 weeks) and later in the fetal liver, spleen, thymus (6 weeks to third trimester), and bone marrow.

Clinical Correlate

Human chorionic gonadotropin (hCG) is a glycoprotein produced by the syncytiotrophoblast. It stimulates progesterone production by the corpus luteum. hCG can be assayed in maternal blood or urine and is the basis for early pregnancy testing. hCG is detectable throughout pregnancy.

- **Low hCG** levels may predict a spontaneous abortion or ectopic pregnancy.

- **High hCG** levels may predict a multiple pregnancy, hydatidiform mole, or gestational trophoblastic disease.

Chapter Summary

- In the second week, implantation is completed with the rapid growth and erosion of the syncytiotrophoblast into the endometrium of the uterus where early utero-placental circulation is established. The inner cell mass of the first week differentiates into the epiblast and hypoblast cells and forms a bilaminar embryonic disk. An amniotic cavity develops from the epiblast and the primary yolk sac replaces the blastocyst cavity.

- The extraembryonic mesoderm and chorion are formed in the second week.

Embryonic Period (Weeks 3–8)

4

Learning Objectives

❏ Solve problems concerning embryonic period

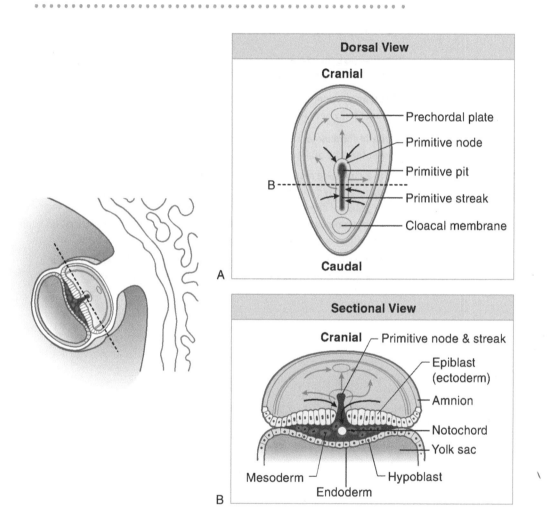

Figure I-4-1. Week 3

- **Gastrulation**—process that produces the 3 primary germ layers: **ecto-derm**, **mesoderm**, and **endoderm**; begins with the formation of the **primitive streak** within the epiblast

- Ectoderm forms **neuroectoderm** and **neural crest cells.**

- Mesoderm forms **paraxial mesoderm** (35 pairs of somites), **intermedi-ate mesoderm**, and **lateral mesoderm.**

- All major organ systems begin to develop during the **embryonic period** (weeks 3–8). By the end of this period, the embryo begins to look human.

- **Third week:** Gastrulation and early development of nervous and cardio-vascular systems; corresponds to first missed period.

Clinical Correlate

Sacrococcygeal teratoma: a tumor that arises from remnants of the primitive streak; often contains various types of tissue (bone, nerve, hair, etc)

Chordoma: a tumor that arises from remnants of the notochord, found either intracranially or in the sacral region

Hydatidiform mole: results from the partial or complete replacement of the trophoblast by dilated villi

- In a **complete mole, there is no embryo;** a haploid sperm fertilizes a blighted ovum and reduplicates so that the karyotype is 46,XX, with all chromosomes of paternal origin. In a **partial mole,** there is a haploid set of maternal chromosomes and usually 2 sets of paternal chromosomes so that the typical karyotype is 69,XXY.

- **Molar pregnancies have high levels of hCG, and 20% develop into a malignant trophoblastic disease, including choriocarcinoma.**

complete ⟹ no ova / 2 sperm
46XX ~~69XX~~

incomplete ⟹ 2 sperm + ova
69XXY

Table I-4-1. Germ Layer Derivatives

Ectoderm	Mesoderm	Endoderm
Surface ectoderm	**Muscle**	**Forms epithelial lining of:**
Epidermis	Smooth	GI track: foregut, midgut, and hindgut
Hair	Cardiac	Lower respiratory system: larynx, trachea, bronchi, and lung
Nails	Skeletal	
Inner ear, external ear	Connective tissue	Genitourinary system: urinary bladder, urethra, and lower vagina
Enamel of teeth	All serous membranes	
Lens of eye	Bone and cartilage	Pharyngeal pouches:
Anterior pituitary (Rathke's pouch)	Blood, lymph, cardiovascular organs	• Auditory tube and middle ear
Parotid gland		• Palatine tonsils
Anal canal below pectinate line	Adrenal cortex	• Parathyroid glands
	Gonads and internal reproductive organs	• Thymus
Neuroectoderm		**Forms parenchyma of:**
Neural tube	Spleen	• Liver
Central nervous system	Kidney and ureter	• Pancreas
Retina and optic nerve	Dura mater	• Submandibular and sublingual glands
Pineal gland		• Follicles of thyroid gland
Neurohypophysis		
Astrocytes		
Oligodendrocytes		
	Notochord	
Neural crest ectoderm	Nucleus pulposus	
Adrenal medulla		
Ganglia		
Sensory—Pseudounipolar Neurons		
Autonomic—Postganglionic Neurons		
Pigment cells		
Schwann cells		
Meninges		
Pia and arachnoid mater		
Pharyngeal arch cartilage		
Odontoblasts		
Parafollicular (C) cells		
Aorticopulmonary septum		
Endocardial cushions		

Yolk sac derivatives:

Primordial germ cells

Early blood cells and blood vessels

Chapter Summary

- The critical events of the third week are gastrulation and early development of the nervous and cardiovascular systems. Gastrulation is the process which establishes 3 primary germ layers that derive from epiblast: ectoderm, mesoderm, and endoderm. Gastrulation begins with the development of the primitive streak and node. The adult derivatives of ectoderm, mesoderm, and endoderm are given in Table I-4-1.

Histology: Epithelia 5

Learning Objectives

❏ Demonstrate understanding of epithelial cells

❏ Use knowledge of epithelium

❏ Interpret scenarios on cytoskeletal elements

❏ Explain information related to cell adhesion molecules

❏ Answer questions about cell surface specializations

Histology is the study of normal tissues. Groups of cells make up tissues, tissues form organs, organs form organ systems, and systems make up the organism. Each organ consists of 4 different types of tissue: epithelial, connective, nervous, and muscular. Only certain aspects of epithelia will be reviewed in the Anatomy Lecture Notes; other aspects of cell biology and histology are reviewed elsewhere.

EPITHELIAL CELLS

Epithelial cells are often polarized: the structure, composition, and function of the apical surface membrane differ from those of the basolateral surfaces. The polarity is established by the presence of tight junctions that separate these 2 regions. Internal organelles are situated symmetrically in the cell. Membrane polarity and tight junctions are essential for the transport functions of epithelia. Many simple epithelia transport substances from one side to the other (kidney epithelia transport salts and sugars; intestinal epithelia transport nutrients, antibodies, etc.). There are 2 basic mechanisms used for these transports:

1. A transcellular pathway through which larger molecules and a combination of diffusion and pumping in the case of ions that pass through the cell, and

2. A paracellular pathway that permits movement between cells.

Tight junctions regulate the paracellular pathway, because they prevent backflow of transported material and keep basolateral and apical membrane components separate.

Epithelial polarity is essential to the proper functioning of epithelial cells; and when polarity is disrupted, disease can develop. For example, epithelia lining the trachea, bronchi, intestine, and pancreatic ducts transport chloride from basolateral surface to lumen via pumps in the basolateral surface and channels in the apical surface. The transport provides a driving force for Na by producing electrical polarization of the epithelium. Thus NaCl moves across, and water follows. In cystic fibrosis the apical Cl channels do not open. Failure of water transport results in thickening of the mucus layer covering the epithelia.

Transformed cells may lose their polarized organization, and this change can be easily detected by using antibodies against proteins specific for either the apical or basolateral surfaces. Loss of polarity in the distribution of membrane proteins may eventually become useful as an early index of neoplasticity.

Epithelia are always lined on the basal side by connective tissue containing blood vessels. Since epithelia are avascular, interstitial tissue fluids provide epithelia with oxygen and nutrients.

Epithelia modify the 2 compartments that they separate by either secreting into or absorbing from them and by selective transport of solutes from one side of the barrier to the other.

Epithelia renew themselves continuously, some very rapidly (skin and intestinal linings), some at a slower rate. This means that the tissue contains stem cells that continuously proliferate. The daughter cells resulting from each cell division either remain in the pool of dividing cells or differentiate.

Epithelial Subtypes

- Simple cuboidal epithelium (e.g., renal tubules, salivary gland acini)
- Simple columnar epithelium (e.g., small intestine)
- Simple squamous epithelium (e.g., endothelium, mesothelium, epithelium lining the inside of the renal glomerular capsule)
- Stratified squamous epithelium
  - Nonkeratinized (e.g., esophagus)
  - Keratinizing (e.g., skin)
- Pseudostratified columnar epithelium (e.g., trachea, epididymis)
- Transitional epithelium (urothelium) (e.g., ureter and bladder)
- Stratified cuboidal epithelium (e.g., salivary gland ducts)

EPITHELIUM

Hematoxylin-and-Eosin Staining

The most common way to stain tissues for viewing in the light microscope is to utilize hematoxylin-and-eosin (H&E) staining.

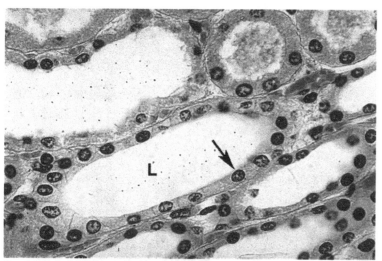

Figure I-5-1. Kidney tubule simple cuboidal epithelium (arrow)
stained with H&E, L-lumen

Hematoxylin is a blue dye which stains basophilic substrates that are the acidic cellular components such as DNA and RNA. Hematoxylin stains nuclei blue, and may tint the cytoplasm of cells with extensive mRNA in their cytoplasm.

Eosin is a pink-to-orange dye which stains acidophilic substrates such as basic components of most proteins. Eosin stains the cytoplasm of most cells and many extracellular proteins, such as collagen, pink.

Epithelial Types

Simple columnar epithelium is found in the small and large intestine.

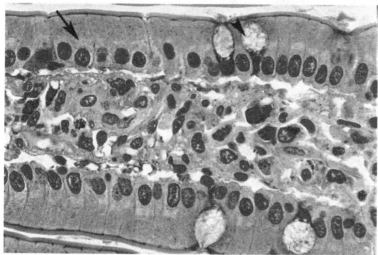

Figure I-5-2. Small Intestine Simple Columnar Epithelium

Enterocytes (arrow), Goblet cells (arrowhead)

Simple squamous epithelium forms an endothelium that lines blood vessels, a mesothelium that forms part of a serous membrane or forms the epithelium lining of the inside of the renal glomerular capsule.

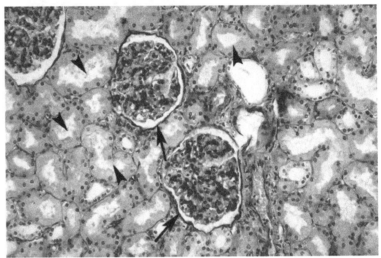

Figure I-5-3. Kidney simple squamous epithelium (arrows),
simple cuboidal epithelium (arrowheads)

Pseudostratified columnar epithelium is found in the nasal cavity, trachea, bronchi, and epididymis.

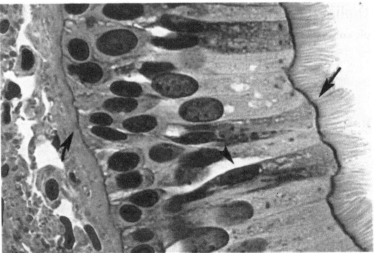

Figure I-5-4. Trachea pseudostratified columnar epithelium with
true cilia (arrow) and goblet cells (arrowhead), basement
membrane (curved arrow)

Transitional epithelium is found in the ureter and bladder.

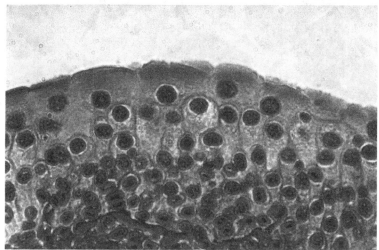

Copyright McGraw-Hill Companies. Used with permission.

Figure I-5-5. Bladder Transitional Epithelium

Stratified squamous epithelium is found in the oral cavity, pharynx, and esophagus (non-keratinized) and in the skin (keratinizing).

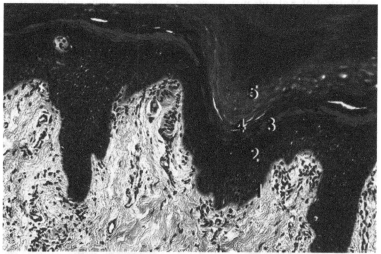

Copyright McGraw-Hill Companies. Used with permission.

Figure I-5-6. Stratified Squamous Epithelium (Thick Skin)

(1) stratum basale (2) stratum spinosum (3) stratum granulosum
(4) stratum lucidum (5) stratum corneum

Simple cuboidal epithelium is the epithelium of the renal tubules and the secretory cells of salivary gland acini.

Stratified cuboidal epithelium is found in the ducts of salivary glands.

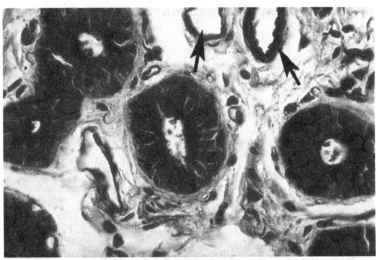

Figure I-5-7. Ducts of salivary gland with stratified cuboidal epithelium small blood vessels with endothelium and smooth muscle (arrows)

Glands

- **Unicellular glands** are goblet cells found in the respiratory and GI epithelium.
- **Multicellular glands** may be exocrine (such as a salivary gland) or endocrine (as in the thyroid gland). All multicellular glands have tubules or acini formed mainly by a simple cuboidal epithelium. Only exocrine glands have ducts, which serve as conduits for glandular secretions to a body surface or to a lumen.

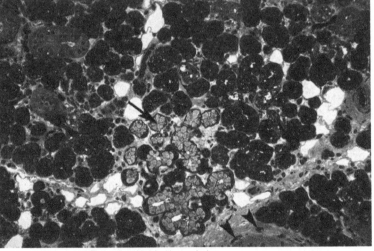

Figure I-5-8. Submandibular gland

This gland is a mixed salivary gland with mucus acini (arrow) and darker staining serous acini; small blood vessels (arrowheads)

CYTOSKELETAL ELEMENTS

Microfilaments

Microfilaments are actin proteins. They are composed of globular monomers of G-actin that polymerize to form helical filaments of F-actin. Actin polymerization is ATP dependent. The F-actin filaments are 7-nm-diameter filaments that are constantly ongoing assembly and disassembly. F-actin has a distinct polarity. The barbed end (the plus end) is the site of polymerization and the pointed end is the site of depolymerization. Tread milling is the balance in the activity at the 2 ends.

In conjunction with myosin, actin microfilaments provide contractile and motile forces of cells including the formation of a contractile ring that provides a basis for cytokinesis during mitosis and meiosis. Actin filaments are linked to cell membranes at tight junctions and at the zonula adherens, and form the core of microvilli.

Intermediate Filaments

Intermediate filaments are 10-nm-diameter filaments that are usually stable once formed. These filaments provide structural stability to cells. There are 4 groups of intermediate filaments:

- **Type I** is keratins. Keratins are found in all epithelial cells.
- **Type II** is intermediate filaments comprising a diverse group.
  - Desmin is found in skeletal, cardiac, and gastrointestinal (GI) tract smooth muscle cells.
  - Vimentin is found in most fibroblasts, fibrocytes, endothelial cells, and vascular smooth muscle.
  - Glial fibrillary acidic protein is found in astrocytes and some Schwann cells.
  - Peripherin is found in peripheral nerve axons.
- **Type III** is intermediate filaments forming neurofilaments in neurons.
- **Type IV** is 3 types of lamins which form a meshwork rather than individual filaments inside the nuclear envelope of all cells.

Clinical Correlate

A first step in the invasion of malignant cells through an epithelium results from a loss of expression of cadherins that weakens the epithelium.

Microtubules

Microtubules consist of 25-nm-diameter hollow tubes. Like actin, microtubules are undergoing continuous assembly and disassembly. They provide "tracks" for intracellular transport of vesicles and molecules. Such transport exists in all cells but is particularly important in axons. Transport requires specific ATPase motor molecules; **dynein** drives retrograde transport and **kinesin** drives anterograde transport. Microtubules are found in **true cilia and flagella,** and utilize dynein to convey motility to these structures. Microtubules form the mitotic spindle during mitosis and meiosis.

Clinical Correlate

Changes in intermediate filaments are evident in neurons in Alzheimer's disease and in cirrhotic liver diseases.

Clinical Correlate

Colchicine prevents microtubule polymerization and is used to prevent neutrophil migration in gout. Vinblastine and vincristine are used in cancer therapy because they inhibit the formation of the mitotic spindle.

CELL ADHESION MOLECULES

Cell adhesion molecules are surface molecules that allow cells to adhere to one another or to components of the extracellular matrix. The expression of adhesion molecules on the surface of a given cell may change with time, altering its interaction with adjacent cells or the extracellular matrix.

Cadherin and selectin are adhesion molecules that are **calcium ion-dependent**. The extracellular portion binds to a cadherin dimer on another cell (trans binding). The cytoplasmic portions of cadherins are linked to cytoplasmic actin filaments by the catenin complex of proteins.

Integrins are adhesion molecules that are **calcium-independent**. They are transmembrane surface molecules with extracellular domains which bind to fibronectin and laminin, that are components of extracellular basement membrane. The cytoplasmic portions of integrins bind to actin filaments. Integrins form a portion of hemidesmosomes but are also important in interactions between leukocytes and endothelial cells.

CELL SURFACE SPECIALIZATIONS

Cell Adhesion

A cell must physically interact via cell surface molecules with its external environment, whether it be the extracellular matrix or **basement membrane**. The basement membrane is a sheet-like structure underlying virtually all epithelia, which consists of **basal lamina** (made of type IV collagen, glycoproteins [e.g., laminin], and proteoglycans [e.g., heparin sulfate]), and **reticular lamina** (composed of reticular fibers). Cell junctions anchor cells to each other, seal boundaries between cells, and form channels for direct transport and communication between cells. The 3 types of junctional complexes include **anchoring, tight,** and **gap junctions**.

Cell Junctions

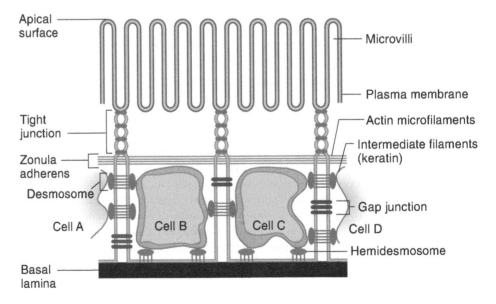

Figure I-5-9. Junctions

Tight junctions (zonula occludens) function as barriers to diffusion and determine cell polarity. They form a series of punctate contacts of adjacent epithelial cells near the apical end or luminal surface of epithelial cells. The major components of tight junctions are occludins (ZO-1,2,3) and claudin proteins. These proteins span between the adjacent cell membranes and their cytoplasmic parts bind to actin microfilaments.

Zonula adherens forms a belt around the entire apicolateral circumference of the cell, immediately below the tight junction of epithelium. Cadherins span between the cell membranes. Like the tight junctions immediately above them, the cytoplasmic parts of cadherins are associated with actin filaments.

Desmosomes (macula adherens) function as anchoring junctions. Desmosomes provide a structural and mechanical link between cells. Cadherins span between the cell membranes of desmosomes and internally desmosomes are anchored to intermediate filaments in large bundles called tonofilaments.

Hemidesmosomes adhere epithelial cells to the basement membrane. The basement membrane is a structure that consists of the basal membrane of a cell and 2 underlying extracellular components, the basal lamina and the reticular lamina. The basal lamina is a thin felt-like extracellular layer composed of predominantly of type IV collagen associated with laminin, proteoglycans, and fibronectin that are secreted by epithelial cells. Fibronectin binds to integrins on the cell membrane, and fibronectin and laminin in turn bind to collagen in the basal lamina. Internally, like a desmosome, the hemidesmosomes are linked to intermediate filaments. Below the basal lamina is the reticular lamina, composed of reticular fibers.

Through the binding of extracellular components of hemidesmosomes to integrins, and thus to fibronectin and laminin, the cell is attached to the basement membrane and therefore to the extracellular matrix components outside the basement membrane. These interactions between the cell cytoplasm and the extracellular matrix have implications for permeability, cell motility during embryogenesis, and cell invasion by malignant neoplasms.

Gap junctions (communicating junctions) function in cell-to-cell communication between the cytoplasm of adjacent cells by providing a passageway for ions such as calcium and small molecules such as cyclic adenosine monophosphate (cAMP). The transcellular channels that make up a gap junction consist of connexons, which are hollow channels spanning the plasma membrane. Each connexon consists of 6 connexin molecules. Unlike other intercellular junctions, gap junctions are not associated with any cytoskeletal filament.

Clinical Correlate

Pemphigus Vulgaris (autoantibodies against desmosomal proteins in skin cells)

- Painful flaccid bullae (blisters) in oropharynx and skin that rupture easily

- Postinflammatory hyperpigmentation

- Treatment: corticosteroids

Bullous Pemphigoid (autoantibodies against basement-membrane hemidesmosomal proteins)

- Widespread blistering with pruritus

- Less severe than pemphigus vulgaris

- Rarely affects oral mucosa

- Can be drug-induced (e.g., middle-aged or elderly patient on multiple medications)

- Treatment: corticosteroids

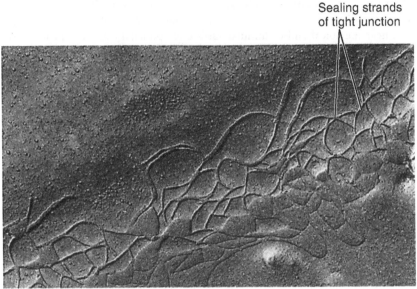

Sealing strands
of tight junction

Figure I-5-10. Freeze-fracture of tight junction

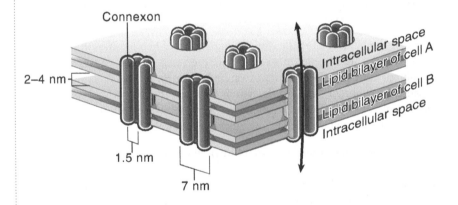

Figure I-5-11. Gap junction

Gap junctions—direct passage for small particles and ions between cells via **connexon** channel proteins

Microvilli

Microvilli contain a core of actin microfilaments and function to increase the absorptive surface area of an epithelial cell. They are found in columnar epithelial cells of the small and large intestine, cells of the proximal tubule of the kidney and on columnar epithelial respiratory cells.

Stereocilia are long, branched microvilli that are found in the male reproductive tract (e.g., epididymis). Short stereocilia cap all sensory cells in the inner ear.

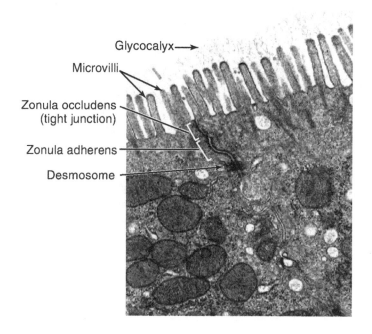

Figure I-5-12. Apical cell surface/cell junctions

Cilia

Cilia contain 9 peripheral pairs of microtubules and 2 central microtubules. The microtubules convey motility to cilia through the ATPase dynein. Cilia bend and beat on the cell surface of pseudostratified ciliated columnar respiratory epithelial cells to propel overlying mucus. They also form the core of the flagella, the motile tail of sperm cells.

Clinical Correlate

Kartagener syndrome is characterized by immotile spermatozoa and infertility. It is due to an absence of dynein that is required for flagellar motility. It is usually associated with chronic respiratory infections because of similar defects in cilia of respiratory epithelium.

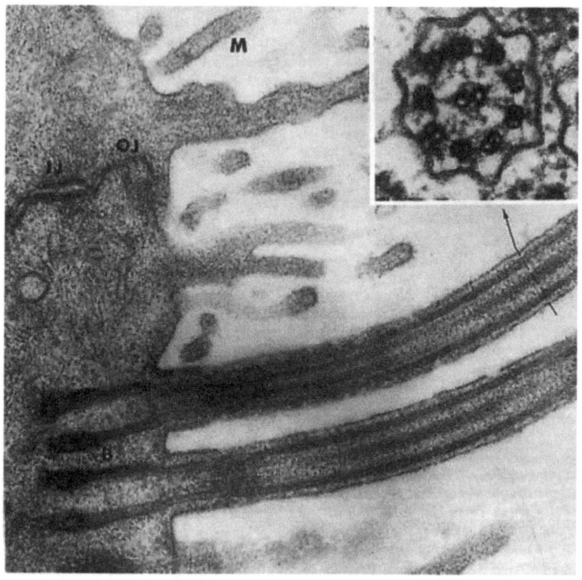

B = Basal body
IJ = Intermediate junction
M = Microvillus
OJ = Occluding junction

Figure I-5-13. Cilia

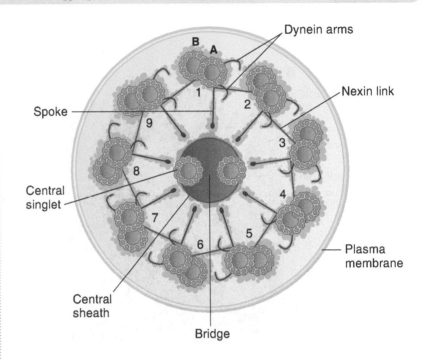

Figure I-5-14. Structure of the axoneme of a cilium

SECTION II

Gross Anatomy

Back and Autonomic Nervous System

1

Learning Objectives

❑ Solve problems concerning vertebral column

❑ Demonstrate understanding of spinal meninges

❑ Use knowledge of spinal nerves

❑ Use knowledge of autonomic nervous system

VERTEBRAL COLUMN

Embryology

During week 4, **sclerotome** cells of the somites (mesoderm) migrate medially to surround the spinal cord and notochord. After proliferation of the caudal portion of the sclerotomes, the vertebrae are formed, each consisting of the caudal part of one sclerotome and the cephalic part of the next.

Vertebrae

The vertebral column is the central component of the axial skeleton which functions in muscle attachments, movements, and articulations of the head and trunk.

- The vertebrae provide a flexible support system that transfers the weight of the body to the lower limbs and also provides protection for the spinal cord.

- The vertebral column (Figure II-1-1) is composed of 32–33 vertebrae (7 cervical, 12 thoracic, 5 lumbar, and the fused 5 sacral, and 3–4 coccygeal), intervertebral disks, synovial articulations (zygapophyseal joints) and ligaments.

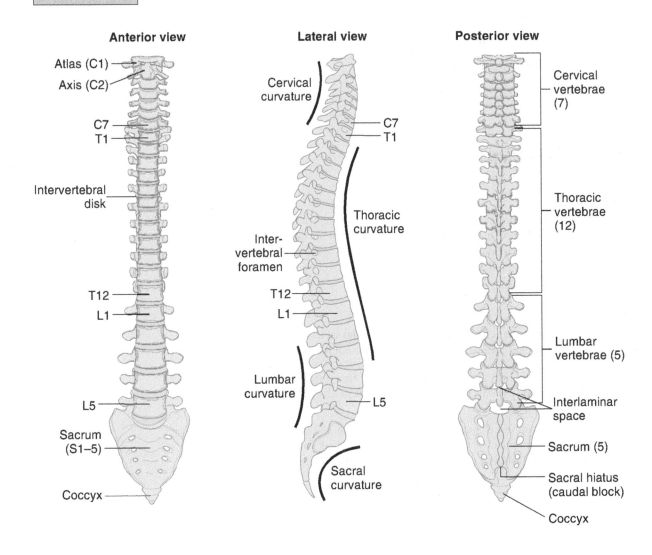

~33 vertebrae

31 spinal nerves

Anterior view

Atlas (C1)
Axis (C2)
C7
T1
Intervertebral disk
T12
L1
L5
Sacrum (S1–5)
Coccyx

Lateral view

Cervical curvature
C7
T1
Inter-vertebral foramen
Thoracic curvature
T12
L1
Lumbar curvature
L5
Sacral curvature

Posterior view

Cervical vertebrae (7)
Thoracic vertebrae (12)
Lumbar vertebrae (5)
Interlaminar space
Sacrum (5)
Sacral hiatus (caudal block)
Coccyx

Figure II-1-1. Vertebral Column

A **typical vertebra** (Figure II-1-2) consists of an anterior **body** and a posterior **vertebral arch** consisting of 2 **pedicles** and 2 **laminae**. The vertebral arch encloses the **vertebral (foramen) canal** that houses the spinal cord. **Vertebral notches** of adjacent pedicles form **intervertebral foramina** that provide for the exit of the spinal nerves. The dorsal projecting **spines** and the lateral projecting **transverse processes** provide attachment sites for muscles and ligaments.

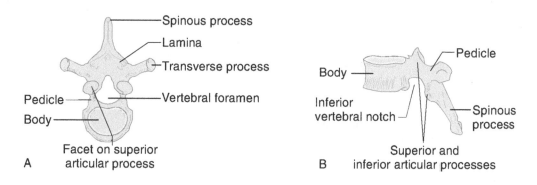

Figure II-1-2. Typical Vertebra

Intervertebral Disks

The **intervertebral disks** (Figure II-1-3) contribute to about 25% of the length of the vertebral column. They form the cartilaginous joints between the vertebral bodies and provide limited movements between the individual vertebrae.

- Each intervertebral disk is numbered by the vertebral body **above** the disk.
- Each intervertebral disk is composed of the following:
  - **Anulus fibrosus** consists of the outer concentric rings of fibrocartilage and fibrous connective tissue. The anuli connect the adjacent bodies and provide limited movement between the individual vertebrae.
  - **Nucleus pulposus** is an inner soft, elastic, compressible material that functions as a shock absorber for external forces placed on the vertebral column. The nucleus pulposus is the postnatal remnant of the **notochord**.

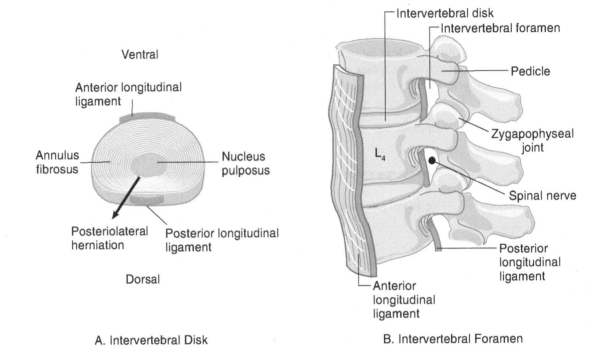

Figure II-1-3. Intervertebral Disks

Clinical Correlate

The herniation of a nucleus pulposus is most commonly in a **posterolateral** direction due to the strength and position of the posterior longitudinal ligament (Figure II-1-3-A).

Ligaments of the Vertebral Column

The vertebral bodies are strongly supported by 2 longitudinal ligaments (Figure II-1-3). Both ligaments are firmly attached to the intervertebral disks and to the bodies of the vertebrae.

- **Anterior longitudinal ligament:** The anterior ligament forms a broad band of fibers that connects the anterior surfaces of the bodies of the vertebrae between the cervical and sacral regions. It prevents **hyperextension** of the vertebrae and is often involved in "whiplash" accidents.

- **Posterior longitudinal ligament:** The posterior ligament connects the posterior surfaces of the vertebral bodies and is located in the vertebral canal. The posterior ligament limits **flexion** of the vertebral column. This ligament causes the herniation of a disk to be positioned **posterolaterally**.

post => Flexion
Ant => Extension

Herniated Disk

The **nucleus pulposus** may herniate through the **anulus fibrosus**. The herniated nucleus pulposus may compress the spinal nerve roots, resulting in pain along the involved spinal nerve (sciatica).

- Herniation usually occurs in the lower lumbar (L4/L5 or L5/S1) or lower cervical (C5/C6 or C6/C7) parts of the vertebral column.

- The herniated disk will usually compress the spinal nerve roots **one number below** (Figure II-1-4) the involved disk (e.g., the herniation of the L4 disk will compress the L5 roots, or herniation of the C7 disk will compress the C8 nerve roots).

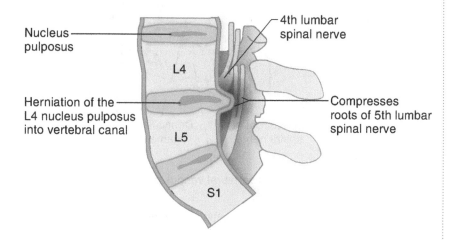

Figure II-1-4. Herniated Intervertebral Disk

Intervertebral Foramen

The intervertebral foramina (Figure II-1-3-B) are formed by successive intervertebral notches and provide for the passage of the **spinal nerve**. The boundaries of the foramina are:

- **Anterior: Bodies** of the vertebrae and **intervertebral disks**
- **Posterior: Zygapophyseal joint** and **articular processes**
- **Superior and inferior: Pedicles** of the vertebrae

SPINAL MENINGES

The spinal cord is protected and covered by 3 connective tissue layers within the vertebral canal: the pia mater, dura mater, and arachnoid (Figure II-1-5).

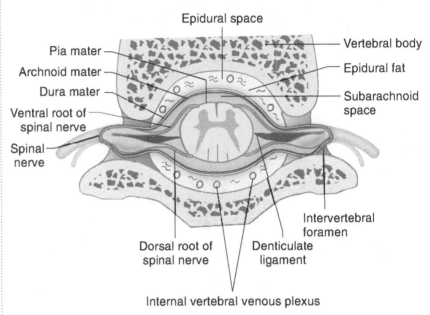

Figure II-1-5. Cross-Section of Vertebral Canal

Pia Mater

The **pia mater** is tightly attached to the surface of the spinal cord and provides a delicate covering of the cord.

- The spinal cord, with its covering of pia mater, terminates at the **L1 or L2 vertebral levels** in the adult.

- There are 2 specializations of the pia mater that are attached to the spinal cord:

  - The **denticulate ligaments** are bilateral thickenings of pia mater that run continuously on the lateral sides of the midpoint of the cord. They separate the ventral and dorsal roots of the spinal nerves and anchor to the dura mater.

  - The **filum terminale** is a continuation of the pia mater distal to the lower end of the spinal cord. The filum terminale is part of the **cauda equina** which is composed of ventral and dorsal roots of lumbar and sacral nerves that extend below the inferior limit of the spinal cord.

Dura Mater

The **dura mater** is a tough, cylindrical covering of connective tissue forming a **dural sac** which envelops the entire spinal cord and cauda equina.

- The dura mater and dural sac terminate inferiorly at the **second sacral vertebra level**.

- Superiorly, the dura mater continues through the foramen magnum and is continuous with the meningeal layer of the cranial dura.

Arachnoid

The **arachnoid** is a delicate membrane which completely lines the inner surface of the dura mater and dural sac. It continues inferiorly and terminates at the **second sacral vertebra**.

Two Spaces Related to the Meninges

The **epidural space** (Figure II-1-5) is located between the inner walls of the vertebral canal and the dura mater. It contains fat and the **internal vertebral venous plexus.** The venous plexus runs the entire length of the epidural space and continues superiorly through the foramen magnum to connect with dural venous sinuses in the cranial cavity.

The **subarachnoid space** (Figure II-1-5) is a pressurized space located between the arachnoid and pia mater layers. It contains **cerebrospinal fluid (CSF)**, which bathes the spinal cord and spinal nerve roots within the dural sac, and terminates at the **second sacral vertebral level**.

Clinical Correlate

The internal vertebral venous plexus is valveless and connects with veins of the pelvis, abdomen, and thorax. It provides a route of metastasis of cancer cells to the vertebral column and the cranial cavity.

Two Important Vertebral Levels

L1 or **L2** vertebrae: inferior limit of the **spinal cord** in adult (**conus medullaris**)

S2 vertebra: inferior limit of the **dural sac** and the **subarachnoid** space (cerebrospinal fluid)

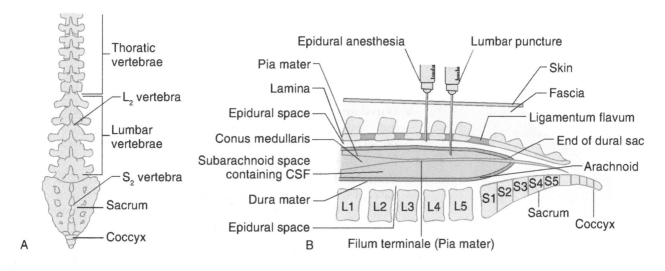

Figure II-1-6. Important Vertebral Levels

SPINAL NERVES

There are 31 pairs of **spinal nerves** (Figure II-1-7) attached to each of the segments of the spinal cord: 8 cervical, 12 thoracic, 5 lumbar, 5 sacral, and 1 coccygeal. The spinal nerves with the cranial nerves form part of the **peripheral nervous system**.

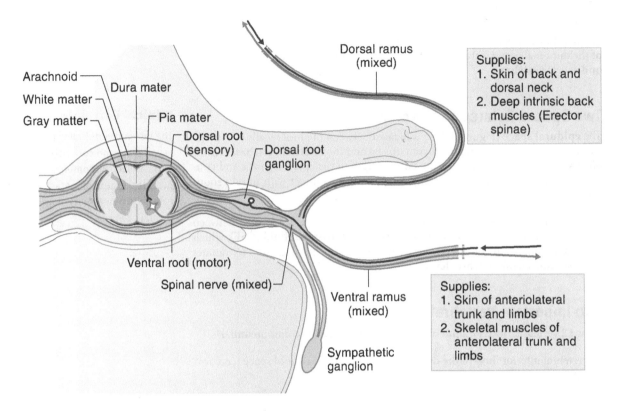

Figure II-1-7. Cross Section of Spinal Cord and Parts of Spinal Nerve

Each spinal nerve is formed by the following components (Figure II-1-7):

- **Dorsal root**: The dorsal root carries **sensory** fibers from the periphery into the dorsal aspect of the spinal cord. On each dorsal root there is a **dorsal root ganglion** (sensory) which contains the pseudounipolar cell bodies of the nerve fibers that are found in the dorsal root.

- **Ventral root**: The ventral root arises from the ventral aspect of the spinal cord and carries axons of **motor** neurons from the spinal cord to the periphery. The cell bodies of the axons in the ventral root are located in the ventral or lateral horns of the spinal- cord gray matter.

- **Spinal nerve**: The spinal nerve is formed by the union of the ventral and dorsal roots. The spinal nerve exits the vertebral column by passing through the intervertebral foramen.

- **Dorsal rami**: The dorsal rami innervate the skin of the dorsal surface of the back, neck, zygapophyseal joints, and intrinsic skeletal muscles of the deep back.

- **Ventral rami**: The ventral rami innervate the skin of the anterolateral trunk and limbs, and the skeletal muscles of the anterolateral trunk and limbs (ventral rami form the brachial and lumbosacral plexuses).

Relationship of Exit of Spinal Nerves and Vertebral Levels

The spinal nerves exit the vertebral column by a specific relationship to the vertebrae as described.

1. The cervical nerves C1–C7 exit the intervertebral foramina **superior** to the pedicles of the same-numbered vertebrae.

2. The C8 nerve exits the intervertebral foramen **inferior** to the C7 pedicle. This is the transition point.

3. All nerves beginning with T1 and below will exit the intervertebral foramina **inferior** to the pedicle of the same-numbered vertebrae.

Lumbar Puncture

A **lumbar puncture** is used to inject anesthetic material in the epidural space or to withdraw CSF from the subarachnoid space.

- A spinal tap is typically performed at the **L4-L5 interspace**.
- A horizontal line drawn at the **top of the iliac crest** marks the level of the L4 vertebra.
- When a lumbar puncture is performed in the midline, the needle passes through the **interlaminar space** of the vertebral column found between the laminae of the lumbar vertebrae (Figure II-1-8).
- The interlaminar spaces are covered by the highly elastic **ligamentum flava**.

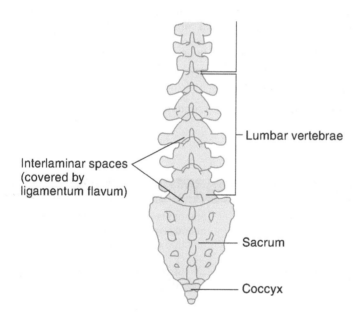

Interlaminar spaces (covered by ligamentum flavum)

Lumbar vertebrae

Sacrum

Coccyx

Figure II-1-8. Interlaminar Spaces

Clinical Correlate

During a lumbar puncture a needle is passed through the interlaminar space while the vertebral column is flexed. The needle passes through the following layers:

- Skin
- Superficial fascia
- Deep fascia
- Supraspinous ligament
- Interspinous ligament
- Interlaminar space
- Epidural space
- Dura
- Arachnoid
- Subarachnoid space

AUTONOMIC NERVOUS SYSTEM

The autonomic nervous system (ANS) is concerned with the motor innervation of smooth muscle, cardiac muscle, and glands of the body.

Anatomically and functionally, the ANS is composed of 2 motor divisions: (1) **sympathetic** and (2) **parasympathetic** (Figure II-1-9). In both divisions, 2 neurons form an autonomic pathway.

- **Preganglionic neurons** have their neuronal cell bodies in the **CNS** (formed by neuroectoderm); their axons exit in cranial and spinal nerves.
- **Postganglionic neurons** have cell bodies in **autonomic ganglia** in the **peripheral nervous system** (PNS) (formed by neural crest cells)

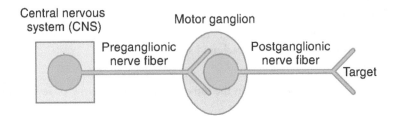

Figure II-1-9. Autonomic Nervous System

Sympathetic Nervous System

The **preganglionic cell bodies** of the sympathetic nervous system are found in the **lateral horn** gray matter of spinal cord segments **T1–L2** (14 segments).

The **postganglionic cell bodies** of the sympathetic system are found in one of 2 types of motor ganglia in the PNS:

- **Chain or paravertebral**
- **Collateral or prevertebral** (found only in abdomen or pelvis)

Table II-1-1. Sympathetic = Thoracolumbar Outflow

Origin (Preganglionic)	Site of Synapse (Postganglionic)	Innervation (Target)
Spinal cord levels T1–L2	Sympathetic chain ganglia (paravertebral ganglia)	Smooth muscle, cardiac muscle and glands of **body wall** and **limbs** (T1–L2), **head** (T1–2) and **thoracic viscera** (T1–5).
Thoracic splanchnic nerves T5–T12	Prevertebral ganglia (collateral) (e.g., celiac, aorticorenal, superior mesenteric ganglia)	Smooth muscle and glands of the **foregut** and **midgut**
Lumbar splanchnic nerves L1–L2	Prevertebral ganglia (collateral) (e.g., inferior mesenteric and pelvic ganglia)	Smooth muscle and glands of the **pelvic viscera** and **hindgut**

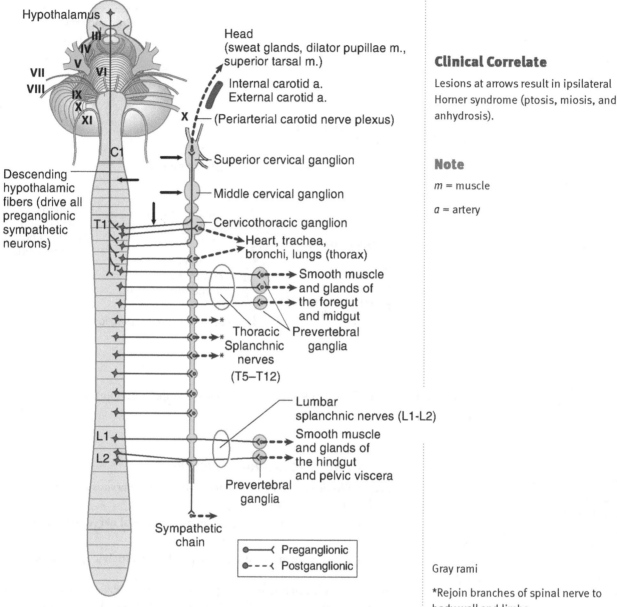

Figure II-1-10. Overview of Sympathetic Outflow

Clinical Correlate

Lesions at arrows result in ipsilateral Horner syndrome (ptosis, miosis, and anhydrosis).

Note

m = muscle

a = artery

Gray rami

*Rejoin branches of spinal nerve to body wall and limbs

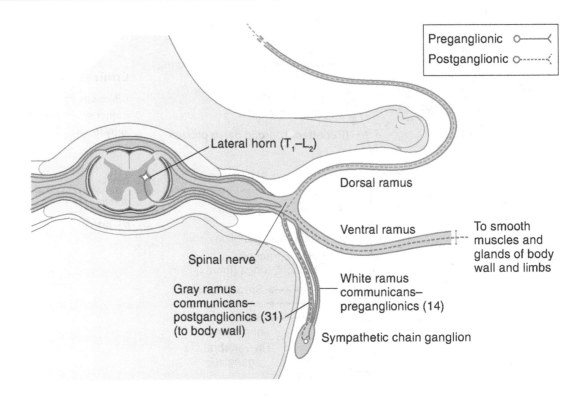

Figure II-1-11. Cross Section of Spinal Cord Showing Sympathetic Outflow

Note

White rami are preganglionic sympathetics that all enter the sympathetic trunk of ganglia. They may synapse with ganglion at point of entry or go up or down and synapse above or below point of entry. If a white ramus does not synapse , it passes through ganglion and becomes a root of a thoracic or lumbar splanchnic nerve.

Parasympathetic Nervous System

The **preganglionic cell bodies** of the parasympathetic nervous system are found in the **CNS** in one of 2 places:

- Gray matter of brain stem associated with **cranial nerves III, VII, IX, and X,** or
- Spinal cord gray in **sacral segments S2 3, and 4 (pelvic splanchnics)**

The **postganglionic cell bodies** of the parasympathetic nervous system are found in **terminal ganglia** in the PNS that are usually located near the organ innervated or in the wall of the organ.

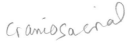

Table II-1-2. Parasympathetic = Craniosacral Outflow

Origin (Preganglionic)	Site of Synapse (Postganglionic)	Innervation (Target)
Cranial nerves III, VII, IX	4 cranial ganglia	Glands and smooth muscle of the **head**
Cranial nerve X	Terminal ganglia (in or near the walls of viscera)	Viscera of the neck, **thorax**, **foregut**, and **midgut**
Pelvic splanchnic nerves S 2, 3, 4	Terminal ganglia (in or near the walls of viscera)	**Hindgut** and **pelvic viscera** (including the bladder, rectum, and erectile tissue)

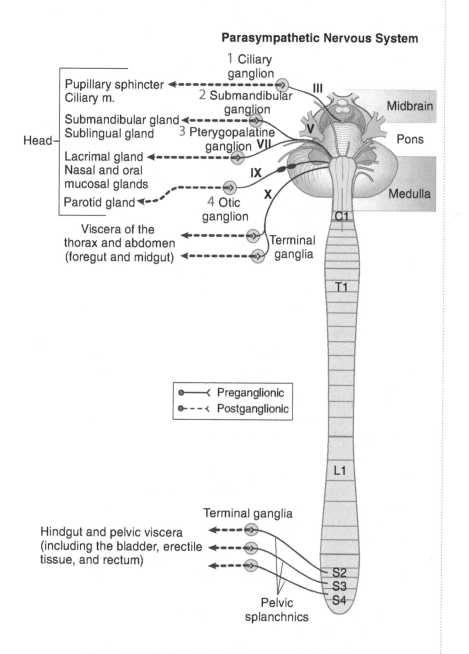

Parasympathetic Nervous System

Figure II-1-12. Overview of Parasympathetic Outflow

Chapter Summary

Vertebral Column

- The vertebral column is composed of a series of cervical, thoracic, lumbar, sacral, and coccygeal vertebrae connected by intervertebral disks and ligaments. The disks consist of an outer core of fibrocartilage, the annulus fibrosus, and an inner part—the nucleus pulposus—which develop from the notochord. Herniation of the nucleus pulposus is usually posterolateral where it can compress a spinal nerve at the intervertebral foramen.

- The spinal nerve exits the vertebral column at the intervertebral foramen. The foramen is bound superiorly and inferiorly by the pedicles of the vertebrae, anteriorly by the vertebral bodies and intervertebral disks, and posteriorly by the zygapophyseal joint.

- The spinal cord is covered by 3 protective layers of meninges: dura mater, arachnoid, and pia mater. The dura and dural sac terminate inferiorly at the second sacral vertebra, and the spinal cord terminates at the second lumbar vertebra. The cauda equina fills the lower part of the dural sac and contains the filum terminale and the ventral and dorsal roots of the lumbar and sacral spinal nerves. Between the arachnoid and pia is the subarachnoid space that contains cerebrospinal fluid (CNS), and between the dura mater and the vertebrae is the epidural space, which contains fat and a plexus of veins. Spinal taps are performed at the level of the L4 vertebra (located at the horizontal level of the iliac crest) to avoid puncturing the spinal cord.

Autonomic Nervous System

- The autonomic nervous system (ANS) provides visceral motor innervation to smooth muscle, cardiac muscle, and glands. The ANS is divided into 2 divisions: sympathetic (thoracolumbar) and parasympathetic (craniosacral). The peripheral distribution of these 2 divisions consists of 2 neurons: preganglionic neuron (cell bodies in the CNS) and postganglionic neuron (cell bodies in motor ganglia in PNS).

- Sympathetic preganglionic cell bodies are found in the lateral horn of the gray matter of spinal cord segments T1–L2. These synapse with postganglionic cell bodies located in either chain (paravertebral) ganglia or collateral (prevertebral) ganglia. Sympathetics to the body wall, head, and thoracic viscera synapse in the chain ganglia. Sympathetics to the foregut and midgut (thoracic splanchnic nerves: T5–T12) and to the hindgut and pelvic viscera (lumbar splanchnic nerves: L1–L2) synapse in collateral ganglia. Interruption of sympathetic innervation to the head results in ipsilateral Horner's syndrome.

- Parasympathetic preganglionic neuron cell bodies are located in the brain stem nuclei of cranial nerves III, VII, IX, X, or in the gray matter of the spinal cord segments S2–S4 (pelvic splanchnics). The preganglionic neurons synapse with postganglionic neurons in terminal ganglia scattered throughout the body. Parasympathetics to the head originate in cranial nerves III, VII, and IX; those to the thorax, foregut, and midgut originate in cranial nerve X; and those to the hindgut and pelvic viscera originate in the S2–S4 cord segments.

Thorax 2

Learning Objectives

❑ Solve problems concerning the chest wall

❑ Use knowledge of embryology of lower respiratory system

❑ Use knowledge of pleura and pleural cavity

❑ Interpret scenarios on respiratory histology

❑ Use knowledge of alveolar ducts, alveolar sacs, and the alveoli

❑ Answer questions about embryology of the heart

❑ Solve problems concerning the mediastinum

❑ Interpret scenarios on heart histology

❑ Solve problems concerning the diaphragm

CHEST WALL

Breast

The breast (mammary gland) is a subcutaneous glandular organ of the superficial pectoral region. It is a modified sweat gland, specialized in women for the production and secretion of milk. A variable amount of fat surrounds the glandular tissue and duct system and is responsible for the shape and size of the female breast.

Cooper ligaments

Cooper ligaments are suspensory ligaments that attach the mammary gland to the skin and run from the skin to the deep fascia.

Arterial supply

There is an extensive blood supply to the mammary tissues. The 2 prominent blood supplies are:

- **Internal thoracic artery (internal mammary)**, a branch of the subclavian artery which supplies the medial aspect of the gland.
- **Lateral thoracic artery**, a branch of the axillary artery which contributes to the blood supply to the lateral part of the gland. On the lateral aspect of the chest wall, the lateral thoracic artery courses with the **long thoracic nerve**, superficial to the serratus anterior muscle.

Clinical Correlate

The presence of a tumor within the breast can distort Cooper ligaments, which results in dimpling of the skin (orange-peel appearance).

Clinical Correlate

During a radical mastectomy, **the long thoracic nerve** (serratus anterior muscle) may be lesioned during ligation of the lateral thoracic artery. A few weeks after surgery, the female may present with a **winged scapula** and weakness in abduction of the arm above 90°. **The thoracodorsal nerve** supplying the latissimus dorsi muscle may also be damaged during mastectomy, resulting in weakness in extension and medial rotation of the arm.

Lymphatic drainage

The lymphatic drainage of the breast is critical due to its important role in metastasis of breast cancer. The lymphatic drainage of the breast follows 2 primary routes (Figure II-2-1):

1. Laterally, most of the lymphatic flow (75%) drains from the nipple and the superior, lateral, and inferior quadrants of the breast to the **axillary nodes**, initially to the **pectoral group**.

2. From the medial quadrant, most lymph drains to the **parasternal nodes**, which accompany the internal thoracic vessels. It is also through this medial route that cancer can spread to the **opposite breast**.

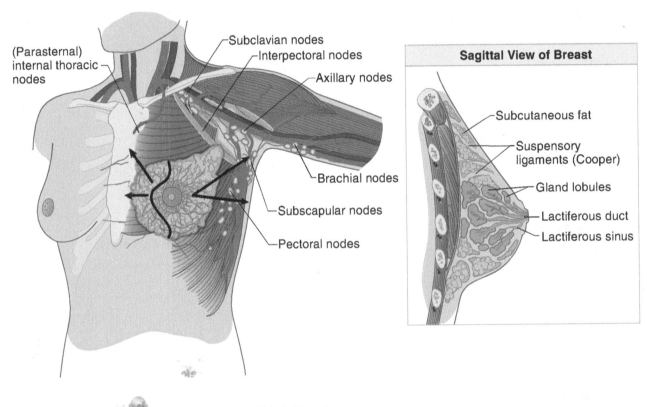

Figure II-2-1. Breast

EMBRYOLOGY OF LOWER RESPIRATORY SYSTEM

During week 4 of development, the lower respiratory system (trachea, bronchi, and lungs) begins to develop as a single **respiratory (laryngotracheal) diverticulum** of endoderm from the ventral wall of the **foregut** (Figure II-2-2).The respiratory epithelium develops from **endoderm** while the muscles, connective tissues, and cartilages develop from **mesoderm**.

- The respiratory diverticulum enlarges distally to form the **lung bud.**
- The diverticulum and lung bud then bifurcates into the 2 **bronchial buds,** which then undergo a series of divisions to form the major part of the bronchial tree (main, secondary, and tertiary bronchi) by the sixth month.

- The tertiary segmental bronchi are related to the bronchopulmonary segments of the lungs.

- To separate the initial communication with foregut, the **tracheoesophageal septum** forms to separate the esophagus from the trachea.

- A critical timeline in lung development is the **25–28th** weeks. By this time, the Type I and II pneumocytes are present and gas exchange and surfactant production are possible. Premature fetuses born during this time can survive with intensive care. The amount of surfactant production is critical.

Clinical Correlate

A **tracheoesophageal fistula** is an abnormal communication between the trachea and esophagus caused by a malformation of the tracheoesophageal septum. It is generally associated with the following:

- **Esophageal atresia** and **polyhydramnios** (increased volume of amniotic fluid)

- Regurgitation of milk

- Gagging and cyanosis after feeding

- Abdominal distention after crying

- **Reflux** of gastric contents into lungs causing pneumonitis

The fistula is most commonly (90% of all cases) located between the esophagus and the **distal third of the trachea** (Figure II-2-3).

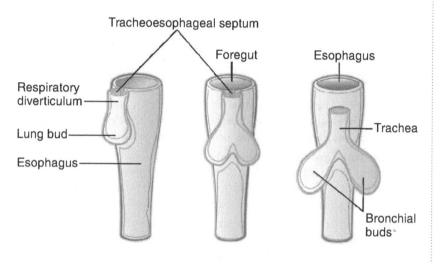

Figure II-2-2. Development of the Lower Respiratory System

Clinical Correlate

Pulmonary hypoplasia occurs when lung development is stunted. This condition has 2 congenital causes: (1) **congenital diaphragmatic hernia** (a herniation of abdominal contents into the thorax, which affects the development of the left lung), or (2) **bilateral renal agenesis** (this causes oligohydramnios, which increases the pressure on the fetal thorax and Potter's sequence). One of the features of Potter's sequence is bilateral pulmonary hypoplasia.

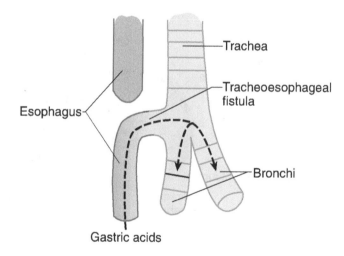

Figure II-2-3. Tracheoesophageal Fistula (Most Common Type)

Clinical Correlate

Passage of instruments through the intercostal space is done in the **lower part** of the space to avoid the intercostal neurovascular structures (as during a thoracentesis).

An intercostal nerve block is done in the **upper portion** of the intercostal space.

ADULT THORACIC CAVITY

The **thoracic cavity** is kidney-shaped on cross section and is bounded anterolaterally by the bony thorax (sternum, ribs, and intercostal spaces) and posteriorly by the thoracic vertebrae. Superiorly, the thoracic cavity communicates through the **thoracic inlet** with the base of the neck. Inferiorly, the **thoracic outlet** is closed by the diaphragm which separates the thoracic from the abdominal cavity.

The thoracic cavity is divided into 2 **lateral compartments** containing the lungs and their covering of serous membranes and a **central compartment** called the **mediastinum** (discussed later) which contains most of the viscera of the thorax (Figure II-2-4B).

Intercostal Spaces

- There are 11 **intercostal spaces** within the thoracic wall (Figure II-2-4A). The spaces are filled in by 3 layers of intercostal muscles and their related fasciae and are bounded superiorly and inferiorly by the adjacent ribs.
- The **costal groove** is located along the inferior border of each rib (upper aspect of the intercostal space) and provides protection for the intercostal nerve, artery, and vein which are located in the groove. The vein is most superior and the nerve is inferior in the groove (VAN).
- The intercostal arteries are contributed to anteriorly from branches of the internal thoracic artery (branch of the subclavian artery) and posteriorly from branches of the thoracic aorta. Thus, the intercostal arteries can provide a potential collateral circulation between the subclavian artery and the thoracic aorta.

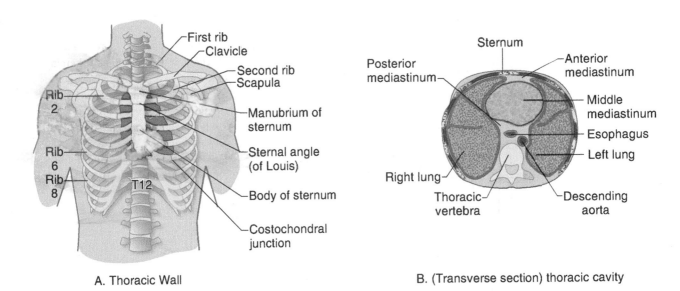

A. Thoracic Wall

B. (Transverse section) thoracic cavity

Figure II-2-4. Thoracic Cavity

PLEURA AND PLEURAL CAVITY

Serous Membranes

Within the thoracic and abdominal cavities there are 3 serous mesodermal-derived membranes which form a covering for the lungs (**pleura**), heart (**pericardium**), and abdominal viscera (**peritoneum**).

Each of these double-layered membranes permits friction-reducing movements of the viscera against adjacent structures.

The outer layer of the serous membranes is referred to as the **parietal layer;** and the inner layer which is applied directly to the surface of the organ, is called the **visceral layer**. The 2 layers are continuous and there is a potential space (pleural cavity) between the parietal and visceral layers containing a thin layer of serous fluid.

Pleura

The **pleura** is the serous membrane that invests the lungs in the lateral compartments of the thoracic cavity (Figure II-2-5). The external **parietal pleura** lines and attaches to the inner surfaces of the chest wall, diaphragm, and mediastinum. The innermost **visceral** layer reflects from the parietal layer at the hilum of the lungs and is firmly attached to and follows the contours of the lung. Visceral and parietal pleura are continuous at the root of the lung.

The **parietal pleura** is regionally named by its relationship to the thoracic wall and mediastinum (Figure II-2-5):

- **Costal parietal pleura** is lateral and lines the inner surfaces of the ribs and intercostal spaces
- **Diaphragmatic parietal pleura** lines the thoracic surface of the diaphragm
- **Mediastinal parietal pleura** is medial and lines the mediastinum. The mediastinal pleura reflects and becomes continuous with the visceral pleura at the hilum.
- **Cervical parietal pleura** extends into the neck above the first rib where it covers the apex of the lung.

The **visceral pleura** tightly invests the surface of the lungs, following all of the fissures and lobes of the lung.

Innervation of Pleura

The **parietal pleura** has extensive **somatic** sensory innervation provided by nerves closely related to different aspects of the pleura.

- The **intercostal nerves** supply the **costal** and peripheral portions of the **diaphragmatic** pleura.
- The **phrenic nerve** supplies the central portion of the **diaphragmatic** pleura and the **mediastinal** pleura.

The **visceral pleura** is supplied by visceral sensory nerves that course with the autonomic nerves.

Clinical Correlate

Respiratory distress syndrome is caused by a deficiency of surfactant (type II pneumocytes). This condition is associated with premature infants, infants of diabetic mothers, and prolonged intrauterine asphyxia. Thyroxine and cortisol treatment increase the production of surfactant.

Surfactant deficiency may lead to **hyaline membrane disease,** whereby repeated gasping inhalations damage the alveolar lining. Hyaline membrane disease is characterized histologically by collapsed alveoli (atelectasis) and eosinophilic (pink) fluid covering the alveoli.

Clinical Correlate

Inflammation of the parietal pleural layers (**pleurisy**) produces sharp pain upon respiration. Costal inflammation produces local dermatome pain of the chest wall via the intercostal nerves; whereby mediastinal irritation produces referred pain via the phrenic nerve to the shoulder dermatomes of C3-5.

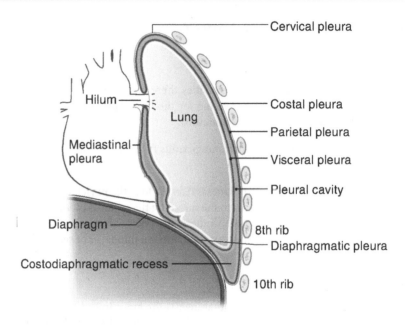

Figure II-2-5. Layers of the Pleura

Clinical Correlate

Open pneumothroax occurs when air enters the pleural cavity following a penetrating wound of the chest cavity. Air moves freely through the wound during inspiration and expiration. During inspiration, air enters the chest wall and the mediastinum will shift toward other side and compress the opposite lung. During expiration, air exits the wound and the mediastinum moves back toward the affected side.

Tension pneumothorax occurs when a piece of tissue covers and forms a flap over the wound. During inspiration, air enters the chest cavity, which results in a shift of the mediastinum toward the other side, compressing the opposite lung. During expiration, the piece of tissue prevents the air from escaping the wound, which increases the pressure and the shift toward the opposite side is enhanced. This severely reduces the opposite lung function and venous return to the heart and can be life-threatening.

Pleural Cavity

The **pleural cavity** is the potential space between the parietal and visceral layers of the pleura (Figure II-2-5). It is a closed space which contains a small amount of serous fluid that lubricates the opposing parietal and visceral layers.

The introduction of air into the pleural cavity may cause the lung to collapse, resulting in a **pneumothorax** which causes shortness of breath and painful respiration. The lung collapses due to the loss of the negative pressure of the pleural cavity during a pneumothroax.

Pleural Reflections

Pleural reflections are the areas where the parietal pleura abruptly changes direction from one wall to the other, outlining the extent of the pleural cavities (Figure II-2-6).

- The sternal line of reflection is where the costal pleura is continuous with the mediastinal pleura posterior to the sternum (from costal cartilages 2–4). The pleural margin then passes inferiorly to the level of the sixth costal cartilage.

- Note that around the chest wall, there are **2 rib interspaces** separating the inferior limit of parietal pleural reflections from the inferior border of the lungs and visceral pleura: between ribs 6–8 in the **midclavicular line**, ribs 8–10 in the **midaxillary line**, and ribs 10–12 at the vertebral column (**paravertebral line**), respectively (Figure II-2-6).

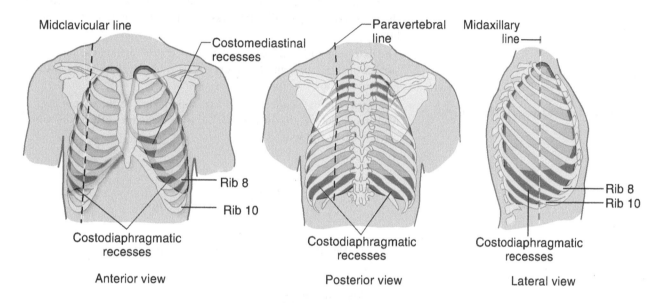

Figure II-2-6. Pleural Reflections and Recesses

Pleural Recesses

Pleural recesses are potential spaces not occupied by lung tissue except during deep inspiration (Figure II-2-6).

- **Costodiaphragmatic recesses** are spaces below the inferior borders of the lungs where costal and diaphragmatic pleura are in contact.

- The **costomediastinal recess** is a space where the left costal and mediastinal parietal pleura meet, leaving a space caused by the cardiac notch of the left lung. This space is occupied by the lingula of the left lung during inspiration.

In A Nutshell

	Visceral Pleura	Parietal Pleura
Midclavicular line	6th rib	8th rib
Midaxillary line	8th rib	10th rib
Paravertebral line	10th rib	12th rib

LUNGS

The lungs and the pleural membranes are located in the lateral compartment of the thoracic cavity. The lungs are separated from each other in the midline by the mediastinum The **hilum** of the lung is on the medial surface and serves for passage of structures in the root of the lung: the pulmonary vessels, primary bronchi, nerves, and lymphatics.

Surfaces and Regions

Each of the lungs has 3 surfaces (Figure II-2-7):

- The **costal surface** is smooth and convex and is related laterally to the ribs and tissues of the chest wall.
- The **mediastinal surface** is concave and is related medially to the middle mediastinum and the heart. The mediastinal surfaces contain the **root** of the lung and a deep **cardiac impression**, more pronounced on the left lung.
- The **diaphragmatic surface** (base) is concave and rests on the superior surface of the diaphragm. It is more superior on the right owing to the presence of the liver.
- The **apex** (cupola) of the lung projects superiorly into the root of the neck above the level of the first rib and is crossed anteriorly by the subclavian artery and vein.

Clinical Correlate

A tumor at the apex of the lung (Pancoast tumor) may result in thoracic outlet syndrome.

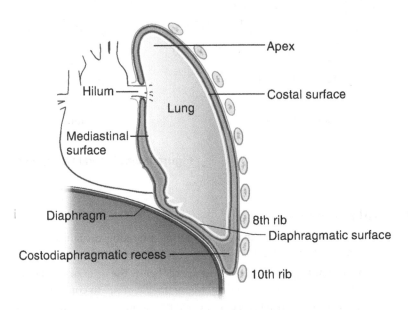

Figure II-2-7. Surfaces of the Lung

Lobes and Fissures

- The **right lung** is divided into 3 lobes (**superior, middle, inferior**) separated by 2 fissures, the **oblique** and **horizontal fissures** (Figure II-2-8). The horizontal fissure separates the superior from the middle lobe and the oblique fissure separates the middle from the inferior lobe.

- The **left lung** is divided into 2 lobes (**superior, inferior**) separated by an **oblique fissure** (Figure II-2-8). The **lingula** of the upper lobe of the left lung corresponds to the middle lobe of the right lung.

- The **horizontal fissure** of the right lung follows the curvature of the **4th rib,** ending medially at the 4th costal cartilage.

- The **oblique fissure** of both lungs projects anteriorly at approximately the **5th intercostal space** in the midclavicular line, ending medially deep to the 6th costal cartilage.

Clinical Correlate

The superior lobe of the **right lung** projects anteriorly on the chest wall **above** the **4th rib** and the middle lobe projects anteriorly **below** the 4th rib.

A small portion of the inferior lobe of both lungs projects **below** the 6th rib anteriorly but primarily projects to the **posterior che**st wall.

Clinical Correlate

To listen to **breath sounds** of the **superior lobes** of the right and left lungs, the stethoscope is placed on the superior area of the anterior chest wall (**above the 4th rib** for the right lung).

For **breath sounds** from the **middle lobe of the right lung**, the stethoscope is placed on the anterior chest wall **inferior to the 4th rib** and medially toward the sternum.

For **the inferior lobe**s of both lungs, **breath sounds** are primarily heard on the **posterior** chest wall.

Clinical Correlate

Aspiration of a foreign body will more often enter the **right primary bronchus,** which is shorter, wider, and more vertical than the left primary bronchus. When the individual is vertical, the foreign body usually falls into the **posterior basal segment** of the **right inferior lobe.**

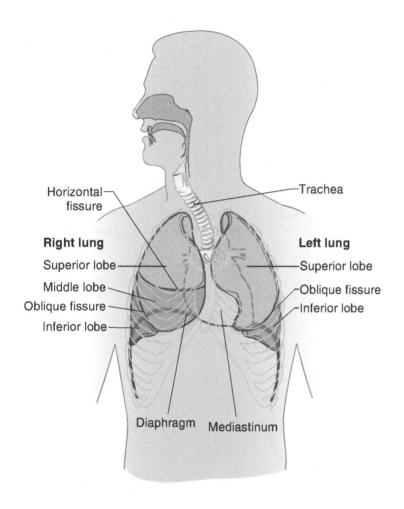

Horizontal fissure

Trachea

Right lung

Superior lobe

Middle lobe

Oblique fissure

Inferior lobe

Left lung

Superior lobe

Oblique fissure

Inferior lobe

Diaphragm   Mediastinum

Figure II-2-8. Lobes and Fissures of Lungs

Lymphatic System

The **lymphatic system** consists of an extensive network of lymph capillaries, vessels, and nodes that drain extracellular fluid from most of the body tissues and organs. The lymph flow will return to the blood venous system by 2 major lymphatic vessels, the **right lymphatic duct** and the **thoracic duct** on the left (Figure II-2-10A). These 2 vessels drain into the junction of the internal jugular and the subclavian veins on their respective sides.

- The **thoracic duct** carries all lymphatic drainage from the body below the diaphragm and on the left side of the trunk and head above the diaphragm (Figure II-2-10B).
- **The right lymphatic duct** drains lymph flow from the right head and neck and the right side of the trunk above the diaphragm (Figure II-2-10B).

Lymphatic Drainage

The lymphatic drainage of the lungs is extensive and drains by way of **superficial** and **deep** lymphatic plexuses. The superficial plexus is immediately deep to the visceral pleura. The deep plexus begins deeply in the lungs and drains through **pulmonary nodes** which follow the bronchial tree toward the hilum.

The major nodes (Figure II-2-9) involved in the lymphatic drainage of these 2 plexuses are:

- **Bronchopulmonary (hilar) nodes** are located at the hilum of the lungs. They receive lymph drainage from both superficial and deep lymphatic plexuses, and they drain into the tracheobronchial nodes.
- **Tracheobronchial nodes** are located at the bifurcation of the trachea, and they drain into the right and left bronchomediastinal nodes and trunk.
- **Bronchomediastinal nodes** and trunk are located on the right and left sides of the trachea, and they drain superiorly into either the right lymphatic duct or the thoracic duct on the left.

Clinical Correlate

The lymphatic drainage from the **lower lobe of the left lung** also drains across the midline into the **right bronchomediastinal** lymphatic trunk and nodes, then continues along the right pathway to the right lymphatic duct. This is important to consider with metastasis of lung cancer.

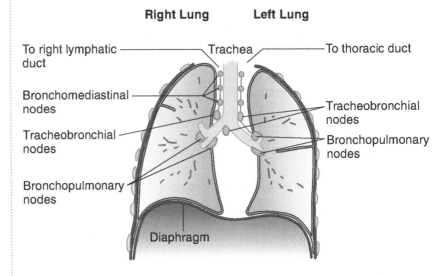

Right Lung   **Left Lung**

To right lymphatic duct — Trachea — To thoracic duct

Bronchomediastinal nodes

Tracheobronchial nodes

Bronchopulmonary nodes

Tracheobronchial nodes

Bronchopulmonary nodes

Diaphragm

Figure II-2-9. Lymphatics of the Lungs

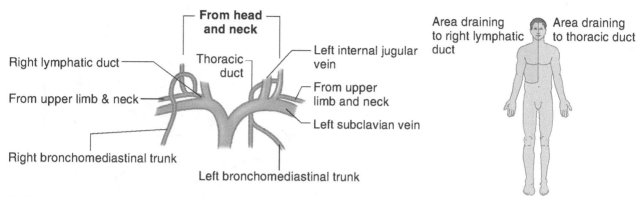

A. Right lymphatic and thoracic ducts

B. General lymphatic drainage

Figure II-2-10.

RESPIRATORY HISTOLOGY

The lung is an organ that functions in the intake of oxygen and exhaling of CO_2. Approximately 14 times each minute, we take in about 500 mL of air per breath. Inspired air will be spread over 120 square meters of the surface area of the lungs. The air–blood barrier has to be thin enough for air to pass across but tough enough to keep the blood cells inside their capillaries.

Lungs are opened to the outside world so that they are susceptible to environmental insults in the form of pollution and infectious bacteria.

The lungs receive the entire cardiac output and are positioned to modify various blood components. The pulmonary endothelium plays an active role in the metabolic transformation of lipoproteins and prostaglandins. **The enzyme that converts angiotensin I to angiotensin II is produced by the lung endothelial cells.**

Clinical Correlate

- Any disease that affects capillaries also affects the extensive capillary bed of the lungs. Bacteria which colonize the lungs may damage the barriers between the alveoli and the capillaries, gaining access to the bloodstream (a common complication of bacterial pneumonia).

- In individuals with allergies, smooth-muscle constriction reduces the diameter of air tubes and results in reduced air intake.

- Lung cancers commonly develop from bronchi (smoking, asbestos, and excessive radiation are the main causes).

- Mesothelioma is a malignant tumor of the pleura (causative agent: asbestos dust).

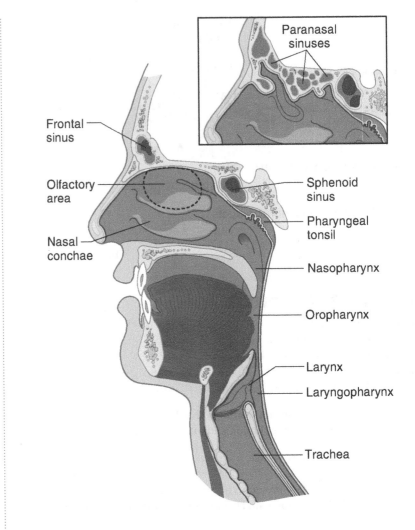

Figure II-2-11. Respiratory Pathways

Table II-2-1. Histologic Features of Trachea, Bronchi, and Bronchioles

	Trachea	Bronchi	Bronchioles
Epithelia	Pseudostratified ciliated columnar (PCC) cells, goblet cells	PCC to simple columnar cells	Ciliated, some goblet cells, Clara cells in terminal bronchioles
Cartilage	16–20 C-shaped cartilaginous rings	Irregular plates	None
Glands	Seromucous glands	Fewer seromucous glands	None
Smooth muscle	Between open ends of C-shaped cartilage	Prominent	Highest proportion of smooth muscle in the bronchial tree
Elastic fibers	Present	Abundant	Abundant

TRACHEA

The **trachea** is a hollow tube, about 10 cm in length (and about 2 cm in diameter), extending from the larynx to its bifurcation at the carina to form a primary bronchus for each lung. The most striking structures of the trachea are the C-shaped hyaline cartilage rings. In the human there are about 16 to 20 of them distributed along the length of the trachea. The rings overlap in the anterior part of the trachea. The free posterior ends of the C-shaped cartilages are interconnected by smooth-muscle cells.

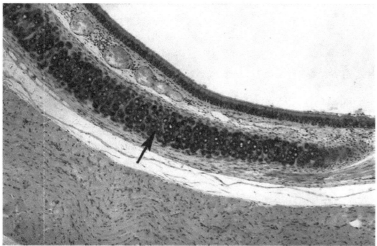

Figure II-2-12. Trachea with a hyaline cartilage ring (arrow)
and pseudostratified columnar epithelium

The trachea is composed of concentric rings of mucosa, submucosa, an incomplete muscularis, and an complete adventitia.

- The mucosa has 3 components: a pseudostratified epithelium, an underlying vascularized loose connective tissue (lamina propria) that contains immune cells, and a thin layer of smooth-muscle cells (muscularis mucosa).

- The submucosa is a vascular service area containing large blood vessels. Collagen fibers, lymphatic vessels and nerves are also present in this layer.

- The outside covering of the trachea, the adventitia, is composed of several layers of loose connective tissue.

The epithelial lining of the trachea and bronchi is pseudostratified columnar in which all cells lie on the same basal membrane but only some reach the luminal surface. The only other place in the body with this epithelium is the male reproductive tract.

Clinical Correlate

If mucosal clearance is ineffective, or the mechanism overwhelmed, infection (pathogenic bacteria) or pneumoconiosis (dust-related disease) may follow.

In cystic fibrosis, the secreted mucus is thick or viscous and the cilia have a difficult time moving it toward the pharynx. Patients with this disease have frequent infections of the respiratory system.

Clinical Correlate

Patients lacking dynein have immotile cilia or **Kartagener syndrome**.

With immotile cilia, patients are subject to many respiratory problems because their cilia cannot move this mucus layer with its trapped bacteria. Males also possess immotile sperm.

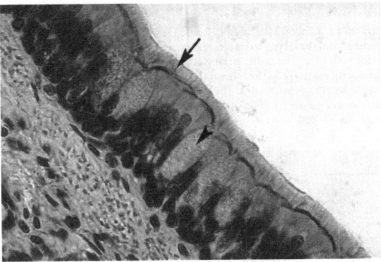

Figure II-2-13. Pseudostratified columnar epithelium with goblet cells (arrowhead) surrounded by ciliated cells (arrow)

Tracheal Epithelial Cell Types

Columnar cells extend from the basal membrane to the luminal surface. These cells contain approximately 200 to 300 apical cilia per cell that are intermingled with microvilli. The cilia are motile and beat to help move the secreted mucus layer over the lining of the trachea and out of the respiratory system.

Goblet cells secrete a polysaccharide mucous material into the lumen of trachea. Mucus production is supplemented by secretions of the submucosal mixed glands. The mucus layer of the respiratory system traps particulate substances (dust, bacteria, and viruses) and absorbs noxious water-soluble gases such as ozone and sulfur dioxide. The mucus sticky layer is moved by the beating cilia toward the pharynx where it is swallowed. This movement is known as the mucociliary escalator system. Most material (dust and bacteria) is trapped in the mucus layer, and is removed and digested.

Pulmonary neuroendocrine (PNE) cells are comparable to the endocrine cells in the gut. These epithelial neuroendocrine cells have been given various names:

- **APUD cells** (Amino-Precursor-Uptake-Decarboxylase), **DNES cells** (Diffuse Neuro Endocrine System) and **K** (Kulchitsky) **cells.** These cells occur in clusters and are often located at airway branch points.

- **Brush cells** may represent goblet cells that have secreted their products or intermediate stages in the formation of goblet or the tall ciliated cells. They have short microvilli on their apical surfaces. Some of these cells have synapses with intraepithelial nerves, suggesting that these cells may be sensory receptors.

Basal cells are stem cells for the ciliated and goblet cells. The stem cells lie on the basal membrane but do not extend to the lumen of the trachea. These cells, along with the epithelial neuroendocrine cells, are responsible for the pseudostratified appearance of the trachea.

BRONCHI

The **bronchial tree** forms a branching airway from the trachea to the bronchioles. When the primary bronchi enter the lung, they give rise to 5 secondary or lobar bronchi—3 for the right lung and 2 for the left. The 5 lobes are further subdivided into 10 tertiary or segmental bronchi in each lung, which form bronchopulmonary segments.

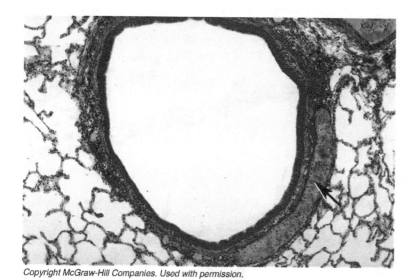

Copyright McGraw-Hill Companies. Used with permission.

Figure II-2-14. Bronchus with a plate of cartilage (arrow)

The epithelial lining of the bronchi is also pseudostratified. It consists of **ciliated columnar cells, basal cells, mucus cells, brush cells** and **neuroendocrine (APUD, DNES, or K) cells**. There are also seromucous glands in the submucosa that empty onto the epithelial surface via ducts. The walls of bronchi contain irregular plates of cartilage and circular smooth-muscle fascicles bound together by elastic fibers. The number of goblet cells and submucosa glands decreases from the trachea to the small bronchi.

Clinical Correlate

The columnar and goblet cells are sensitive to irritation. The ciliated cells become taller, and there is an increase in the number of goblet cells and submucosal glands.

Intensive irritation from smoking leads to a squamous metaplasia where the ciliated epithelium becomes a squamous epithelium. This process is reversible.

Clinical Correlate

Bronchial metastatic tumors arise from Kulchitsky cells.

Clinical Correlate

Cystic fibrosis that results in abnormally thick mucus is in part due to defective chloride transport by Clara cells.

BRONCHIOLES

The **wall of a bronchiole** does not contain cartilage or glands. The smooth-muscle fascicles are bound together by elastic fibers. The epithelium is still ciliated, but is a simple cuboidal or columnar epithelium rather than pseudostratified. The epithelial lining of the airway is composed of **ciliated cells** (goblet and basal cells are absent in the terminal bronchioles) and an additional type called the **Clara cell.**

Clara cells (also called bronchiolar secretory cells) are nonciliated and **secrete a serous solution similar to surfactant**. They aid in the **detoxification of airborne toxins**, and serve as a **stem cell for the ciliated cells** and for themselves. The number of Clara cells increases in response to increased levels of pollutants like cigarette smoke. **Clara cells are most abundant in the terminal bronchioles, where they make up about 80 % of the epithelial cell lining**; they are also involved with chloride ion transport into the lumens of the terminal bronchioles.

Clinical Correlate

Chronic obstructive pulmonary disease (COPD) affects the bronchioles and includes emphysema and asthma.

- Emphysema is caused by a loss of elastic fibers and results in chronic airflow obstruction.

- Asthma is a chronic process characterized by a reversible narrowing of airways.

- Asthma is reversible; emphysema is not.

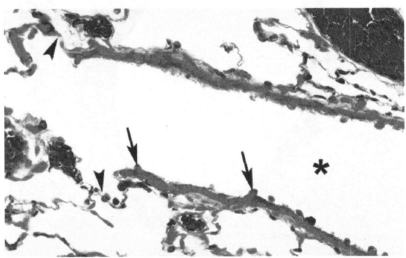

Copyright McGraw-Hill Companies. Used with permission.

Figure II-2-15. Terminal bronchiole lumen (asterisk) with epithelium containing ciliated cells and Clara cells (arrows)

Terminal Bronchioles

The **terminal bronchiole** is the last conducting bronchiole. This bronchiole is followed by **respiratory bronchioles** which are periodically interrupted by alveoli in their walls. The goblet cells are absent from the epithelial linings of the respiratory bronchioles, but are still lined with a sparse ciliated cuboidal epithelium that prevent the movement of mucous into the alveoli. After the last respiratory bronchiole, the wall of the airway disappears and air enters the alveoli.

ALVEOLAR DUCTS, ALVEOLAR SACS, AND THE ALVEOLI

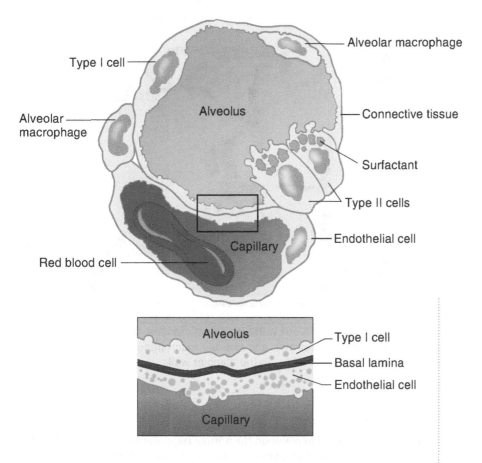

Figure II-2-16. Alveolus and blood–air barrier

The **alveolar ducts and sacs** have little or no walls and consist almost entirely of alveoli. The alveoli constitute 80 to 85% of the volume of the normal lung. There are 300 million alveoli in the lungs. Each alveolus is approximately 200 microns in diameter. The cuboidal epithelium of the respiratory bronchioles and the alveolar ducts are continuous with the squamous cells lining the alveoli.

The **type I pneumocyte** is the major cell lining cell of the alveolar surfaces (also called small alveolar cell or alveolar type I cell).

- These cells represent only 40% of the alveolar lining cells, but are spread so thinly that they cover about 90 to 95% of the surface.
- Primarily involved in gas exchange
- These cells are post-mitotic.

The **type II pneumocyte** is the other major alveolar cell (also called the great alveolar cell because of its size). Other names for this cell type include granular pneumocyte, septal cell, corner cell, niche cell, and alveolar type II.

- Though they constitute 60% of the cells lining the alveoli, they form only 5 to 10% of the surface.
- Produce and secrete surfactant

- They are large, round cells with "myelin figures" in their apical cytoplasm which represent the remnants of surfactant after histological processing.
- The type II cells serve as stem cells for themselves and the type I cell.

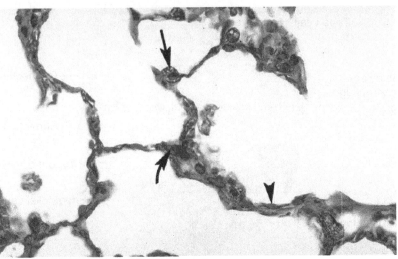

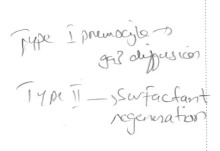

Copyright McGraw-Hill Companies. Used with permission.

Figure II-2-17. Alveoli with type I pneumocytes (arrowhead), type II pneumocytes (arrow), and alveolar macrophage (curved arrow) in the alveolar wall.

Clinical Correlate

Corticosteroids induce the fetal synthesis of surfactant. High insulin levels in diabetic mothers antagonize the effects of corticosteroids.

Infants of diabetic mothers have a higher incidence of respiratory distress syndrome.

Surfactant

Surfactant is essential to maintain the normal respiratory mechanics of the alveoli. Production of surfactant in the fetus is essential for the survival of the neonate as it takes its first breath. Surfactant is composed of a mixture of phospholipids and surfactant proteins whose function is to aid in the spreading of the surfactant at the alveolar air–water interface. The phospholipids act as a detergent which lowers the surface tension of the alveoli and prevents alveolar collapse during expiration.

Most surfactant is recycled back to Type II cells for reutilization; some of it undergoes phagocytosis by macrophages.

Alveolar Wall

In the **alveolar wall** under the alveolar epithelium is a rich network of capillaries arising from pulmonary arteries. The alveolar wall contains a variety of cells and extracellular fibers. The cells include fibroblasts, macrophages, myofibroblasts, smooth-muscle cells, and occasional mast cells. Type I and II collagens, as well as elastic fibers, are in the septa. Type I collagen is present primarily in the walls of the bronchi and bronchioles. Twenty percent of the mass of the lung consists of collagen and elastic fibers. Elastic fibers are responsible for the stretching and recoiling activities of the alveoli during respiration. These microscopic elements are responsible for the recoil of the lungs during expiration.

Gas exchange occurs between capillary blood and alveolar air across the blood–gas barrier. This barrier consists of surfactant, the squamous Type I pneumocytes, a shared basal lamina, and capillary endothelium. The distance between the lumen of the capillary and the lumen of the alveolus can be as thin as 0.1 microns. There are openings in the wall of most alveoli that form the **pores of Kohn**. These pores are thought to be important in collateral ventilation. The diameter of these alveolar pores can be as large as 10 to 15 microns.

Alveolar Macrophages

The **alveolar macrophages** are derived from monocytes that exit the blood vessels in the lungs. The resident alveolar macrophages can undergo limited mitoses to form additional macrophages. These cells can reside in the interalveolar septa as well as in the alveoli. Alveolar macrophages that patrol the alveolar surfaces may pass through the pores of Kohn.

There are about 1 to 3 macrophages per alveolus. Alveolar macrophages vary in size from 15 to 40 microns in diameter. These macrophages represent the last defense mechanism of the lung. Macrophages can pass out of the alveoli to the bronchioles and enter the lymphatics or become trapped in the moving mucus layer and propelled toward the pharynx to be swallowed and digested.

EMBRYOLOGY OF THE HEART

Formation of Heart Tube

The heart begins to develop from splanchnic **mesoderm** in the latter half of the third week within the cardiogenic area of the cranial end of the embryo. **Neural crest cells** migrate into the developing heart and play an important role in cardiac development. The cardiogenic cells condense to form a pair of primordial heart tubes which will fuse into a single **heart tube** (Figure II-2-18) during body folding.

- The heart tube undergoes dextral looping (bends to the right) and rotation.
- The upper truncus arteriosus (ventricular) end of the tube grows more rapidly and folds downward and **ventrally** and to the right.
- The atria and sinus venosus lower part of the tube fold upward and **dorsally** and to the left. These foldings begin to place the chambers of the heart in their postnatal anatomic positions (Figure II-2-18).

Adult structures derived from dilatations of the primitive heart

The primitive heart tube forms 4 dilatations and a cranial outflow tract, the truncus arteriosus. The fates of these are shown in Table II-2-2.

Clinical Correlate

Alveolar macrophages have several other names: **dust cells** because they have phagocytosed dust or cigarette particles, and **heart failure cells** because they have phagocytosed blood cells that have escaped into the alveolar space during congestive heart failure.

↙ haemosiderin loaded ↗

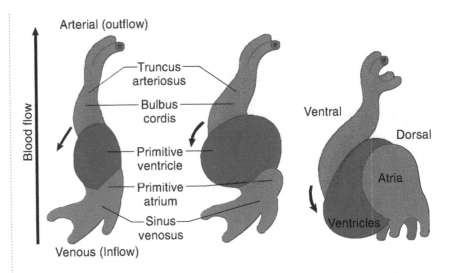

Figure II-2-18. Development of the Heart Tube

Table II-2-2. Adult Structures Derived From the Dilatations of the Primitive Heart

Embryonic Dilatation	Adult Structure
Truncus arteriosus (neural crest)	Aorta; Pulmonary trunk; Semilunar values
Bulbus cordis	Smooth part of right ventricle **(conus arteriosus)** Smooth part of left ventricle **(aortic vestibule)**
Primitive ventricle	Trabeculated part of right ventricle Trabeculated part of left ventricle
Primitive atrium*	Trabeculated part of right atrium (pectinate muscles) Trabeculated part of left atrium (pectinate muscles)
Sinus venosus (the only dilation that does not become subdivided by a septum)	Right—Smooth part of right atrium **(sinus venarum)** Left—Coronary sinus and oblique vein of left atrium

*The **smooth-walled part** of the **left atrium** is formed by incorporation of parts of the **pulmonary veins** into its wall. The **smooth-walled part** of the **right atrium** is formed by the incorporation of the **right sinus venosus**.

Fetal Circulation

Venous systems associated with the fetal heart

There are 3 major venous systems that flow into the sinus venosus end of the heart tube.

- **Viteline (omphalomesenteric) veins** drain deoxygenated blood from the yolk stalk; they will coalesce and form the veins of the liver (sinusoids, hepatic portal vein, hepatic vein) and part of the inferior vena cava.
- **Umbilical vein** carries oxygenated blood from the placenta.
- **Cardinal veins** carry deoxygenated blood from the body of the embryo; they will coalesce and contribute to some of the major veins of the body (brachiocephalic, superior vena cava, inferior vena cava, azygos, renal).

Arterial systems associated with the fetal heart

During fetal circulation, oxygenated blood flood from the placenta to the fetus passes through the **umbilical vein**. Three **vascular shunts** develop in the fetal circulation to bypass blood flow around the liver and lungs (Figure II-2-19).

1. The **ductus venosus** allows oxygenated blood in the umbilical vein to bypass the sinusoids of the liver into the inferior vena cava and to the right atrium. From the right atrium, oxygenated blood flows mostly through the foramen ovale into the left atrium then left ventricle and into the systemic circulation.
2. The **foramen ovale** develops during atrial septation to allow oxygenated blood to bypass the pulmonary circulation. Note that this is a **right-to-left** shunting of blood during fetal life.
3. During fetal circulation, the superior vena cava drains deoxygenated blood from the upper limbs and head into the right atrium. Most of this blood flow is directed into the right ventricle and into the pulmonary trunk. The **ductus arteriosus** opens into the underside of the aorta just **distal** to the origin of the left subclavian artery and shunts this deoxygenated blood from the pulmonary trunk to the aorta to bypass the pulmonary circulation.

The shunting of blood through the foramen ovale and through the ductus arteriosus (right to left) during fetal life occurs because of a **right-to-left pressure gradient**.

Pressure Gradients

Fetal

   R → L

Postnatal

   L → R

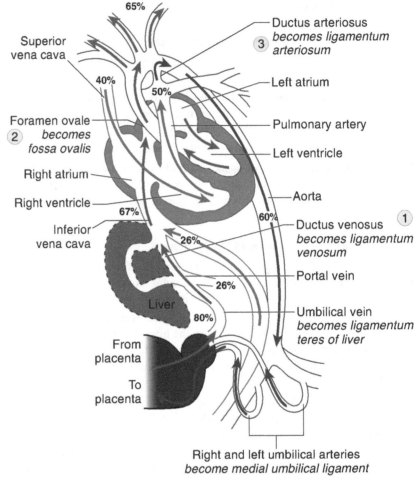

Figure II-2-19. Fetal Circulation and Shunts

Postnatal circulation

Following birth, these 3 shunts will close because of changes in the pressure gradients and in oxygen tensions. The umbilical vein closes and reduces blood flow into the right atrium. The ductus venosus also closes. Lung expansion reduces pulmonary resistence and results in increased flow to the lungs and increased venous return to the left atrium.

- Closure of the foramen ovale occurs as a result of the increase in left atrial pressure and reduction in right atrial pressure.
- Closure of the ductus venosus and ductus arteriosus occurs over the next several hours as a result of the contraction of smooth muscles in its wall and increased oxygen tension.
- The release of bradykinin and the immediate drop of prostaglandin E at birth also facilitate the closure of the ductus arteriosus.

The changes which occur between pre- and postnatal circulation are summarized in Table II-2-3.

Table II-2-3. Adult Vestiges Derived from the Fetal Circulatory System

Changes After Birth	Remnant in Adult
Closure of right and left umbilical arteries	Medial umbilical ligaments
Closure of the umbilical vein	Ligamentum teres of liver
Closure of ductus venosus	Ligamentum venosum
Closure of foramen ovale	Fossa ovalis
Closure of ductus arteriosus	Ligamentum arteriosum

SEPTATION OF THE HEART TUBE

Except for the **sinus venosus** of the embryonic heart tube that initially develops into right and left horns, the ventricular, atrial, and truncus parts of the heart tube, which are originally a common chamber, will undergo septation into a right and left heart structure. The septation of the atria and ventricles occurs simultaneously beginning in week 4 and is mostly finished in week 8. Most of the common congenital cardiac anomalies result from defects in the formation of these septa.

Atrial Septation

During fetal life, blood is shunted from the right to the left atrium via the foramen ovale (FO). Note that during fetal circulation, right atrial pressure is higher than left due to the large bolus of blood directed into the right atrium from the placenta and to high pulmonary resistance.

The FO has to remain open and functional during the entire fetal life to shunt oxygenated blood from the right atrium into the left atrium.

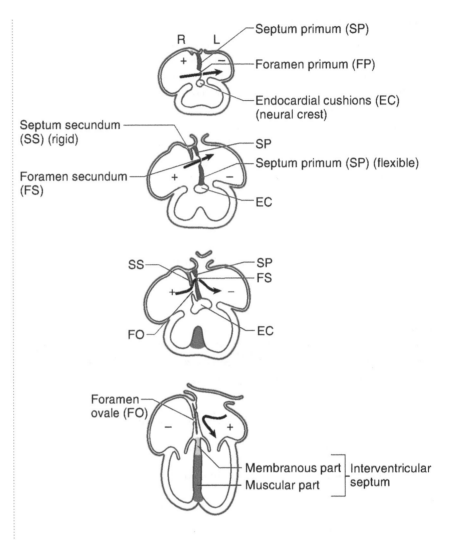

Figure II-2-20. Formation of Atrial Septum

The **common atrium** (Figure II-2-20) is divided into right and left atria by a series of events involving 2 septa and 2 foramina, beginning in week 4. The structures involved in the septation are listed below:

- The flexible **septum primum** (SP) grows inferiorly from the roof of the common atrium toward the **endocardial cushions**, a centrally located mass of mesoderm in the developing heart. Initially, the SP does not reach and fuse with the endocardial cushions. The endocardial cushions form the right and left atrioventricular canals and contribute to the formation of the atrioventricular valves, membranous part of the interventricular septum, and aorticopulmonary septum. **Neural crest cells** migrate into the cushions and facilitate their development.

- The **foramen primum** (FP) is located between the inferior edge of the SP and the endocardial cushion; it is obliterated when the SP later fuses with the endocardial cushions.

- The **foramen secundum** (FS) forms within the upper part of the SP just before the FP closes to maintain the right-to-left shunting of oxygenated blood that entered the right atrium via the inferior vena cava.

- The rigid **septum secundum** (SS) forms to the right of the SP from the roof of the atrium, descends, and partially covers the FS. It does not fuse with the endocardial cushions.
- The **foramen ovale** (FO) is the opening between SP and SS.

Closure of the FO normally occurs immediately after birth and is caused by increased left atrial pressure resulting from changes in the pulmonary circulation and decreased right atrial pressure that have been caused by the closure of the umbilical vein (Figure II-2-21).

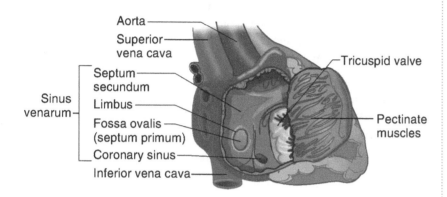

Figure II-2-21. Postnatal Atrial Septum

Atrial Septal Defects

Atrial septal defect (ASD) is one of several congenital heart defects. It is more common in female births than in male. Postnatally, ASDs result **in left-to-right shunting** and are **non-cyanotic conditions**.

Two clinically important ASDs are the **secundum** and **primum** types.

1. **Secundum-type ASD** (Figure II-2-22) is the most common ASD. It is caused by either an excessive resorption of the SP or an underdevelopment and reduced size of the SS or both. This ASD results in variable openings between the right and left atria in the central part of the atrial septum above the limbus. If the ASD is small, clinical symptoms may be delayed as late as age 30.

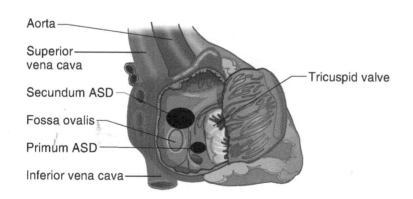

Figure II-2-22. Secundum and Primum Atrial Septal Defect

In A Nutshell

Postnatal Shunts

- **Right-to-left** shunts are **cyanotic conditions**.
- **Left-to-right** shunts are **non-cyanotic conditions**.

Clinical Correlate

Ventricular septal defect (VSD) is the most common of the congenital heart defects, being more common in males than in females. The most common VSD is a **membranous ventricular septal defect**, associated with the failure of **neural crest** cells to migrate into the endocardial cushions.

Clinical Correlate

Membranous VSD

A membranous VSD is caused by the failure of the membranous interventricular (IV) septum to develop, and it results in **left-to-right shunting** of blood through the IV foramen. Patients with left-to-right shunting complain of **excessive fatigue upon exertion**. Left-to-right shunting of blood is **noncyanotic** but causes increased blood flow and pressure to the lungs (pulmonary hypertension). Pulmonary hypertension causes marked proliferation of the tunica intima and media of pulmonary muscular arteries and arterioles. Ultimately, the pulmonary resistance becomes higher than systemic resistance and causes **right-to-left shunting** of blood and late **cyanosis**. At this stage, the condition is called **Eisenmenger complex**.

2. **Primum type ASD** is less common than secundum ASD and results from a failure of the septum premium to fuse with the endocardial cushions, and may be combined with defects of the endocardial cushions. Primum ASDs occur in the lower aspect of the atrial wall, usually with a normal formed fossa ovalis. If the endocardial cushion is involved, a primum ASD can also be associated with a defect of the membranous interventricular septum and the atrioventricular valves.

Ventricular Septation

The development of the **interventricular (IV) septum** begins in the fourth week and is usually completed by the end of the seventh week. Unlike atrial septation, the IV septum will develop and close completely by the eighth week without any shunting between the ventricles.

The adult IV septum consists of 2 parts: a large, **muscular component** forming most of the septum; and a thin, **membranous part** forming a small component at the superior aspect of the septum (Figure II-2-23A).

The **muscular IV septum** (Figure II-2-23B) develops in the floor of the ventricle, ascends, and partially separates the right and left ventricles, leaving the **IV foramen**.

The **membranous IV septum** closes the IV foramen. It forms by the fusion of the following:

- Right conotruncal ridge
- Left conotruncal ridge
- Endocardial cushion (**neural crest cells** are associated with the endocardial cushion and conotruncal ridges)

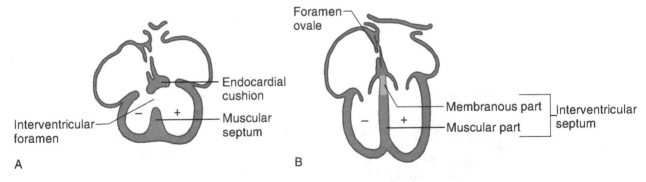

Figure II-2-23. Interventricular Septum

Patent Ductus Arteriosus

A **patent ductus arteriosus** (PDA) (Figure II-2-24) occurs when the ductus arteriosus (a connection between the pulmonary trunk and aorta) fails to close after birth. PDA is common in premature infants and in cases of maternal rubella infection.

- Postnatally, a PDA causes a **left-to-right** shunt (from aorta to pulmonary trunk) and is **non-cyanotic**. The newborn presents with a machine-like murmur.

- Normally, the ductus arteriosus closes within a few hours after birth via smooth-muscle contraction to form the **ligamentum arteriosum**. Prostaglandin E (PGE) and low oxygen tension sustain patency of the ductus arteriosus in the fetal period.

- PGE is used to keep the PDA open in certain heart defects (transposition of great vessels).

- PGE inhibitor (e.g., indomethacin), acetylcholine, histamine, and catecholamines promote closure of the ductus arteriosus in a premature birth.

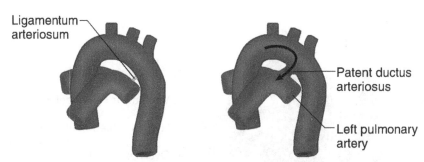

Ligamentum arteriosum

Patent ductus arteriosus

Left pulmonary artery

A. Normal obliterated ductus arteriosus   B. Patent ductus arteriosus

Figure II-2-24. Ductus Arteriosus

Septation of the Truncus Arteriosus

The **septation of the truncus arteriosus** occurs during the eighth week. **Neural crest cells** migrate into the conotruncal and bulbar ridges of the truncus arteriosus, which grow in a **spiral fashion** and fuse to form the **aorticopulmonary (AP) septum**. The AP septum divides the truncus arteriosus into the **aorta** and **pulmonary trunk** (Figure II-2-25).

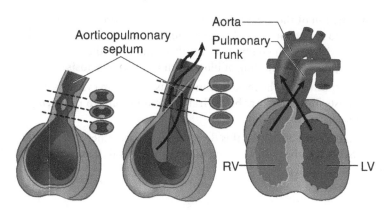

Aorticopulmonary septum

Aorta

Pulmonary Trunk

RV   LV

Figure II-2-25. Formation of the Aorticopulmonary Septum

Truncus arteriosus defects

Three classic **cyanotic congenital heart abnormalities** occur with defects in the development of the aorticopulmonary septum and are related to the failure of neural crest cells to migrate into the truncus arteriosus:

1. **Tetralogy of Fallot** (Figure II-2-26) is the **most common** cyanotic congenital heart defect. Tetralogy occurs when the AP septum fails to align properly and shifts anteriorly to the right. This causes **right-to-left** shunting of blood with resultant **cyanosis** that is usually present sometime after birth. Imaging typically shows a boot-shaped heart due to the enlarged right ventricule.

   - There are 4 major defects in Tetralogy of Fallot:
     - Pulmonary stenosis (most important)
     - Overriding aorta (receives blood from both ventricles)
     - Membranous interventricular septal defect
     - Right ventricular hypertrophy (develops secondarily)

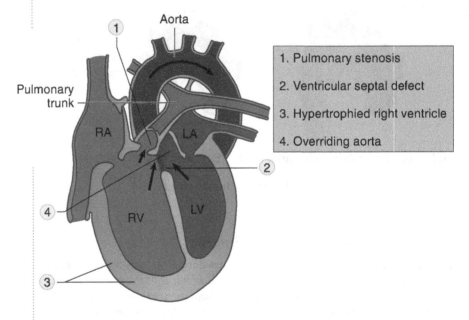

1. Pulmonary stenosis
2. Ventricular septal defect
3. Hypertrophied right ventricle
4. Overriding aorta

Figure II-2-26. Tetralogy of Fallot

2. **Transposition of the great vessels** (Figure II-2-27) occurs when the AP septum fails to develop in a spiral fashion and results in the aorta arising from the right ventricle and the pulmonary trunk arising from the left ventricle. This causes **right-to-left** shunting of blood with resultant **cyanosis**.

   - Transposition is the most common cause of severe cyanosis that persists immediately at birth. Transposition results in producing 2 closed circulation loops.
   - Infants born alive with this defect usually have other defects (PDA, VSD, ASD) that allow mixing of oxygenated and deoxygenated blood to sustain life.

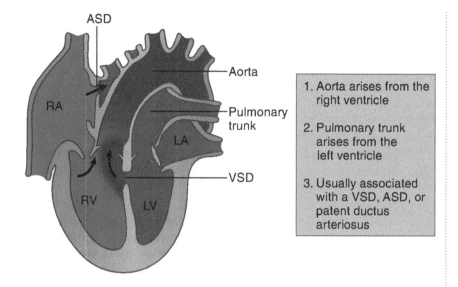

1. Aorta arises from the right ventricle

2. Pulmonary trunk arises from the left ventricle

3. Usually associated with a VSD, ASD, or patent ductus arteriosus

Figure II-2-27. Transposition of the Great Vessels

3. **Persistent truncus arteriosus** (Figure II-2-28) occurs when there is only partial development of the AP septum. This results in a condition where only one large vessel leaves the heart that receives blood from both the right and left ventricles. This causes **right-to-left** shunting of blood with resultant **cyanosis**. This defect is <u>always accompanied</u> by a membranous VSD.

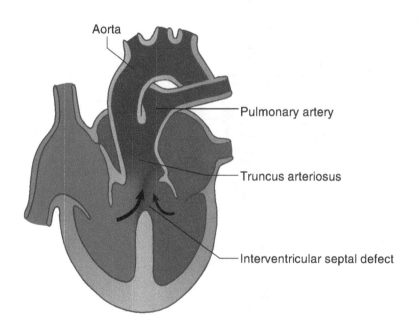

Figure II-2-28. Persistent Truncus Arteriosus

In A Nutshell

Non-cyanotic congenital (left-to-right) heart defects at birth:

- Atrial septal defect
- Ventricular septal defects
- Patent ductus arteriosus

Cyanotic congenital (right-to-left) heart defects at birth

- Transposition of great vessels
- Tetralogy of Fallot
- Persistent truncus arteriosus

MEDIASTINUM

General Features

The mediastinum (Figure II-2-29) is the central, midline compartment of the thoracic cavity. It is bounded anteriorly by the sternum, posteriorly by the 12 thoracic vertebrae, and laterally by the pleural cavities.

- Superiorly, the mediastinum is continuous with the neck through the **thoracic inlet**; and inferiorly, is closed by the diaphragm. The mediastinum contains most of the viscera of the thoracic cavities except from the lungs (and pleura) and the sympathetic trunk.

- The sympathetic trunks are primarily located paravertebrally, just outside the posterior mediastinum. However, the greater, lesser, and least thoracic splanchnic nerves, which convey preganglionic sympathetic fibers to the collateral (prevertebral) ganglia below the diaphragm, enter the posterior mediastinum after leaving the sympathetic trunks.

- The mediastinum is divided into **superior** and **inferior** mediastina by a plane passing from the **sternal angle (of Louis)** anteriorly to the intervertebral disc between T4 and T5 posteriorly. The sternal angle and plane are **important clinical landmarks**. The inferior mediastinum is classically subdivided into **anterior, middle, and posterior** mediastina.

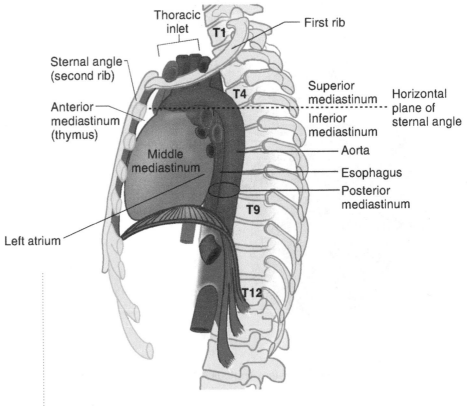

Figure II-2-29. Divisions of the Mediastinum

Anterior Mediastinum

The anterior mediastinum is the small interval between the sternum and the anterior surface of the pericardium. It contains fat and areolar tissue and the inferior part of the **thymus gland**. A tumor of the thymus (**thymoma**) can develop in the anterior or superior mediastina

Posterior Mediastinum

The **posterior mediastinum** is located between the posterior surface of the pericardium and the T5-T12 thoracic vertebrae. Inferiorly, it is closed by the diaphragm.

There are 4 vertically oriented structures coursing within the posterior mediastinum:

- **Thoracic (descending) aorta**
  - Important branches are the **bronchial, esophageal,** and **posterior intercostal arteries**
  - Passes through the **aortic hiatus** (with the thoracic duct) at the T12 vertebral level to become the abdominal aorta

- **Esophagus**
  - Lies immediately posterior to the left primary bronchus and the **left atrium,** forming an important radiological relationship
  - Covered by the **anterior and posterior esophageal plexuses** which are derived from the left and right vagus nerves, respectively
  - Passes through the **esophageal hiatus** (with the vagal nerve trunks) at the T10 vertebral level
  - Is constricted (1) at its origin from the pharynx, (2) posterior to the arch of the aorta, (3) posterior to the left primary bronchus, and (4) at the esophageal hiatus of the diaphragm.

- **Thoracic duct**
  - Lies posterior to the esophagus and between the thoracic aorta and azygos vein
  - Ascends the posterior and superior mediastina and drains into the junction of the left subclavian and internal jugular veins
  - Arises from the cisterna chyli in the abdomen (at vertebral level L1) and enters the mediastinum through the **aortic hiatus** of the diaphragm

- **Azygos system of veins**
  - Drains the posterior and thoracic lateral wall
  - Communicates with the inferior vena cava in the abdomen and terminates by arching over the root of the right lung to empty into the **superior vena cava** above the pericardium
  - Forms a **collateral venous circulation** between the inferior and superior vena cava

Middle Mediastinum

The middle mediastinum contains the heart and great vessels and pericardium and will be discussed later.

Superior Mediastinum

The **superior mediastinum** (Figure II-2-29) is located between the manubrium of the sternum, anteriorly, and the thoracic vertebrae 1-4, posteriorly. As with all mediastina, the parietal pleura and the lungs form the lateral boundary. The thoracic inlet connects superiorly with the neck and the horizontal plane through the sternal angle forms the inferior boundary.

- The superior mediastinum contains the thymus, great arteries and veins associated with the upper aspect of the heart, trachea, and esophagus.
- The vagus and phrenic nerves and the thoracic duct (Figure II-2-30) also course through the mediastinum.
- Note that the pulmonary trunk and arteries are located completely in the middle mediastinum and are not found in the superior mediastinum.

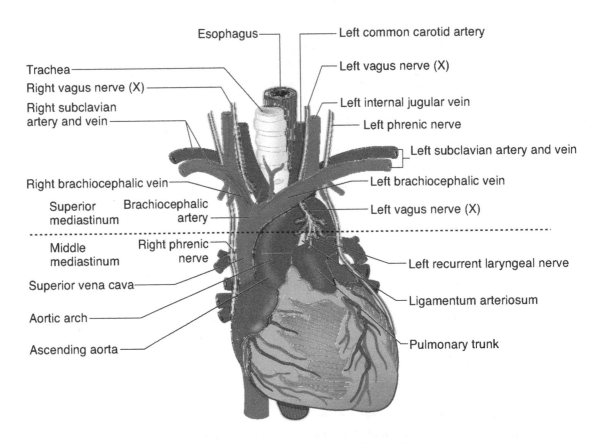

Figure II-2-30. Structures of the Mediastinum

The relationships of these structures in the superior mediastinum are best visualized in **a ventral to dorsal** orientation between the sternum anteriorly and the vertebrae posteriorly:

- **Thymus**: Located posterior to the manubrium, usually atrophies in the adult and remains as fatty tissue
- **Right and left brachiocephalic veins**: Right vein descends almost vertically and the left vein obliquely crosses the superior mediastinum posterior to the thymic remnants.
  - The 2 veins join to form the **superior vena cava** posterior to the **right first costal cartilage**.
  - The superior vena cava descends and drains into the right atrium **deep to the right third costal cartilage**.
- **Aortic arch and its 3 branches**: Aortic arch begins and ends at the plane of the sternal angle and is located just **inferior** to the left brachiocephalic vein. As a very important radiological landmark, the origins of the 3 branches of the aortic arch (**brachiocephalic, left common carotid, and left subclavian**) are directly **posterior** to the left brachiocephalic vein.
- **Trachea**: Lies posterior to the aortic arch and bifurcates at the level of T4 vertebra to form the right and left primary bronchi. The **carina** is an internal projection of cartilage at the bifurcation.
- **Esophagus**: Lies posterior to the trachea and courses posterior to the left primary bronchus to enter the posterior mediastinum

In addition to these structures, the superior mediastinum also contains the **right and left vagus** and **phrenic nerves** and the superior end of the **thoracic duct.**

Vagus nerves

- Right and left vagus nerves contribute to the pulmonary and cardiac plexuses.
- In the neck, the right vagus nerve gives rise to the **right recurrent laryngeal nerve**, which passes under the right subclavian artery to ascend in the groove between the esophagus and the trachea to reach the larynx. **Note:** The right recurrent laryngeal nerve is not in the mediastinum.
- The left vagus nerve gives rise to the **left recurrent laryngeal nerve** in the superior mediastinum, which passes under the aortic arch and ligamentum arteriosum to ascend to the larynx (Figure II-2-31).

Thoracic duct

The thoracic duct is the largest lymphatic channel in the body. It returns lymph to the venous circulation at the junction of the left internal jugular vein and the left subclavian vein.

Phrenic nerves

Phrenic nerves arise from the ventral rami of **cervical nerves 3, 4, and 5**. The nerves are the sole motor supply of the diaphragm and convey sensory information from the central portion of both the superior and inferior portions of the diaphragm and parietal pleura. Both phrenic nerves pass through the middle mediatstinum lateral between the fibrous pericardium and pleura, and anterior to the root of the lung.

Clinical Correlate

The **left recurrent laryngeal nerve** (Figure II-2-30) curves under the aortic arch distal to the ligamentum arteriosum where it may be damaged by pathology (e.g., malignancy or aneurysm of the aortic arch), resulting in paralysis of the left vocal folds. The right laryngeal nerve is not affected because it arises from the right vagus nerve in the root of the neck and passes under the subclavian artery.

Either the right or the left recurrent laryngeal nerve may be lesioned with thyroid gland surgery.

Coarctation of the Aorta

Coarctation of the aorta is a narrowing of the aorta distal to the origin of the left subclavian artery. Two types are usually identified based on if the constriction is found proximal or distal to the opening of the ductus arteriosus (DA).

- **Preductal coarctation** (infantile type) is less common and occurs proximal to the DA (Figure II-2-31A). The DA usually remains patent and provides blood flow via the DA to the descending aorta and the lower parts of the body.

- **Postductal coarctation** (adult type) is more common and occurs distal to the DA (Figure II-2-31B). In postductal coarctation, the DA usually closes and obliterates.

  – This results in the intercostal arteries providing collateral circulation between the internal thoracic artery and the thoracic aorta to provide blood supply to the lower parts of the body (Figure II-2-31C).

  – These patients will be hypertensive in the upper body (head, neck, and upper limbs) and hypotensive with weak pulses in the lower limbs.

  – Enlargement of the intercostal arteries results in **costal notching** on the lower border of the ribs, evident in imaging.

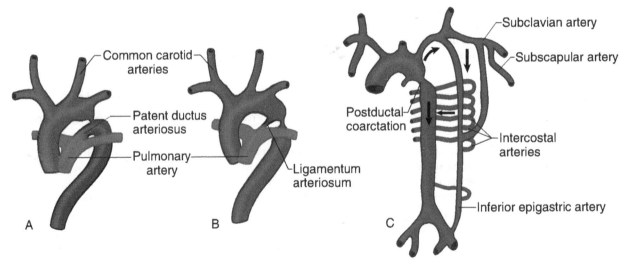

Figure II-2-31. Coarctation of the Aorta: (A) Preductal; (B) Postductal; (C) Collateral Circulation

Middle Mediastinum

The middle mediastinum contains the pericardium, the heart, parts of the **great vessels**, and the phrenic nerves.

Pericardium

The pericardium (Figure II-2-32) is the serous sac covering the heart and is the only one of the 3 serous membranes that has 3 layers: an outer **fibrous layer** and a double-layered **parietal and visceral serous** layers.

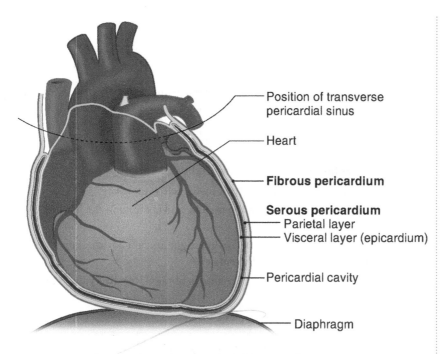

Figure II-2-32. Layers of the Pericardium

The **fibrous pericardium** surrounds the entire heart and the great vessels at the upper aspect of the heart. It is firmly attached below to the central tendon of the diaphragm and superiorly to the adventitia of the great vessels at the plane of the sternal angle (level of the second rib). The fibrous pericardium is very strong and maintains the position of the heart within the middle mediastinum.

The **serous pericardium** is double-layered and formed by the outer **parietal layer** that lines the inner aspect of the fibrous pericardium and the inner **visceral layer** (epicardium) that covers the surface of the heart. The reflection between these 2 serous layers is at the base of the great vessels.

The **pericardial cavity** is the potential space between the parietal and visceral layers containing a small amount of serous fluid that allows free movement of the beating heart. The pericardial cavity is expanded to form 2 sinuses:

- **The transverse pericardial sinus** is a space posterior to the ascending aorta and pulmonary trunk and anterior to the superior vena cava and pulmonary veins. Note that it separates the great arteries from the great veins. The transverse sinus is useful in cardiac surgery to allow isolation of the aorta and pulmonary trunk.

- The **oblique pericardial sinus** is the blind, inverted, U-shaped space posterior to the heart and bounded by reflection of serous pericardium around the 4 pulmonary veins and the inferior vena cava as they enter the heart.

Clinical Correlate

Cardiac tamponade is the pathological accumulation of fluids (serous or blood) within the pericardial cavity. The fluid compresses the heart and restricts venous filling during diastole and reduces cardiac output. A **pericardiocentesis** is performed with a needle at the **left infrasternal angle** through the cardiac notch of the left lung to remove the fluid.

HEART

External Features of the Heart

The heart lies obliquely within the middle mediastinum, mostly posterior to the sternum. Externally, the heart can be described by its **borders** and **surfaces**.

Borders of the heart (Figure II-2-33)

- The **right border** is formed by the **right atrium**.
- The **left border** is mainly formed by the **left ventricle**.
- The **apex** is the tip of the **left ventricle**. and is found in the left fifth intercostal space.
- The superior border is formed by the right and left auricles plus the conus arteriosus of the right ventricle.
- The inferior border is formed at the diaphragm, mostly by the right ventricle.

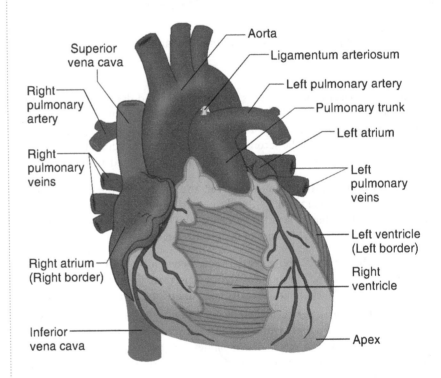

Figure II-2-33. Sternocostal View of the Heart

Surfaces of the heart (Figure II-2-34)

- The **anterior (sternocostal)** surface is formed primarily by the **right ventricle**.
- The **posterior surface** is formed primarily by the left **atrium.**
- The **diaphragmatic** surface is formed primarily by the **left ventricle.**

Sulci of the heart (Figure II-2-34)

There are 3 main sulci (**coronary** and the **anterior and posterior interventricular**) that course on the surfaces of the heart and contain the major vessels of the heart and epicardial fat.

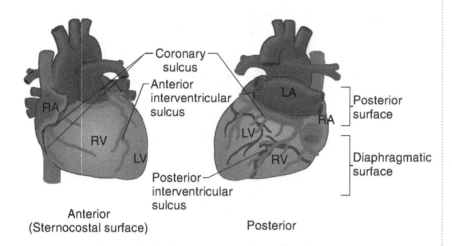

Figure II-2-34. Surfaces of Heart with Sulci

Surface projections

Surface projections of the heart may be traced on the anterior chest wall (Figure II-2-35).

- The **upper right** aspect of the heart is deep to the **third right costal cartilage.**

- The **lower right** aspect of the heart is deep to the **sixth right costal cartilage.**

- **The upper left aspect** of the heart is deep to the **left second costal cartilage**

- The **apex** of the heart is in the **left fifth intercostal space** at the midclavicular line.

- The **right border** extends between the margin of the third right costal cartilage to the sixth right costal cartilage just to the right of the sternum.

- The **left border** extends between the fifth left intercostal space to the second left costal cartilage.

- The **inferior border** extends from the sixth right costal cartilage to the fifth left intercostal space at the midclavicular line.

- The **superior border** extends from the inferior margin of the second left costal cartilage to the superior margin of the third right costal cartilage.

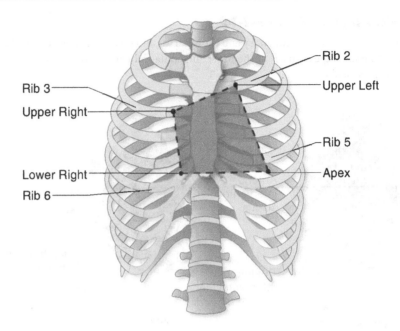

Figure II-2-35. Surface Projections of the Heart

Internal Features of the Heart

Chambers of the Heart

1. Right atrium

The right atrium (Figure II-2-36) receives venous blood from the entire body with the exception of blood from the pulmonary veins.

- **Auricle**

  The auricle is derived from the fetal atrium; it has rough myocardium known as pectinate muscles.

- **Sinus Venarum**

  The sinus venarum is the smooth-walled portion of the atrium, which receives blood from the superior and inferior venae cavae. It developed from the **sinus venosus**.

- **Crista Terminalis**

  The crista terminalis is the vertical ridge that separates the smooth from the rough portion (pectinate muscles) of the right atrium; it extends longitudinally from the superior vena cava to the inferior vena cava. The **SA node** is in the upper part of the crista terminalis.

- **Fossa Ovalis**

  The fossa ovalis is close to the foramen ovale, an opening in the inter-atrial septum which allows blood entering the right atrium from the inferior vena cava to pass directly to the left side of the heart.

- **Tricuspid Valve**

  The right AV (tricuspid) valve communicates with the right ventricle.

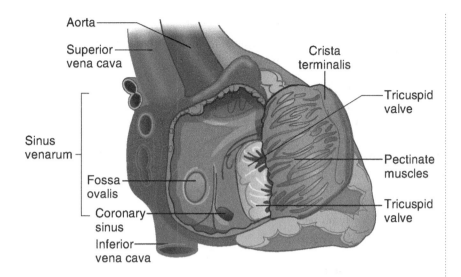

Figure II-2-36. Inside the Right Atrium

2. Left atrium

The left atrium receives oxygenated blood from the lungs via the pulmonary veins. There are 4 openings: the upper right and left and the lower right and left pulmonary veins.

- **Bicuspid Valve**

  The left AV orifice is guarded by the mitral (bicuspid) valve; it allows oxygenated blood to pass from the left atrium to the left ventricle.

3. Right ventricle

The right ventricle (Figure II-2-37) receives blood from the right atrium via the tricuspid valve; outflow is to the pulmonary trunk via the pulmonary semilunar valve.

- **Trabeculae Carneae**

  The trabeculae carneae are ridges of myocardium in the ventricular wall.

- **Papillary Muscles**

  The papillary muscles project into the cavity of the ventricle and attach to cusps of the AV valve by the strands of the chordae tendineae.

- **Chordae Tendineae**

  The chordae tendineae are fibrous cords between the papillary muscles and the valve leaflets that control closure of the valve during contraction of the ventricle.

- **Infundibulum**

  The infundibulum is the smooth area of the right ventricle leading to the pulmonary valve.

- **Septomarginal Trabecula (moderator band)**

  This is a band of cardiac muscle between the interventricular septum and the anterior papillary muscle that conducts part of the cardiac conduction system.

4. Left Ventricle

Blood enters from the left atrium through the mitral valve and is pumped out to the aorta through the aortic valve (Figure II-2-37).

- **Trabeculae Carneae**

  The trabeculae carneae are ridges of myocardium in the ventricular wall, normally thicker than those of the right ventricle.

- **Papillary Muscles**

  The papillary muscles, usually 2 large ones, are attached by the chordae tendineae to the cusps of the bicuspid valve.

- **Chordae Tendinae**

  Same as right ventricle.

- **Aortic Vestibule**

  The aortic vestibule leads to the aortic semilunar valve and ascending aorta.

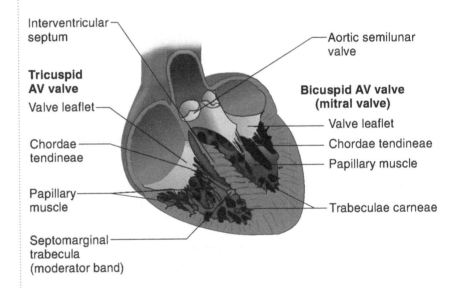

Figure II-2-37. Right and Left Ventricles

HEART HISTOLOGY

Cardiac muscle is striated in the same manner as skeletal muscle, but it differs in being composed of smaller cells (fibers) with only one or 2 nuclei. The nuclei are located centrally, instead of peripherally.

Layers of the Heart Wall

The heart wall is composed of 3 distinct layers: an outer epicardium, a middle myocardium and an inner endocardium. The epicardium, or visceral layer of serous pericardium, consists of a simple squamous epithelium (mesothelium) and its underlying connective tissue. The connective tissue contains a large number of fat cells and the coronary vessels. The muscular wall of the heart is the myocardium and is composed mainly of cardiac muscle cells. The endocardium, which lines the chambers of the heart, is composed of a simple squamous epithelium, the endothelium, and a thin layer of connective tissue. Cardiac muscle is striated like skeletal muscle, but these cells are smaller, with centrally placed nuclei. Cardiac muscle has a similar but somewhat less well developed T-tubule system compared to skeletal muscle that is located at the Z-line.

Intercalated Discs

Intercalated discs are special junctional complexes that join myocardial cells. The intercalated discs appear as dark, transverse lines in the light microscope. These disks contain gap junctions and adhering junctions. These junctions permit the spread of electrical (gap) and mechanical (adhering) effects through the walls of the heart, synchronizing activity and for the pumping action of the heart chambers. While intercalated discs allow coordinated action of the myocardial cells, the squeezing and twisting movements of the heart chambers (particularly the left ventricle) during systole are due to the disposition of cardiac myocytes.

Purkinje cells are modified cardiac muscle cells with fewer contractile filaments. They are specialized for electrical impulse conduction rather than contraction. Purkinje cells are found in the conduction system of the heart.

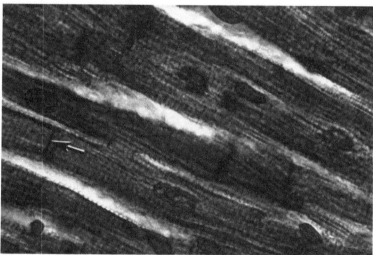

Figure II-2-38. Cardiac muscle cells with centrally placed nuclei and intercalated disks (arrow)

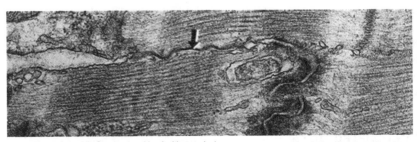

Figure II-2-39. EM of part of an intercalated disk with gap junction (arrow) adjacent to an adhering junction with intracellular density.

Auscultation of Heart Valves

Points of auscultation of the **semilunar valves** (aortic and pulmonary) and the **atrioventricular valves** (tricuspid and mitral or bicuspid) are shown in Figure II-2-40. The first heart sound occurs at the closure of the atrioventricular valves at the beginning of systole and the second heart sound occurs at the closure of the aortic and pulmonary semilunar valves at the end of systole.

Valves of the Heart

1. Atrioventricular

    Right Heart: Tricuspid

    Left Heart: Bicuspid

2. Semilunar

    Aortic (3 cusps)

    Pulmonary (3 cusps)

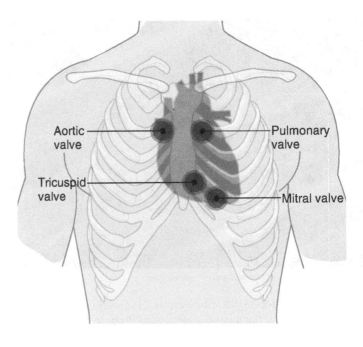

Figure II-2-40. Surface Projections of the Heart

Heart Murmurs

Murmurs in valvular heart disease result when there is **valvular insufficiency or regurgitation** (the valves fail to close completely) or **stenosis** (narrowing of the valves). The **aortic and mitral valves** are more commonly involved in valvular heart disease.

For most of ventricular systole, the mitral valve should be closed and the aortic valve should be open, so that "common **systolic** valvular defects" include **mitral insufficiency** and **aortic stenosis**. For most of ventricular diastole, the mitral valve should be open and the aortic valve should be closed, so that "common **diastolic** valvular defects" include **mitral stenosis** and **aortic insufficiency**.

A heart murmur is heard downstream from the valve. Thus, stenosis is orthograde direction from valve and insufficiency is retrograde direction from valve.

Auscultation sites for mitral and aortic murmurs are shown in Figure II-2-41.

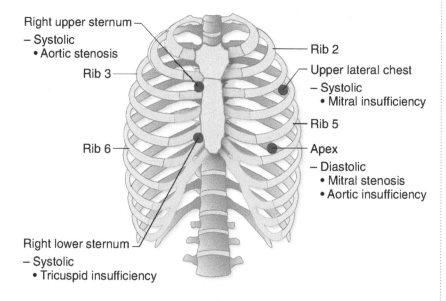

Figure II-2-41. Auscultation of Heart Murmurs

Table II-2-4. Heart Murmurs

	Stenosis	Insufficiency
A-V Valves Tricuspid (right) Mitral (left)	Diastolic Murmur	Systolic Murmur
Outflow Valves Pulmonic (right) Aortic (left)	Systolic Murmur	Diastolic Murmur

Arterial Supply of the Heart

The blood supply to the myocardium is provided by branches of the **right and left coronary arteries**. These 2 arteries are the only branches of the ascending aorta and arise from the **right and left aortic sinuses of the ascending aorta**, respectively. Blood flow enters the coronary arteries during diastole.

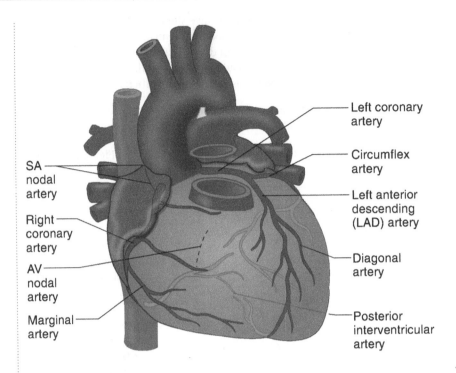

Figure II-2-42. Arterial Supply to the Heart

Clinical Correlate

In myocardial infarction, the left anterior descending artery is obstructed in 50% of cases, the right coronary in 30%, and the circumflex artery in 20% of cases.

Right coronary artery

The **right coronary artery** (Figure II-2-42) courses in the coronary sulcus and supplies major parts of the right atrium and the right ventricle.

The branches of the right coronary include the following:

- **Sinoatrial (SA) nodal artery:** One of the first branches of the right coronary, it encircles the base of the superior vena cava to supply the **SA node**.
- **Atrioventricular (AV) nodal artery:** It arises from the distal end of the right coronary artery as it forms the posterior interventricular artery and penetrates the interatrial septum to supply the **AV node**.
- **Posterior interventricular artery**: It is the terminal distribution of the right coronary artery and courses in the posterior interventricular sulcus to supply parts of the right and left ventricles and, importantly, **the posterior third** of the interventricular septum.

Left coronary artery

The **left coronary artery** (Figure II-2-42) travels a short course between the left auricle and ventricle, and divides into 2 branches: **anterior interventricular or left anterior descending (LAD) artery** and **circumflex artery**.

- The **anterior interventricular artery** descends in the anterior interventricular sulcus and provides branches to the (1) **anterior left ventricle wall**, (2) **anterior two-thirds of the interventricular septum**, (3) **bundle of His**, and (4) **apex**. The LAD is the most common site of coronary occlusion.

- The **circumflex artery** courses around the left border of the heart in the coronary sulcus and supplies (1) the **left border of the heart** via the **marginal branch** and (2) ends on the posterior aspect of the left ventricle and supplies the **posterior-inferior** left ventricular wall.

Venous Drainage of the Heart

The major cardiac veins (Figure II-2-43) draining the heart course in the sulci and accompany the arteries but do not carry the same names. The major veins are the following:

- **Coronary sinus**

  The coronary sinus is the main vein of the coronary circulation; it lies in the posterior coronary sulcus. It drains to an opening in the right atrium (Figure II-2-43). It develops from the **left sinus venosus**.

- **Great cardiac vein**

  The great cardiac vein lies in the anterior interventricular sulcus with the LAD artery. It is the main tributary of the coronary sinus.

- **Middle cardiac vein**

  The middle cardiac vein lies in the posterior interventricular sulcus with the posterior interventricular artery. It joins the coronary sinus.

- **Venae cordis minimae (thebesian veins) and anterior cardiac veins**

  The venae cordis minimae and anterior cardiac veins open directly to the chambers of the heart.

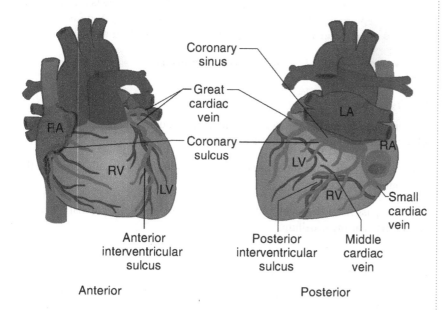

Figure II-2-43. Venous Drainage of the Heart

Conducting System of the Heart

The **cardiac conduction system is** a specialized group of myocardial cells that initiates the periodic contractions of the heart due to their ability to depolarize at a faster rate than other cardiac myocytes. Electrical activity spreads through the walls of the atria from the SA node and is quickly passed by way of internodal fibers to the atrioventricular node. From the atrioventricular node, activity passes through the bundle of His and then down the right and left bundle branches in the interventricular septum. The bundle branches reach additional specialized cardiac muscle fibers known as Purkinje fibers in the ventricular walls.

- The Purkinje fibers run in several bundles along the endocardial surface and initiate ventricle activity starting at the apex of the ventricles.
- Purkinje fibers have a large cross section, a cytoplasm with few contractile fibrils and a large content of glycogen.

SA node

The SA node initiates the impulse for contraction of heart muscle (and is therefore termed the "pacemaker" of the heart). It is located at the superior end of the crista terminalis, where the superior vena cava enters the right atrium (Figure II-2-44).

The SA node is supplied by the SA nodal branch of the **right coronary artery**.

Impulse production is speeded up by sympathetic nervous stimulation; it is slowed by parasympathetic (vagal) stimulation.

AV node

The AV node receives impulses from the SA node. The AV node is located in the interatrial septum near the opening of the coronary sinus. The AV node slows the impulse so that it reaches the ventricles after it has reached the atria.

The AV node is supplied by the **right coronary artery**.

Bundle of His

The **bundle of His** originates in the AV node. It conducts impulses to the right and left ventricles. It is supplied by the **LAD artery**.

In the right ventricle, the moderator band (septomarginal trabecula) contains the right bundle branch.

Impulses pass from the right and left bundle branches to the papillary muscles and ventricular myocardium.

Innervation

The cardiac plexus is a combination of sympathetic and parasympathetic (vagal) fibers.

- **Sympathetic** stimulation increases the heart rate. Nerves that sense **pain** associated with coronary artery ischemia (angina) follow the **sympathetic pathways** back into spinal cord segments T1–T5.
- **Parasympathetic** stimulation slows the heart rate. Sensory nerves that carry the afferent limb of cardiac **reflexes** travel with the **vagus nerve**.

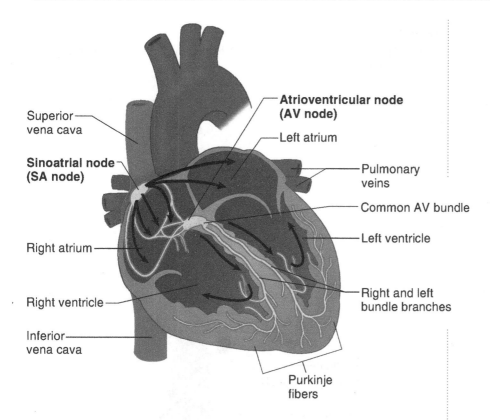

Figure II-2-44. Cardiac Conduction System

DIAPHRAGM

Composition

The diaphragm is composed of a muscular portion and a central tendon. It is dome-shaped, and descends upon contraction of its muscular portion. It is innervated by the **phrenic nerves** that arise from spinal cord segments **C3 through C5**.

Apertures in the Diaphragm

Caval hiatus

Located to the right of the midline at the level of T8, within the central tendon (Figure II-2-45)

Transmits the inferior vena cava and some branches of the right phrenic nerve

Esophageal hiatus

Located to the left of the midline at the level of T10, within the muscle of the right crus

Transmits the esophagus and the anterior and posterior vagus trunks

Aortic hiatus

Located in the midline at the level of T12, behind the 2 crura. Transmits the aorta and the thoracic duct.

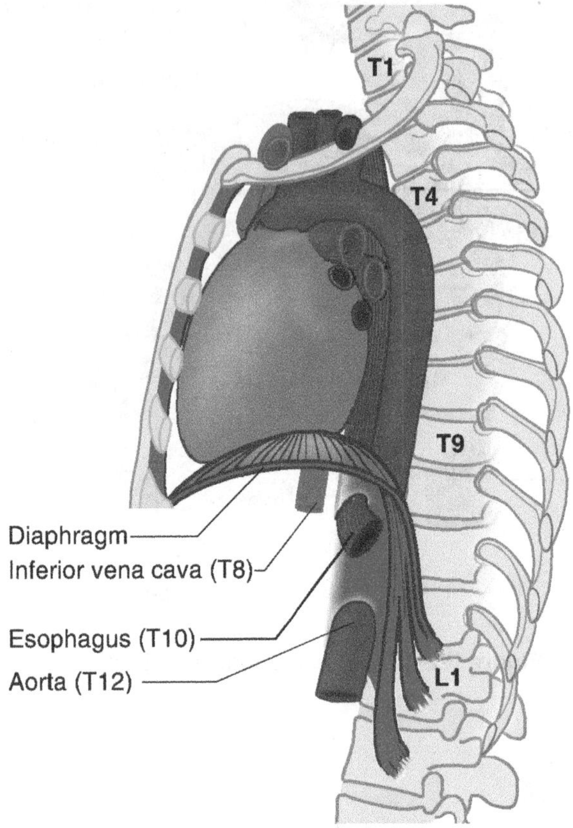

Clinical Correlate

Pain Referral

Because the innervation to the diaphragm (motor and sensory) is primarily from C3 through C5 spinal nerves, pain arising from the diaphragm (e.g., subphrenic access) is referred to these dermatomes in the shoulder region.

Clinical Correlate

A **congenital diaphragmatic hernia** is a herniation of abdominal contents into the plural cavity due to the failure of the **pleuroperitoneal membranes** to develop properly. The hernia is most commonly found on the left posterolateral side and causes pulmonary hypoplasia.

An **esophageal hiatal hernia** is a herniation of the stomach into the pleural cavity due to an abnormally large esophageal hiatus to the diaphragm. This condition renders the esophagogastric sphincter incompetent so that contents reflux into the esophagus.

Figure II-2-45. The Diaphragm

The diaphragm is formed by the fusion of tissues from 4 different sources:

1. The septum transversum gives rise to the central tendon of the diaphragm.
2. The pleuroperitoneal membranes give rise to parts of the tendinous portion of the diaphragm.
3. The dorsal mesentery of the esophagus gives rise to the crura of the diaphragm.
4. The body wall contributes muscle to the periphery of the diaphragm.

RADIOLOGY

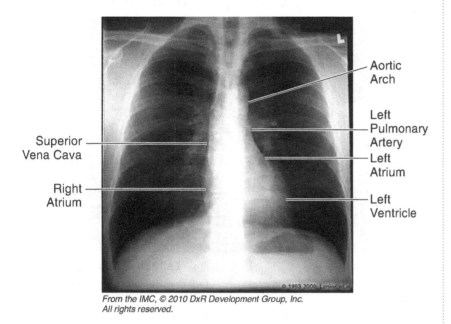

Figure II-2-46. Anterior Projection of Chest, Male

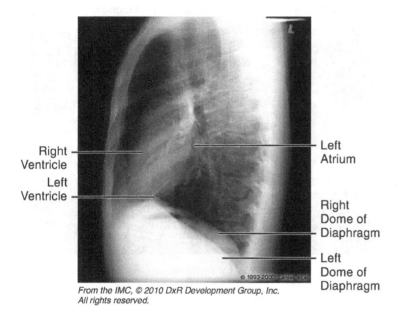

Figure II-2-47. Lateral Projection of Chest, Male

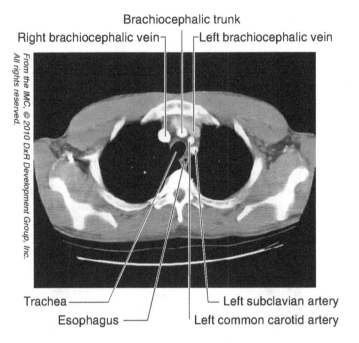

Figure II-2-48. Chest: CT, T2

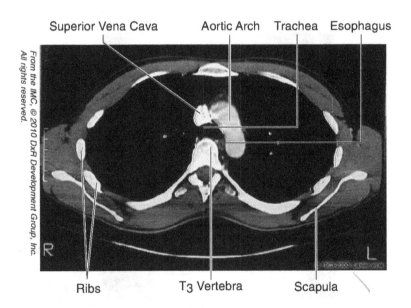

Figure II-2-49. Chest: CT, T3

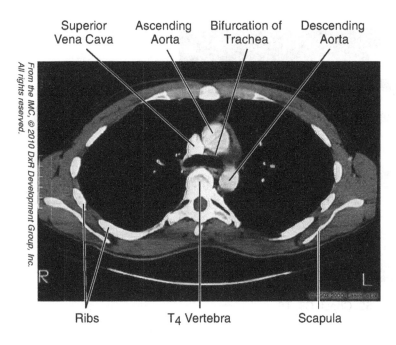

Superior Vena Cava   Ascending Aorta   Bifurcation of Trachea   Descending Aorta

Ribs   T4 Vertebra   Scapula

Figure II-2-50. Chest: CT, T4

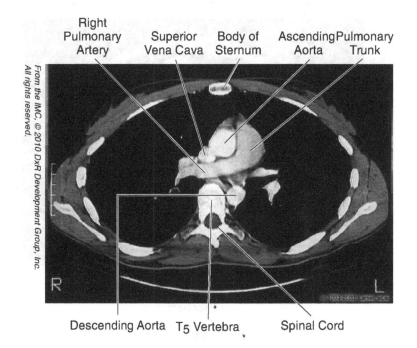

Right Pulmonary Artery   Superior Vena Cava   Body of Sternum   Ascending Aorta   Pulmonary Trunk

Descending Aorta   T5 Vertebra   Spinal Cord

Figure II-2-51. Chest: CT, T5

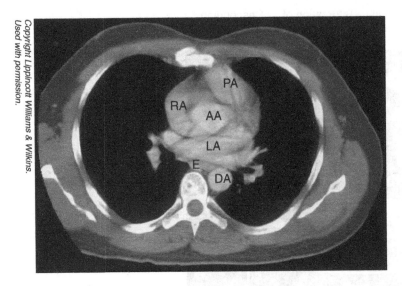

PA = pulmonary artery
RA = right atrium
AA = ascending aorta
LA = left atrium
E = esophagus
DA = descending aorta

Figure II-2-52. Chest: CT, T5

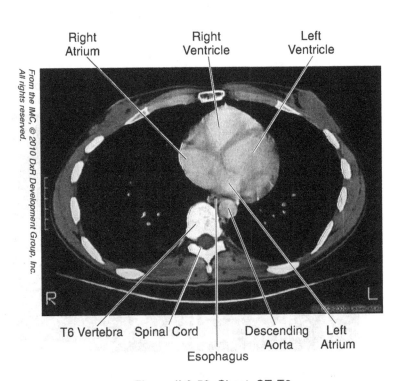

Right
Atrium

Right
Ventricle

Left
Ventricle

T6 Vertebra   Spinal Cord   Descending   Left
Aorta   Atrium

Esophagus

Figure II-2-53. Chest: CT, T6

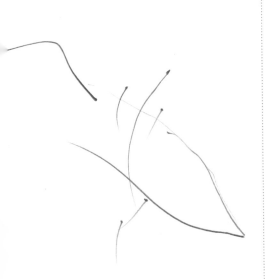

Chapter Summary

- The chest wall is formed by 12 thoracic vertebrae, 12 pairs of ribs, and the sternum. An important landmark on the anterior chest wall is the sternal angle found where the 2nd rib articulates with the sternum.

- The respiratory system develops as an endodermal outgrowth of the foregut. The tracheoesophageal septum separates the lung buds from the foregut. Improper development of this septum will produce an abnormal communication between the trachea and esophagus, a tracheoesophageal fistula.

- The lungs are surrounded by the pleura, which is divided into the parietal pleura lining, the inner surface of the thoracic cavity, and the visceral pleura that is attached to the surface of the lung. Between these 2 layers is the pleural cavity containing a small amount of serous fluid. The lungs demonstrate costal, mediastinal, and diaphragmatic surfaces and an apex that projects through the thoracic inlet into the root of the neck. Oblique and horizontal fissures divide the lungs into lobes.

- The nasal cavities have 2 major areas: respiratory and olfactory.

- **The respiratory area** is lined by pseudostratified, ciliated columnar epithelium. Goblet cells are present as well. **The olfactory area** is in the posterosuperior area and contains bipolar neurons. Olfactory neurons are constantly replenished. **Paranasal sinuses** are located in the frontal, maxillary, ethmoid, and sphenoidal bones. They communicate with the nasal cavities. The **nasopharynx** is composed of stratified, squamous nonkeratinized epithelium. The **pharyngeal tonsil** is an aggregate of nodular and diffuse lymphatic tissue within the posterior wall of the nasopharynx.

- Histologic features of the trachea, bronchi, and bronchioles are described in Table II-2-1. **Respiratory bronchioles** contain alveoli and branch to form alveolar ducts, which terminate in alveolar sacs and are lined by squamous alveolar epithelium. **Alveoli** are terminal, thin-walled sacs of the respiratory tree responsible for gaseous exchange. They contain 2 kinds of cells.

  - **Type I cells** provide a thin surface for gaseous exchange

  - **Type II cells** produce surfactant.

  Alveolar macrophages (dust cells) are located on the surface of alveoli and within the interalveolar connective tissue. They are derived from monocytes.

- Heart development begins with the formation of a primitive heart tube, which develops from the lateral plate mesoderm in the third week. The arterial end of the heart tube is called the truncus arteriosus and will develop into the aorta and pulmonary trunk. The sinus venosus at the venous end of the heart tube will develop into the coronary sinus and the smooth part of the right atrium. The primitive atrial and ventricle chambers divide into right and left chambers following development of interatrial and interventricular septae. Ventricular septal defects result from failure of the membranous septum to develop. Failure of the foramen ovale to close at birth results in atrial septal defects. Fetal circulation involves 3 shunts: ductus venosus, ductus arteriosus, and the foramen ovale. After birth these shunts shut down following changes in the circulatory system.

(Continued)

Chapter Summary

- The thoracic cavity is divided into the superior mediastinum above the plane of the sternal angle and the inferior mediastinum (anterior, middle, and posterior mediastina) below that sternal plane. The superior mediastinum contains the superior vena cava, aortic arch and its branches, trachea, esophagus, thoracic duct, and the vagus and phrenic nerves. The anterior mediastinum is anterior to the heart and contains remnants of the thymus. The middle mediastinum contains the heart and great vessels and the posterior mediastinum containing the thoracic aorta, esophagus, thoracic duct, azygos veins, and vagus nerve. The inferior vena cava passes through the diaphragm at the caval hiatus at the level of the 8th thoracic vertebra, the esophagus through the esophageal hiatus at the 10th thoracic vertebra, and the aorta course through the aortic hiatus at the level of the 12th thoracic vertebra.

- Covering the heart is the pericardium formed by an outer, tough fibrous layer and a doubled-layered serous membrane divided into parietal and visceral layers. The pericardial cavity is located between these 2 serous layers and includes the transverse and oblique pericardial sinuses.

- The external surface of the heart consists of several borders: the right border formed by the right atrium, the left border formed by the left ventricle, the base formed by the 2 atria, and the apex at the tip of the left ventricle. The anterior surface is formed by the right ventricle, the posterior surface formed mainly by the left atrium, and a diaphragmatic surface is formed primarily by the left ventricle.

- Arterial supply to the heart muscle is provided by the right and left coronary arteries, which are branches of the ascending aorta. The right coronary artery supplies the right atrium, the right ventricle, the sinoatrial and atrioventricular nodes, and parts of the left atrium and left ventricle. The distal branch of the right coronary artery is the posterior interventricular artery that supplies, in part, the posterior aspect of the interventricular septum.

- The left coronary artery supplies most of the left ventricle, the left atrium, and the anterior part of the interventricular septum. The 2 main branches of the left coronary artery are the anterior interventricular artery and the circumflex artery.

- Venous drainage of the heart is provided primarily by the great cardiac and middle cardiac veins and the coronary sinus, which drains into the right atrium.

- Sympathetic innervation increases the heart rate while the parasympathetics slows the heart rate. These autonomics fibers fire upon the conducting system of the heart.

  - The sinoatrial node initiates the impulse for cardiac contraction.

  - The atrioventricular node receives the impulse from the sinoatrial node and transmits that impulse to the ventricles through the bundle of His. The bundle divides into the right and left bundle branches and Purkinje fibers to the 2 ventricles.

Abdomen, Pelvis, and Perineum

Learning Objectives

- ❏ Explain information related to inguinal region and canal
- ❏ Answer questions about embryology of the GI system
- ❏ Solve problems concerning peritoneum
- ❏ Answer questions about GI histology, innervation, and immune functions
- ❏ Solve problems concerning arterial supply and venous drainage to abdominal viscera
- ❏ Explain information related to posterior abdominal body wall
- ❏ Answer questions about urinary histology and function
- ❏ Use knowledge of male and female reproductive histology
- ❏ Demonstrate understanding of radiology of the abdomen and pelvis

ANTERIOR ABDOMINAL WALL

Surface Anatomy

Linea Alba

The linea alba is a shallow groove that runs vertically in the median plane from the xiphoid to the pubis. It separates the right and left rectus abdominis muscles. The components of the rectus sheath intersect at the linea alba.

Linea Semilunaris

The linea semilunaris is a curved line defining the lateral border of the rectus abdominis, a bilateral feature.

Planes and Regions

The anterior abdominal wall is divided into 9 regions separated by several planes and lines (Figure II-3-1).

Subcostal plane

The subcostal plane (horizontal) passes through the inferior margins of the 10th costal cartilages at the level of the third lumbar vertebra.

Transpyloric plane

The transpyloric plane passes through the L1 vertebra, being half the distance between the pubis and the jugular notch. The plane passes through several important abdominal landmarks useful for radiology: pylorus of the stomach (variable), fundus of gallbladder, neck and body of the pancreas, hila of kidneys, first part of the duodenum, and origin of the superior mesenteric artery

Midclavicular lines

The midclavicular lines (vertical) are the 2 planes that pass from the midpoint of the clavicle to the midpoint of the inguinal ligament on each side.

RH: right hypochondrium

LH: left hypochondrium

RL: right lumbar

LL: left lumbar

RI: right inguinal

LI: left inguinal

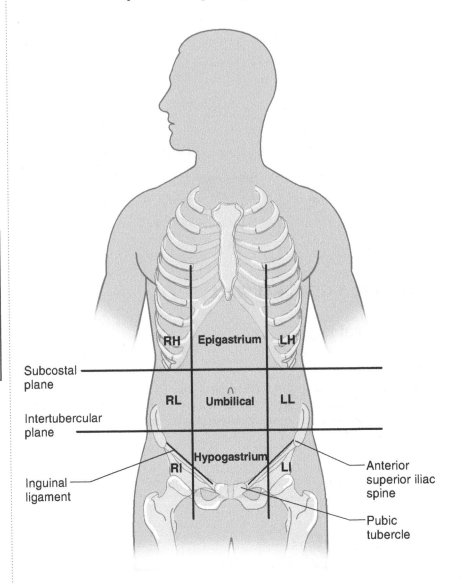

Figure II-3-1. Regions and Planes of the Abdomen

MUSCLES AND FASCIAE OF ANTERIOR BODY WALL

The anterolateral abdominal body wall is a multilayer of fat, fasciae, and muscles (with their aponeuroses) that support and protect the abdominal contents. Three flat abdominal muscles are arranged in layers and the rectus abdominis is oriented vertically adjacent to the midline, extending between the costal margin and the pubis. Abdominal muscles are important in respiration, defecation, micturition, childbirth, etc. The layers of tissue that make up the abdominal wall are described superficial to deep.

Layers of Anterior Abdominal Wall

Skin

Superficial fascia: The superficial fascia of the anterior abdominal wall below the umbilicus consists of 2 layers:

- **Camper** (fatty) fascia is the outer, subcutaneous layer of superficial fascia that is variable in thickness owing to the presence of fat.

- **Scarpa** (membranous) fascia is the deeper layer of superficial fascia devoid of fat. It is continuous into the perineum with various perineal fascial layers (Colles' fascia, dartos fascia of the scrotum, superficial fascia of the clitoris or penis).

Muscles

External abdominal oblique muscle and aponeurosis (Figure II-3-3): This is the most superficial of the 3 flat muscles of the abdominal wall. Its contributions to the abdominal wall and inguinal region are the following:

- **Inguinal ligament** is the inferior rolled under aponeurotic fibers of the external oblique that extend between the anterior superior iliac spine and the pubic tubercle. Medially, the fibers of the inguinal ligament form a flattened, horizontal shelf called the **lacunar ligament** that attaches deeply to the pectineal line of the pubis and continues as the pectineal ligament. Lacunar ligament forms the medial border of a femoral hernia.

- **Superficial inguinal ring** is a vertical triangular cleft in the external oblique aponeurosis that represents the medial opening of the inguinal canal just superior and lateral to the pubic tubercle. It transmits the structures of the female and male inguinal canals.

- **External spermatic fascia** is the outer layer of the 3 coverings of the spermatic cord formed at the superficial inguinal ring in males.

- **Rectus sheath**: The external aponeuroses contribute to the anterior layer of the rectus sheath.

In A Nutshell

Anterior Abdominal Wall Layers

- Skin
- Superficial fascia
  - Camper (fatty)
  - Scarpa (fibrous)
- External oblique
- Internal oblique
- Transversus abdominis
- Transversalis fascia
- Extraperitoneal connective tissue
- Parietal peritoneum

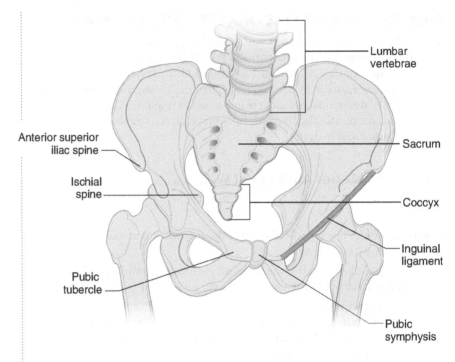

Figure II-3-2. Osteology of the Abdominopelvic Cavity

Internal abdominal oblique muscle and aponeurosis: This middle layer of the 3 flat muscles originates, in part, from the lateral two-thirds of the inguinal ligament. The internal oblique fibers course medially and arch over the inguinal canal in parallel with the arching fibers of the transversus abdominis muscle. The contributions of the internal abdominal oblique to the abdominal wall and inguinal region are the following:

> **Conjoint tendon (falx inguinalis)** is formed by the combined arching fibers of the internal oblique and the transversus abdominis muscles that insert on the pubic crest posterior to the superficial inguinal ring.
>
> **Rectus sheath**: The internal aponeuroses contribute to the layers of the rectus sheath.
>
> **Cremasteric muscle and fascia** represent the middle layer of the spermatic fascia covering the spermatic cord and testis in the male. It forms in the inguinal canal.

Transversus abdominis muscle and aponeurosis: This is the deepest of the flat muscles. The transversus muscle originates, in part, from the lateral one-third of the inguinal ligament and arches over the inguinal canal with the internal oblique fibers to contribute to the **conjoint tendon**. The aponeuroses of the transversus muscle also contribute to the layers of the rectus sheath. Note that it does not contribute to any of the layers of the spermatic fasciae.

Abdominopelvic Fasciae and Peritoneum

Transversalis fascia: This fascia forms a continuous lining of the entire abdominopelvic cavity. Its contributions to the inguinal region include the following (Figure II-3-3):

- **Deep inguinal ring** is formed by an outpouching of the transversalis fascia immediately above the midpoint of the inguinal ligament and represents the lateral and deep opening of the inguinal canal. The **inferior epigastric vessels** are **medial** to the deep ring.
- **Internal spermatic fascia** is the deepest of the coverings of the spermatic cord formed at the deep ring in the male.
- **Femoral sheath** is an inferior extension of the transversalis fascia deep to the inguinal ligament into the thigh containing the femoral artery and vein and the femoral canal (site of femoral hernia).
- **Rectus sheath:** The transversalis fascia contributes to the posterior layer of the rectus sheath.

Extraperitoneal connective tissue: This is a thin layer of loose connective tissue and fat surrounding the abdominopelvic cavity, being most prominent around the kidneys. The **gonads** develop from the urogenital ridge within this layer.

Parietal peritoneum: This is the outer serous membrane that lines the abdominopelvic cavity.

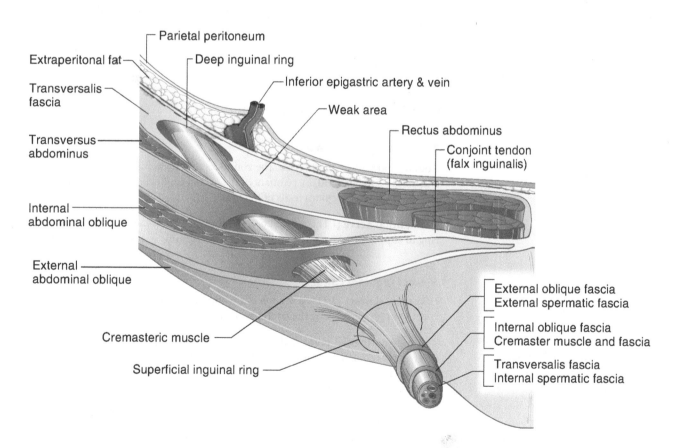

Figure II-3-3. Layers of Anterolateral Abdominal Wall and Inguinal Canal

Nerves, Blood Vessels, and Lymphatics of Abdominal Wall

Innervation of the skin and musculature of the anterior abdominal wall is via branches of the ventral primary rami of the lower 6 thoracic spinal nerves (includes the subcostal nerve), plus the iliohypogastric and ilioinguinal branches of the ventral primary rami of L1.

The major **arterial blood supply** to the anterior wall is derived from the superior epigastric branch of the internal thoracic artery, as well as the inferior epigastric and the deep circumflex iliac branches of the external iliac artery.

Venous drainage from the anterior wall is to the superficial epigastric, the lateral thoracic veins superiorly and the great saphenous vein inferiorly.

Lymph drainage from tissues of the anterior wall is to axillary nodes superiorly and to superficial inguinal nodes inferiorly.

INGUINAL REGION AND CANAL

The **inguinal canal** (Figure II-3-3) is the oblique passage way (approximately 4 cm long) in the lower aspect of the anterior abdominal wall running parallel and superior to the medial half of the inguinal ligament. Clinically, the inguinal region is important because it is the area where inguinal hernias occur.

The entrance into the canal is the **deep inguinal ring**, located just lateral to the inferior epigastric vessels and immediately superior to the midpoint of the inguinal ligament.

The **superficial inguinal ring** is the medial opening of the canal superolateral to the pubic tubercle.

Contents of the Inguinal Canal

1. Female Inguinal Canal

Round ligament of the uterus: The round ligament extends between the uterus and the labia majora and is a remnant of the caudal genital ligament and the homologue of the gubernaculum testis of the male.

Ilioinguinal nerve (L1) is a branch of the lumbar plexus that exits the superficial ring to supply the skin of the anterior part of the mons pubis and labia majora.

2. Male Inguinal Canal

Ilioinguinal nerve (L1) is a branch of the lumbar plexus that exits the superficial ring to supply the skin of the lateral and anterior scrotum.

The spermatic cord is formed during descent of the testis and contains structures that are related to the testis. The cord begins at the deep ring and courses through the inguinal canal and exits the superficial ring to enter the scrotum. The spermatic cord is covered by 3 layers of spermatic fascia: external, middle, and internal. The cord contains the following:

- **Testicular artery:** A branch of the abdominal aorta that supplies the testis.
- **Pampiniform venous plexus:** An extensive network of veins draining the testis located within the scrotum and spermatic cord. The veins of the plexus coalesce to form the testicular vein at the deep ring. The venous plexus assists in the regulation of the temperature of the testis.

Clinical Correlate

A **varicocele** develops when blood collects in the pampiniform venous plexus and causes dilated and tortuous veins. This may result in swelling and enlargement of the scrotum or enlargement of the spermatic cord above the scrotum. Varicoceles are more prominent when standing because of the blood pooling into the scrotum. A varicocele will reduce in size when the individual is horizontal.

- **Vas deferens** (ductus deferens) and its artery
- **Autonomic nerves**
- **Lymphatics:** Lymphatic drainage of the testis will drain into the lumbar (aortic) nodes of the lumbar region and not to the superficial inguinal nodes which drain the rest of the male perineum.

Fascial Layers of Spermatic Cord

There are 3 fascial components derived from the layers of the abdominal that surround the spermatic cord (Figure II-3-3):

1. **External spermatic fascia** is formed by the aponeuroses of the **external abdominal oblique** muscle at the superficial ring.

2. **Middle or cremasteric muscle and fascia** are formed by fibers of the **internal abdominal oblique** within the inguinal canal The cremasteric muscle elevates the testis and helps regulate the thermal environment of the testis.

3. **Internal spermatic fascia** is formed by the **transversalis fascia** at the deep ring.

Boundaries of the Inguinal Canal

Roof

Formed by fibers of the internal abdominal oblique and the transverse abdominis muscles arching over the spermatic cord (Figure II-3-3)

Anterior Wall

Formed by aponeurosis of the external abdominal oblique throughout the inguinal canal and the internal abdominal oblique muscle laterally

Floor

Formed by **inguinal ligament** throughout the entire inguinal canal and the lacunar ligament at the medial end

Posterior Wall: The posterior wall is divided into lateral and medial areas:

- **Medial area** is formed and reinforced by the fused aponeurotic fibers of the internal abdominal oblique and transversus abdominis muscles (**conjoint tendon**).
- **Lateral area** is formed by the **transversalis fascia** and represents the **weak area** of the posterior wall.
- **Inferior epigastric artery and vein** ascend the posterior wall just lateral to the weak area and just medial to the deep ring.

Descent of the Testes

The testis develops from the mesoderm of the urogenital ridge within the extra-peritoneal connective tissue layer.

- During the last trimester, the testis descends the posterior abdominal wall inferiorly toward the deep inguinal ring guided by the fibrous **gubernaculum.**
- An evagination of the parietal peritoneum and the peritoneal cavity extends into the inguinal canal called the **processus vaginalis**

Clinical Correlate

Cancers of the **penis** and **scrotum** will metastasize to the **superficial inguinal lymph nodes**, and **testicular** cancer will metastasize to the **aortic (lumbar) nodes**.

Clinical Correlate

In males, a **cremasteric reflex** can be demonstrated by lightly touching the skin of the upper medial thigh, resulting in a slight elevation of the testis. The sensory fibers of the reflex are carried by the L1 fibers of the **ilioinguinal nerve** and the motor response is a function of the genital branch of the **genitofemoral nerve** that innervates the cremasteric muscle.

Clinical Correlate

Failure of one or both of the testes to descend completely into the scrotum results in **cryptorchidism,** which may lead to sterility if bilateral.

(Figure II-3-4). The open connection of the processus vaginalis with the peritoneal cavity closes before birth.

- A portion of the processus vaginalis remains patent in the scrotum and surrounds the testis as the **tunica vaginalis.**

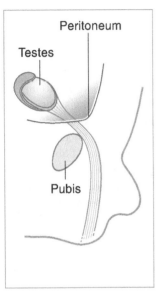
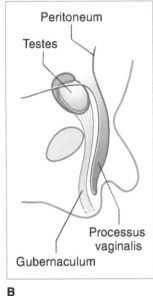
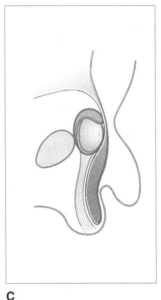
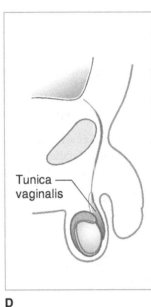

A   **B**   **C**   **D**

Figure II-3-4. Descent of the Testes

Inguinal Hernias

Herniation of abdominal viscera can occur in one of several weak aspects of the abdominal wall (e.g. inguinal, femoral, umbilical, or diaphragmatic). Inguinal hernias are the most common of the abdominal hernias and occur more frequently in males due to the inherent weakness of the male inguinal canal. Inguinal hernias occur superior to the inguinal ligament.

Two types of inguinal hernias are described (Figure II-3-5).

1. **Indirect inguinal hernias** result when abdominal contents protrude through the deep inguinal ring **lateral** to the inferior epigastric vessels.
   - After passing through the inguinal canal and superficial ring, the viscera can continue and coil in the scrotum.
   - Indirect hernias follow the route taken by the testis and are found **within** the spermatic cord.
   - They are covered by the 3 layers of spermatic fascia.

2. During a **direct inguinal hernia**, the abdominal contents protrude through the weak area of the posterior wall of the inguinal canal **medial** to the inferior epigastric vessels (in the **inguinal [Hesselbach's] triangle**).
   - Direct hernias rupture through the posterior wall of the inguinal canal and are usually found on the surface of the spermatic cord and bulge at the superficial ring.
   - They may be covered by only the external layer of spermatic fascia.

Note that both direct and indirect hernias exit through the superficial ring but only indirect hernias pass through the deep ring.

Clinical Correlate

Direct inguinal hernias usually pass through the **inguinal (Hasselbach's) triangle:**

- **Lateral border:** inferior epigastric vessels
- **Medial border:** rectus abdominis muscle
- **Inferior border:** inguinal ligament

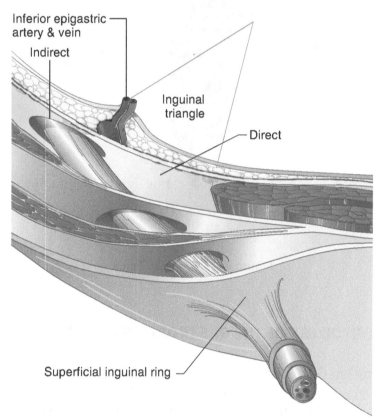

Inferior epigastric artery & vein

Indirect

Inguinal triangle

Direct

Superficial inguinal ring

Figure II-3-5. Inguinal Hernia

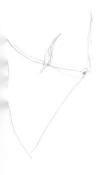

Femoral Hernias

Most often occur in women (Figure II-3-6)

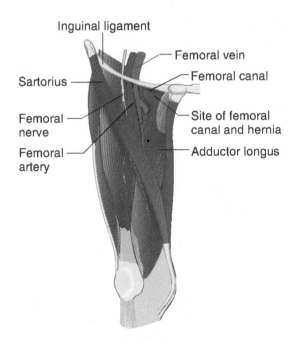

Femoral sheath contains femoral artery, vein, and canal

Inguinal ligament

Femoral vein

Femoral canal

Sartorius

Femoral nerve

Site of femoral canal and hernia

Femoral artery

Adductor longus

Figure II-3-6. Femoral Hernia

EMBRYOLOGY OF THE GASTROINTESTINAL SYSTEM

Primitive Gut Tube

- The primitive gut tube is formed by incorporation of the **yolk sac** into the embryo during 2 body foldings: **head to tail (cranial-caudal)** and **lateral foldings** (Figure II-3-7A).
- The epithelial lining of the mucosa of the primitive gut tube is derived from **endoderm**. The lamina propria, muscularis mucosae, submucosa, muscularis externa, and adventitia/serosa are derived from **mesoderm**.
- The primitive gut tube is divided into **the foregut, midgut, and hindgut,** each supplied by a specific artery and autonomic nerves (Table II-3-1).

Table II-3-1. Adult Structures Derived from Each of the 3 Divisions of the Primitive Gut Tube

Foregut	Midgut	Hindgut
Artery: celiac	**Artery:** superior mesenteric	**Artery:** inferior mesenteric
Parasympathetic innervation: vagus nerves	**Parasympathetic innervation:** vagus nerves	**Parasympathetic innervation:** pelvic splanchnic nerves
Sympathetic innervation: • Preganglionics: thoracic splanchnic nerves, T5–T9 • Postganglionic cell bodies: celiac ganglion	**Sympathetic innervation:** • Preganglionics: thoracic splanchnic nerves, T9–T12 • Postganglionic cell bodies: superior mesenteric ganglion	**Sympathetic innervation:** • Preganglionics: lumbar splanchnic nerves, L1–L2 • Postganglionic cell bodies: inferior mesenteric ganglion
Referred Pain: Epigastrium	**Referred Pain:** Umbilical	**Referred Pain:** Hypogastrium
Foregut Derivatives	**Midgut Derivatives**	**Hindgut Derivatives**
Esophagus Stomach Duodenum (first and second parts) Liver Pancreas Biliary apparatus Gallbladder	Duodenum (second, third, and fourth parts) Jejunum Ileum Cecum Appendix Ascending colon Transverse colon (proximal two-thirds)	Transverse colon (distal third—splenic flexure) Descending colon Sigmoid colon Rectum Anal canal (above pectinate line)

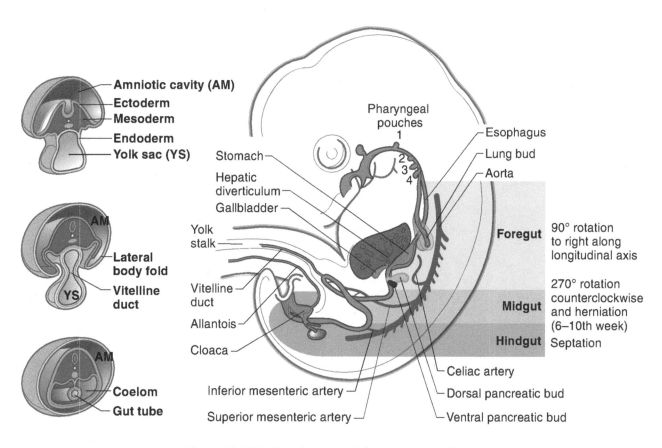

Figure II-3-7A. Development of Gastrointestinal Tract

In A Nutshell

The lower respiratory tract, liver and biliary system, and pancreas all develop from an **endodermal outgrowth of the foregut.**

Development and Rotation of Foregut

After body foldings and the formation of the gut tube, the foregut is suspended from the dorsal body wall by the **dorsal embryonic mesentery** and from the ventral body wall by the **ventral embryonic mesentery** (Figure II-3-7B). Note that the **liver** develops in the ventral embryonic mesentery, and the **spleen** and dorsal pancreatic bud develop in the dorsal embryonic mesentery.

- The abdominal foregut rotates 90° (clockwise) around its longitudinal axis. The original left side of the stomach before rotation becomes the ventral surface after rotation and its anterior and posterior borders before rotation will become the **lesser and greater curvatures**, respectively.

- Foregut rotation results in the liver, lesser omentum (ventral embryonic mesentery), pylorus of the stomach, and duodenum moving to the **right**; and the spleen, pancreas, and greater omentum (dorsal embryonic mesentery) moving to the **left** (Figure II-3-7B).

- The ventral embryonic mesentery will contribute to the **lesser omentum** and **the falciform ligament**, both of which attach to the liver.

- The dorsal embryonic mesentery will contribute to the **greater omentum** and the **gastro-splenic** and **splenorenal** ligaments, all of which attach to the spleen or the greater curvature of the stomach.

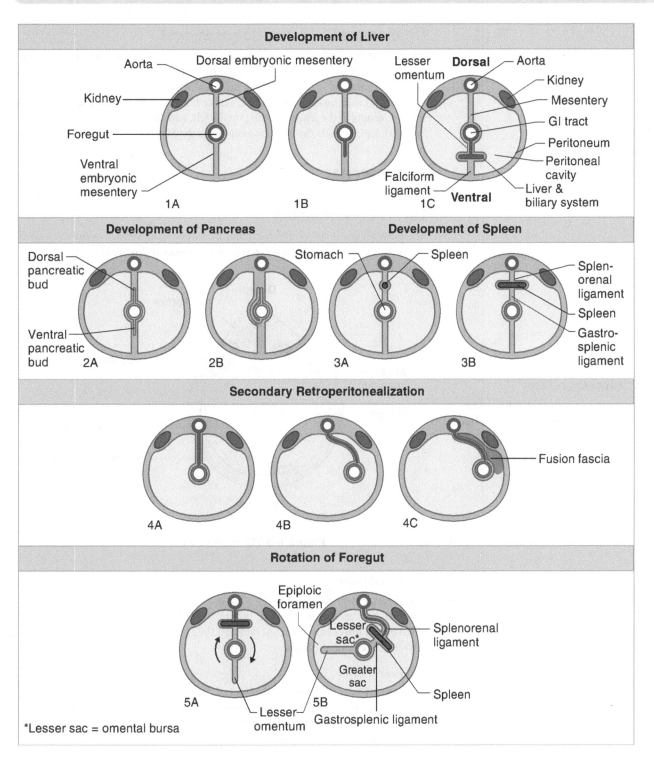

Figure II-3-7B. Cross-Sectional View of Foregut Development and Rotation

Development and Rotation of Midgut

The midgut originally develops from the cranial and caudal intestinal loops. During the sixth to the tenth week the midgut herniates into the umbilical cord. During herniation into and return from the umbilical cord, the midgut undergoes a 270° counterclockwise rotation around the axis of the **superior mesenteric artery**. This rotation results in the jejunum being on the left, and the ileum and cecum being on the right. It also causes the colon to assume the shape of an inverted "U."

270° anti clock

PERITONEUM

Layers of Peritoneum

The peritoneum is the serous membrane related to the viscera of the abdominal cavity. It is divided into 2 layers: **parietal** and **visceral** (Figure II-3-7C).

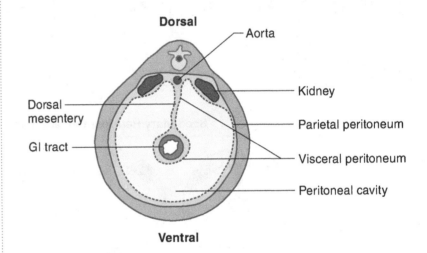

Figure II-3-7C. Peritoneum

Clinical Correlate

Inflammation of the parietal peritoneum (peritonitis) results in sharp pain that is localized over the area.

1. Parietal Layer

The parietal layer lines the body wall and covers the retroperitoneal organs on one surface. Parietal peritoneum is very sensitive to somatic pain and is innervated by the lower intercostal nerves and the ilioinguinal and the iliohypogastric nerves of the lumbar plexus.

2. Visceral Layer

The visceral layer encloses the surfaces of the intraperitoneal organs. The visceral peritoneum usually forms double-layered peritoneal membranes (mesenteries) that suspend parts of the GI tract from the body wall. The mesenteries allow for the passage of vessels, nerves, and lymphatics to reach the GI tract.

Different terms describe the postnatal remnants of mesenteries in the abdomen (Figures II-3-8 and II-3-9) and include the following:

- **Omentum:** Lesser and greater omenta attach to the lesser or greater curvatures of the stomach, respectively.
- **Mesocolon:** Transverse and sigmoid mesocolon attach to the transverse colon or the sigmoid colon, respectively.
- **Ligaments:** Reflections of mesenteries between organs or the body wall, named according to their attachments

Peritoneal Cavity

The peritoneal cavity is the potential space located between the parietal and visceral peritoneal layers. The 90° rotation and the shift of the embryonic mesenteries divides the peritoneal cavity into 2 sacs (Figures II-3-7B and II-3-9).

- **The lesser sac (omental bursa)** is a cul-de-sac formed posterior to the stomach and the lesser omentum
- **The greater sac** is formed by the larger area of the remaining peritoneal cavity. The only communication between the lesser sac and the greater sac is the **epiploic foramen (of Winslow)**.

Intraperitoneal versus Retroperitoneal Organs

The abdominal viscera are classified according to their relationship to the peritoneum (Table II-3-2).

- **Intraperitoneal organs** are suspended by a mesentery and are almost completely enclosed in visceral peritoneum. These organs are mobile.
- **Retroperitoneal organs** are partially covered on one side with parietal peritoneum and are immobile or fixed organs. Many retroperitoneal organs were originally suspended by a mesentery and become secondarily retroperitoneal.

Secondary Retroperitonealization: Parts of the gut tube (most of the duodenum, pancreas, ascending colon, descending colon, part of rectum) fuse with the body wall by way of fusion of visceral peritoneum with parietal peritoneum. This results in these organs becoming secondarily retroperitoneal and the visceral peritoneum covering the organ being renamed as the parietal peritoneum. The vessels within the mesentery of these gut structures become secondarily retroperitoneal.

Table II-3-2. Intraperitoneal and Retroperitoneal Organs

Major Intraperitoneal Organs (suspended by a mesentery)	Major Secondary Retroperitoneal Organs (lost a mesentery during development)	Major Primary Retroperitoneal Organs (never had a mesentery)
Stomach	Duodenum, 2nd and 3rd parts	Kidneys
Liver and gallbladder		Adrenal glands
Spleen	Head, neck, and body of pancreas	Ureters
Duodenum, 1st part	Ascending colon	Aorta
Tail of pancreas	Descending colon	Inferior vena cava
Jejunum	Upper rectum	Lower rectum
Ileum		Anal canal
Appendix		
Transverse colon		
Sigmoid colon		

Epiploic Foramen (of Winslow)

The **epiploic foramen** is the opening between omental bursa and greater peritoneal sac (Figures II-3-7B, II-3-8, and II-3-9). The boundaries of the epiploic foramen are the following:

Anteriorly: Hepatoduodenal ligament and the hepatic portal vein

Posteriorly: Inferior vena cava

Superiorly: Caudate lobe of the liver

Inferiorly: First part of the duodenum

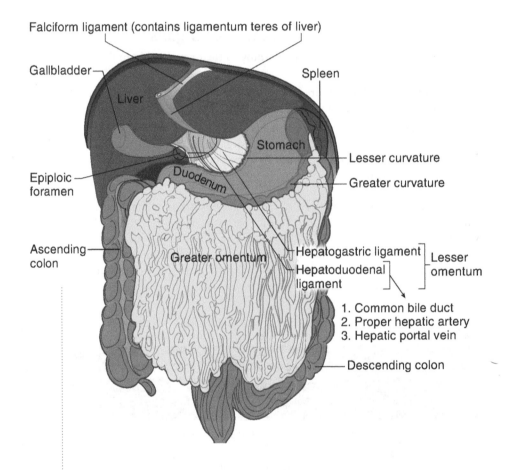

Figure II-3-8. Peritoneal Membranes

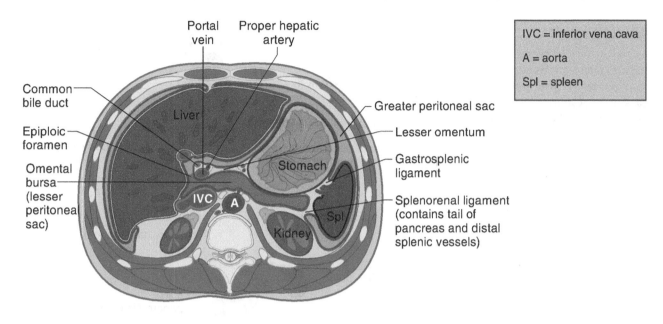

IVC = inferior vena cava

A = aorta

Spl = spleen

Figure II-3-9. Greater and Lesser Peritoneal Sacs

DEVELOPMENT OF ABDOMINAL VISCERA

Liver

The hepatic diverticulum develops as an outgrowth of the **endoderm** of the foregut in the region of the duodenum near the border between the foregut and the midgut (Figure II-3-7A).

- This diverticulum enters the ventral embryonic mesentery and distally becomes the liver and gallbladder and proximately becomes the biliary duct system.
- The part of the ventral embryonic mesentery between the liver and gut tube becomes the **lesser omentum**, and the part between the liver and ventral body wall becomes the **falciform ligament**.

Pancreas

The pancreas develops from 2 pancreatic diverticula (buds), which evaginate from the **endodermal** lining of the foregut in the region of duodenum (Figure II-3-10).

- The ventral bud rotates around the gut tube to fuse with the dorsal bud, together to form a single pancreas.
- The **dorsal pancreatic bud** forms the **neck, body, and tail of the pancreas**.
- The **ventral pancreatic bud** forms the **head and uncinate process**.

Clinical Correlate

A defect in the rotation and fusion of the ventral and dorsal buds results in an **annular pancreas** which can **constrict or obstruct** the duodenum and result in **polyhydramnios**.

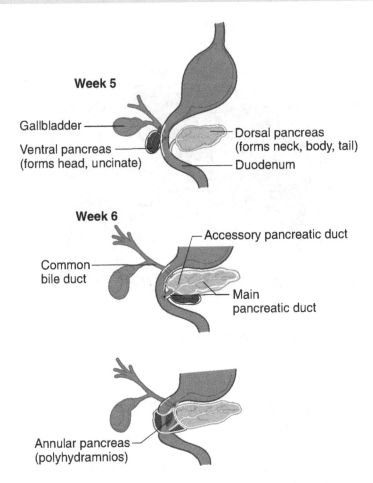

Figure II-3-10. Development of the Pancreas and Duodenum

Spleen

The spleen develops from **mesoderm** within the dorsal embryonic mesentery (Figure II-3-7B). The embryonic mesentery between the spleen and the gut tube becomes the **gastrosplenic ligament**. The mesentery between the spleen and the dorsal body wall becomes the **splenorenal ligament**.

CONGENITAL ABNORMALITIES OF THE GUT TUBE

Hypertrophic Pyloric Stenosis

Occurs when the muscularis externa hypertrophies, causing a narrow pyloric lumen. This condition is associated with **polyhydramnios**; projectile, nonbilious vomiting; and a small knot at the right costal margin.

Extrahepatic Biliary Atresia

Occurs when the lumen of the biliary ducts is occluded owing to incomplete re-canalization. This condition is associated with jaundice, white-colored stool, and dark-colored urine.

Annular Pancreas

Occurs when the ventral and dorsal pancreatic buds form a ring around the duo-denum, thereby causing an obstruction of the duodenum and polyhydramnios

Duodenal Atresia

Occurs when the lumen of the duodenum is occluded owing to failed recanaliza-tion. This condition is associated with **polyhydramnios**, bile-containing vomitus, and a distended stomach.

Omphalocele

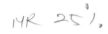

An omphalocele occurs when the midgut loop fails to return to the abdominal cavity and remains in the umbilical stalk.

- The viscera herniate through the **umbilical ring** and are contained in a **shiny sac** of amnion at the base of the umbilical cord.
- Omphalocele is often associated with multiple anomalies of the heart and nervous system with a high mortality rate (25%).

Gastroschisis

Gastroschisis occurs when the abdominal viscera herniate through the body wall directly into the amniotic cavity, usually to the right of the umbilicus.

- This is a defect in the closure of the lateral body folds and a weakness of the anterior wall.
- Note that the viscera do not protrude through the umbilical ring and are not enclosed in a sac of amnion.

Ileal (Meckel) Diverticulum

Occurs when a remnant of the vitelline duct persists, thereby forming a blind pouch on the antimesenteric border of the ileum. This condition is often asymp-tomatic but occasionally becomes inflamed if it contains ectopic gastric, pancre-atic, or endometrial tissue, which may produce ulceration. They are found 2 feet from the ileocecal junction, are 2 inches long, and appear in 2% of the population.

Vitelline Fistula

Occurs when the vitelline duct persists, thereby forming a direct connection between the intestinal lumen and the outside of the body at the umbilicus. This condition is associated with drainage of meconium from the umbilicus.

Malrotation of Midgut

Occurs when the midgut undergoes only partial rotation and results in abnormal position of abdominal viscera. This condition may be associated with **volvulus** (twisting of intestines).

Colonic Aganglionosis (Hirschsprung Disease)

Results from the failure of **neural crest** cells to form the myenteric plexus in the sigmoid colon and rectum. This condition is associated with loss of peristalsis and immobility of the hindgut, fecal retention and abdominal distention of the transverse colon (megacolon).

ABDOMINAL VISCERA

Liver

The liver has 2 surfaces: a superior or **diaphragmatic** surface and an inferior or a **viscera**l surface (Figure II-3-11). It lies mostly in the right aspect of the abdominal cavity and is protected by the rib cage. The liver is invested by visceral peritoneum:

- The reflection of visceral peritoneum between the diaphragmatic surface of the liver and the diaphragm forms the **falciform ligament**, which continues onto the liver as the coronary ligament and the right and left triangular ligaments.
- The extension of visceral peritoneum between the visceral surface of the liver and the first part of the duodenum and the lesser curvature of the stomach forms the **hepatoduodena**l **and hepatogastric ligaments** of the **lesser omentum**, respectively.

The liver is divided into 2 lobes of unequal size as described below (Figure II-3-11).

- Fissures for the ligamentum teres and the ligamentum venosum, the porta hepatis, and the fossa for the gallbladder further subdivide the right lobe into the right lobe proper, the quadrate lobe, and the caudate lobe.
- The quadrate and caudate lobes are anatomically part of the right lobe but functionally part of the left. They receive their blood supply from the left branches of the portal vein and hepatic artery and secrete bile to the left hepatic duct.

The liver has a central hilus, or porta hepatis, which receives venous blood from the **portal vein** and arterial blood from the **hepatic artery**.

- The central hilus also transmits the common bile duct, which collects bile produced by the liver.
- These structures, known collectively as the portal triad, are located in the hepatoduodenal ligament, which is the right free border of the lesser omentum.

The **hepatic veins** drain the liver by collecting blood from the liver sinusoids and returning it to the inferior vena cava.

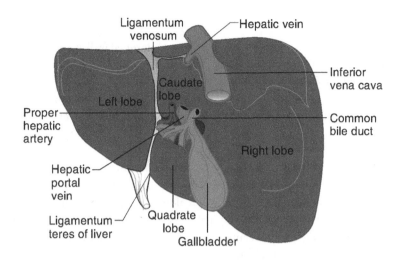

Figure II-3-11. Visceral Surface of the Liver

Gallbladder

The gallbladder lies in a fossa on the visceral surface of the liver to the right of the quadrate lobe. It stores and concentrates bile, which enters and leaves through the cystic duct.

- The cystic duct joins the common hepatic duct to form the **common bile duct** (Figure II-3-12).
- The common bile duct descends in the hepatoduodenal ligament, then passes posterior to the first part of the duodenum (Figure II-3-12). The common bile duct penetrates the head of the pancreas where it joins the main pancreatic duct and forms the **hepatopancreatic ampulla**, which drains into the second part of the duodenum at the **major duodenal papilla**.

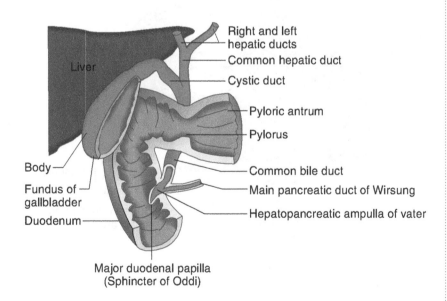

Figure II-3-12. Biliary Ducts

Pancreas

The pancreas horizontally crosses the posterior abdominal wall at approximately at the level of the transpyloric plane (Figure II-3-13). The gland consists of 4 parts: **head, neck, body, and tail.**

- The head of the pancreas rests within the C-shaped area formed by the duodenum and is traversed by the common bile duct. The head of the pancreas includes the **uncinate process** which is crossed by the superior mesenteric vessels.

- Posterior to the neck is the site of formation of the hepatic portal vein.

- The body passes to the left and passes anterior to the aorta and the left kidney. The splenic artery undulates along the superior border of the body of the pancreas with the splenic vein coursing posterior to the body.

- The tail of the pancreas enters the **splenorenal ligament** to reach the hilum of the spleen. The tail is the only part of the pancreas that is **intraperitoneal.**

The main **pancreatic duct** (Figures II-3-12 and II-3-13) courses through the body and tail of the pancreas to reach the head of the pancreas, where it joins with the common bile duct to form the hepatopancreatic ampulla.

The head of the pancreas receives its blood supply from the **superior and inferior pancreaticoduodenal branches** of the gastroduodenal and superior mesenteric arteries, respectively. This region is important for **collateral circulation** because there are anastomoses between these branches of the celiac trunk and superior mesenteric artery.

The neck, body, and tail of the pancreas receive their blood supply from the **splenic artery**.

Clinical Correlate

Carcinoma of the pancreas commonly occurs in the **head of the pancreas** and may constrict the main **pancreatic duct** and the **common bile duct**. Obstruction of the bile duct may result in **jaundice**.

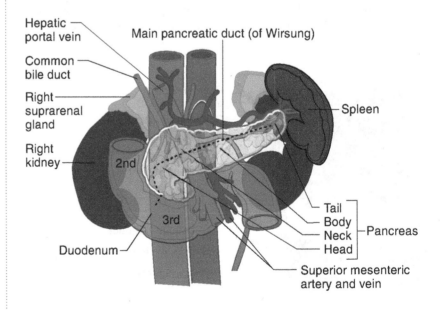

Figure II-3-13. Adult Pancreas

Spleen

The spleen is a peritoneal organ in the upper left quadrant that is deep to the left 9th, 10th, and 11th ribs The visceral surface of the spleen is in contact with the left colic flexure, stomach, and left kidney. Inasmuch as the spleen lies above the costal margin, a normal-sized spleen is not palpable.

The splenic artery and vein reach the hilus of the spleen by traversing the **spleno-renal ligament**.

Stomach

The stomach has a right **lesser curvature**, which is connected to the porta hepatis of the liver by the lesser omentum (hepatogastric ligament), and a left **greater curvature** from which the greater omentum is suspended (Figure II-3-8).

The cardiac region receives the esophagus; and the dome-shaped upper portion of the stomach, which is normally filled with air, is the fundus. The main central part of the stomach is the body. The pyloric portion of the stomach has a thick muscular wall and narrow lumen that empties into the duodenum approximately in the transpyloric plane (L1 vertebra).

Duodenum

The duodenum is C-shaped, has 4 parts, and is located retroperitoneal except for the first part.

- The first part is referred to as the duodenal cap (bulb). The gastroduodenal artery and the common bile duct descend posterior to the first part.
- The second part (descending) receives the **common bile duct** and main **pancreatic duct** (Figures II-3-10 and II-3-12) at the hepatopancreatic ampulla (of Vater). Smooth muscle in the wall of the duodenal papilla is known as the sphincter of Oddi.
- Note that the foregut terminates at the point of entry of the common bile duct; the remainder of the duodenum is part of the midgut.

Jejunum and Ileum

The jejunum begins at the duodenojejunal junction and comprises 2/5 of the remaining small intestine. The beginning of the ileum is not clearly demarcated; it consists of the distal 3/5 of the small bowel.

The jejunoileum is suspended from the posterior body wall by the mesentery proper. Although the root of the mesentery is only 6 inches long, the mobile part of the small intestine is approximately 22 feet in length.

Colon

Cecum

The cecum is the first part of the colon, or large intestine, and begins at the ileocecal junction. It is a blind pouch, which often has a mesentery and gives rise to the vermiform appendix. The appendix has its own mesentery, the mesoappendix.

Clinical Correlate

The spleen may be lacerated with a fracture of the **9th, 10th, or 11th rib on the left side**.

Clinical Correlate

A **sliding hiatal hernia** occurs when the cardia of the stomach herniates through the esophageal hiatus of the diaphragm. This can damage the vagal trunks as they pass through the hiatus.

Ascending colon

The ascending colon lies retroperitoneally and lacks a mesentery. It is continuous with the transverse colon at the right (hepatic) flexure of colon.

Transverse colon

The transverse colon has its own mesentery called the **transverse mesocolon**. It becomes continuous with the descending colon at the left (splenic) flexure of colon. The midgut terminates at the junction of the proximal two-thirds and distal one-third of the transverse colon.

Descending colon

The descending colon lacks a mesentery. It joins the sigmoid colon where the large bowel crosses the pelvic brim.

Sigmoid colon

The sigmoid colon is suspended by the **sigmoid mesocolon**. It is the terminal portion of the large intestine and enters the pelvis to continue as the rectum.

Rectum

The superior one-third of the rectum is covered by peritoneum anteriorly and laterally. It is the fixed, terminal, straight portion of the hindgut.

Anal Canal

- The **anal canal** is about 1.5 inches long and opens distally at the anus. The anal canal is continuous with the rectum at the pelvic diaphragm where it makes a 90-degree posterior bend (anorectal flexure) below the rectum.
- The **puborectalis component** of the pelvic diaphragm pulls the flexure forward, helping to maintain fecal continence.
- The **internal anal sphincter** is circular smooth muscle that surrounds the anal canal. The **sympathetics** (lumbar splanchnics) **increase** the tone of the muscle and the **parasympathetics** (pelvic splanchnics) **relax** the muscle during defecation.
- The **external anal sphincter** is circular voluntary skeletal muscle surrounding the canal that is voluntarily controlled by the inferior rectal branch of the **pudendal nerve** and **relaxes** during defecation.
- The anal canal is divided in an upper and lower parts separated by the **pectinate line**, an elevation of the mucous membrane at the distal ends of the anal columns. A comparison of the features of the anal canal above and below the pectinate line is shown in Table II-3-3.

Table II-3-3. Comparison of Features Above and Below the Pectinate Line

Above	Below
Visceral (ANS) sensory innervation	Somatic sensory innervation
Portal venous drainage	Caval venous drainage
Drain to iliac lymph nodes	Drain to superficial inguinal nodes
Internal hemorrhoids (painless)	External hemorrhoids (painful)
Endoderm	Ectoderm

Abbreviations: ANS, autonomic nervous system

GASTROINTESTINAL HISTOLOGY

The alimentary or gastrointestinal (GI) tract is a muscular tube that runs from the oral cavity to the anal canal. The GI tract walls are composed of 4 layers: mucosa, submucosa, muscularis externa, and serosa.

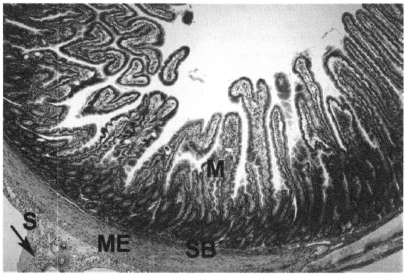

Copyright McGraw-Hill Companies. Used with permission.

Figure II-3-14. Organization of the GI tract

Mucosa (M) submucosa (SB), muscularis externa (ME),
serosa or visceral peritoneum (S), mesentery (arrow)

Mucosa

The **mucosa** is the innermost layer and has 3 components.

- The **epithelium** lining the lumen varies in different regions depending on whether the function is primarily conductive and protective (stratified squamous; in the pharynx and esophagus), or secretory and absorptive (simple columnar; stomach and intestine).
- The **lamina propria** is a layer of areolar connective tissue that supports the epithelium and attaches it to the underlying muscularis mucosae. Numerous capillaries form extensive networks in the lamina propria (particularly in the small intestine).

Within the lamina propria are blind-ended lymphatic vessels (lacteals) that carry out absorbed nutrients and white blood cells (particularly lymphocytes). The GALT (gut- associated lymphoid tissue), responsible for IgA production, is located within the lamina propria.

- The **muscularis mucosa** is a thin smooth-muscle layer that marks the innermost edge of the mucosa. The muscle confers some motility to the mucosa and facilitates discharge of secretions from glands. In the small intestine, a few strands of smooth muscle may run into the lamina propria and up to the tips of villi.

Submucosa

The **submucosa** is a layer of loose areolar connective tissue that attaches the mucosa to the muscularis externa and houses the larger blood vessels and mucus-secreting glands.

Muscularis Externa

The **muscularis externa** is usually comprised of 2 layers of muscle: an inner circular and an outer longitudinal. The muscularis externa controls the lumen size and is responsible for peristalsis. The muscle is striated in the upper third of the esophagus and smooth elsewhere.

Serosa

The **serosa** (or peritoneum of anatomy) is composed of a mesothelium (a thin epithelium lining the thoracic and abdominal cavities) and loose connective tissue. In the abdominal cavity, the serosa surrounds each intestinal loop and then doubles to form the mesentery within which run blood and lymphatic vessels.

INNERVATION

The GI tract has both intrinsic and extrinsic innervation. The intrinsic innervation is entirely located within the walls of the GI tract. The **intrinsic** system is capable of autonomous generation of peristalsis and glandular secretions. An interconnected network of ganglia and nerves located in the submucosa forms the Meissner's plexus and controls much of the intrinsic motility of the lining of the alimentary tract. Auerbach's plexus contains a second network of neuronal ganglia, and is located between the 2 muscle layers of the muscularis externa. All GI-tract smooth muscle is interconnected by gap junctions.

The **extrinsic** autonomic innervation to the GI tract is from the parasympathetic (stimulatory) and sympathetic (inhibitory) axons that modulate the activity of the intrinsic innervation. Sensory fibers accompany the parasympathetic nerves and mediate visceral reflexes and sensations, such as hunger and rectal fullness. Visceral pain fibers course back to the CNS with the sympathetic innervation. Pain results from excessive contraction and or distention of the smooth muscle. Visceral pain is referred to the body wall dermatomes that match the sympathetic innervation to that GI tract structure.

IMMUNE FUNCTIONS

The lumen of the GI tract is normally colonized by abundant bacterial flora. The majority of the bacteria in the body—comprising about 500 different species—

Clinical Correlate

Hirschsprung disease or aganglionic megacolon is a genetic disease present in approximately 1 out of 5,000 live births. It may result from mutations that affect the migration of neural crest cells into the gut. This results in a deficiency of terminal ganglion cells in Auerbach's plexus and affects of digestive tract motility, particularly in the rectum (peristalsis is not as effective and constipation results).

are in our gut, where they enjoy a rich growth medium within a long, warm tube. Most of these bacteria are beneficial (vitamins B$_{12}$ and K production, additional digestion, protection against pathogenic bacteria) but a few species of pathogenic microbes appear at times. Our gut has defense mechanisms to fight these pathogens (GALT and Paneth cells).

REGIONAL DIFFERENCES

Major differences lie in the general organization of the mucosa (glands, folds, villi, etc.) and in the types of cells comprising the epithelia and associated glands in the GI tract.

Table II-3-4. Histology of Specific Regions

Region	Major Characteristics	Mucosal Cell Types at Surface	Function of Surface Mucosal Cells
Esophagus	• Nonkeratinized stratified squamous epithelium • Skeletal muscle in muscularis externa (upper 1/3) • Smooth muscle (lower 1/3)	—	—
Stomach (body and fundus)	*Rugae:* shallow pits; deep glands	Mucus cells Chief cells Parietal cells Enteroendocrine (EE) cells	Secrete mucus; form protective layer against acid; tight junctions between these cells probably contribute to the acid barrier of the epithelium. Secrete pepsinogen and lipase precursor Secrete HCl and intrinsic factor Secrete a variety of peptide hormones
Pylorus	Deep pits; shallow, branched glands	Mucous cells Parietal cells EE cells	Same as above Same as above High concentration of gastrin
Small intestine	Villi, plicae, and crypts	Columnar absorptive cells	Contain numerous microvilli that greatly increase the luminal surface area, facilitating absorption
Duodenum	Brunner glands, which discharge alkaline secretion	Goblet cells Paneth cells EE cells	Secrete acid glycoproteins that protect mucosal linings Contains granules that contain lysozyme. May play a role in regulating intestinal flora High concentration of cells that secrete cholecystokinin and secretin
Jejunum	Villi, well developed plica, crypts	Same cell types as found in the duodenal epithelium	Same as above
Ileum	Aggregations of lymph nodules called Peyer's patches	M cells found over lymphatic nodules and Peyer's patches	Endocytose and transport antigen from the lumen to lymphoid cells
Large intestine	Lacks villi, crypts	Mainly mucus-secreting and absorptive cells	Transports Na$^+$ (actively) and water (passively) out of lumen

Oral Cavity

The epithelium of the oral cavity is a stratified squamous epithelium. Mucous and serous secretions of the salivary glands lubricate food, rinse the oral cavity, moisten the food for swallowing and provide partial antibacterial protection. Secretions of IgA from plasma cells within the connective tissue are transported through the gland epithelia to help protect against microbial attachment and invasion.

Esophagus

The esophagus is also lined by a stratified squamous epithelium. In the lower part of the esophagus there is an abrupt transition to the simple columnar epithelium of the stomach. Langerhans cells—macrophage-like antigen-presenting cells—are present in the epithelial lining. The muscularis externa of the esophagus consists of striated muscle in the upper third, smooth muscle in the distal third, and a combination of both in the middle third.

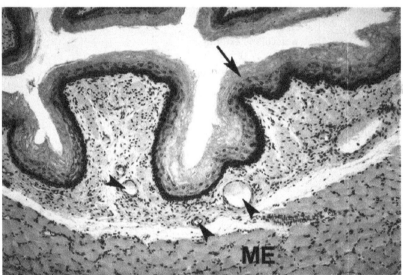

Copyright McGraw-Hill Companies. Used with permission.

Figure II-3-15. Esophagus with non-keratinizing stratified squamous epithelium (arrow) and a thin lamina propria with vessels (arrowheads)

The underlying muscularis externa (ME) is skeletal muscle from the upper half of the esophagus

Stomach

The stomach has 3 distinct histological areas: the cardia, body, and pyloric antrum. The mucosa of the stomach is thrown into folds (rugae) when empty, but disappears when the stomach is full. The surface is lined by a simple columnar epithelium. The stomach begins digestion by initiating the chemical and enzymatic breakdown of ingested food. Proteins are initially denatured by the acidic gastric juice before being hydrolyzed to polypeptide fragments by the enzyme pepsin. The chyme consists of denatured and partially broken-up food particles suspended in a semi-fluid, highly acidic medium.

Gastric pits form numerous deep tubular invaginations that line the inner surface of the stomach. The gastric pits are closely spaced; they penetrate into the thickness of the mucosa and extend into gastric glands. The transition between pits and glands is marked by the isthmus, where there is a narrowing of the lumen, and by a change in cellular composition of the epithelium. The glands are coiled in the cardiac and pyloric regions of the stomach and straight in the fundus and body regions. Glands in the body of the stomach deliver gastric juice (containing HCl and enzymes, rennin and lipase) to each pit, and from there to the stomach lumen. There are about 5 million glands in the stomach, secreting some 2 liters of fluid per day.

Mucus-secreting cells are located on the inner surface of the stomach, in the pit and in the neck, the transitional region between pits and glands. These cells produce a thick layer of mucus which covers and protects the stomach. The mucus falls into 2 categories: the surface mucus is composed of neutral glycoproteins, while the mucus secreted by the neck mucus cells is composed of acidic glycoproteins. In cardiac and pyloric regions, mucus cells are also the major cell type in the glands.

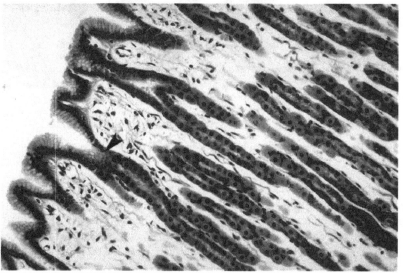

Figure II-3-16. Cardia part of the stomach with gastric pits and coiled gastric glands.

Stem cells that regenerate all stomach cells are located at the isthmus (arrowhead)

Oxyntic or parietal cells secrete 0.1N HCl into the stomach lumen and bicarbonate ions into the lamina propria (a byproduct of the acid production) in response to histamine, gastrin, and acetylcholine. These cells also secrete intrinsic factor (a glycoprotein necessary for absorption of vitamin B_{12}).

- Vitamin B_{12} is required for production of erythrocytes; deficiencies result in pernicious anemia and a disruption of peripheral and central nervous system myelin (see subacute combined degeneration in *Neuroscience* section).

Parietal cells, located in the upper regions of the gastric glands, have a broader base and narrower apex. Their structure varies greatly depending on their functional state.

Clinical Correlate

Acetylcholine and gastrin increase HCL secretion by parietal cells. Histamine potentiates both by binding to the histamine H_2 receptor. Cimetidine and H_2 antagonists inhibit histamine.

Clinical Correlate

Infection by *Helicobacter pylori* affects the gastric mucosal lining and allows pepsin, HCl, and proteases to erode the mucosa.

Hematemesis and melena are common clinical findings.

Chief or **peptic cells** secrete pepsinogen, an enzyme precursor that is stored in secretory (zymogen) granules before its induced secretion. Pepsinogen is inactive and protects the peptic cells from autodigestion. Low pH, in the stomach lumen, converts pepsinogen to pepsin.

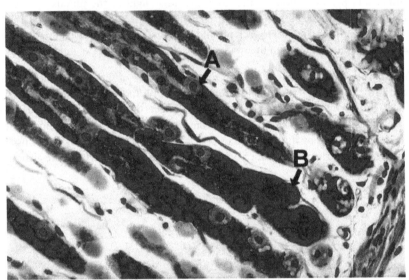

Figure II-3-17. Stomach near the base of gastric glands

Pale-staining parietal cells (A) and chief cells (B) are shown.

The **enteroendocrine cells** or APUD cells (amine precursor uptake and decarboxylation) are present throughout the GI tract and are also found in the respiratory tract. They constitute a diffuse neuroendocrine system that collectively accounts for more cells than all other endocrine organs in the body. Enteroendocrine cells are dispersed throughout the GI tract so that they can receive and transmit local signals.

The **stem cells** responsible for the regeneration of all types of cells in the stomach epithelium are **located in the isthmus**. Their mitotic rate can be influenced by the presence of gastrin and by damage (aspirin, alcohol, bile salt reflux). Renewal of many gastric epithelial cells occurs every 4–7 days.

- Although the stem cells are capable of differentiating into any of the stomach cell types, there is evidence that the position of the cell along the gland influences its fate.
- In contrast to the short life span (4–5 days) of the cells near the acidic environment, the chief cells—deep within the glands—may have a life span greater than 190 days.

Small Intestine

The small intestine is tubular in shape and has a total length of about 21 feet. The effective internal surface area of the small intestine is greatly increased by the plicae circulares, villi and microvilli.

Plicae circulares (circular folds or valves of Kerckring) are foldings of the inner surface that involve both mucosa and sub-mucosa. Plicae circulares increase the surface area by a factor of 3.

Villi arise above the muscularis mucosae and they include the lamina propria and epithelium of the mucosa. Villi increase the surface area by a factor of 10.

Microvilli of the absorptive epithelial cells increase the surface area by a factor of 20–30. The surface area of microvilli is increased even further by the presence surface membrane glycoproteins, constituting the glycocalyx to which enzymes are bound.

The luminal surface of the small intestine is perforated by the openings of numerous tubular invaginations (the crypts of Lieberkühn) analogous to the glands of the stomach. The crypts penetrate through the lamina propria and reach the muscularis mucosae.

The small intestine completes digestion, absorbs the digested food constituents (amino acids, monosaccharides, fatty acids) and transports it into blood and lymphatic vessels.

The **duodenum** is the proximal pyloric end of the small intestine. Distal to the duodenum is the **jejunum**, and then the **ileum**.

In the small intestine, the chyme from the stomach is **mixed** with mucosal cell secretions, exocrine pancreatic juice, and bile.

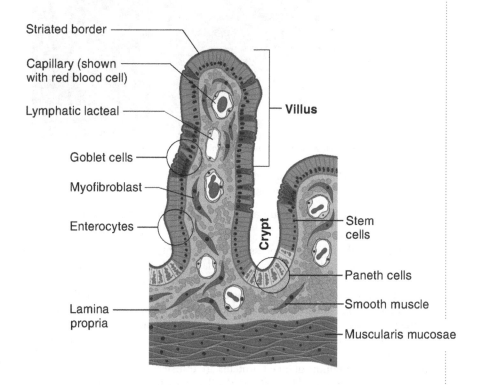

Striated border

Capillary (shown with red blood cell)

Lymphatic lacteal

Villus

Goblet cells

Myofibroblast

Enterocytes

Crypt

Stem cells

Paneth cells

Smooth muscle

Lamina propria

Muscularis mucosae

Figure II-3-18. Small Intestine Mucosal Histology

Clinical Correlate

Any compromise of the mucous protection can lead to significant damage and irritation of the gastrointestinal tract, leading to gastritis, duodenitis, or even peptic ulcer disease.

Clinical Correlate

Peristalsis is activated by the **parasympathetic system.** For those suffering from decreased intestinal motility manifesting as constipation (paralytic ileus, diabetic gastroparesis), dopaminergic and cholinergic agents are often used (e.g., metoclopramide).

Mucus production occurs in surface epithelial cells throughout the GI tract, by **Brunner glands** in the duodenum and **goblet cells** in the mucosa throughout the intestine.

Mucus functions include lubrication of the GI tract, binding bacteria, and trapping immunoglobulins where they have access to pathogens.

The **rate of mucus** secretion is increased by cholinergic stimulation, chemical irritation, and physical irritation.

In the **duodenum,** the acidic chyme from the stomach is neutralized by the neutral or alkaline mucus secretions of glands located in the submucosal or Brunner's glands. The duodenum also receives digestive enzymes and bicarbonate from the pancreas and bile from the liver (via gallbladder) through the bile duct, continuing the digestive process.

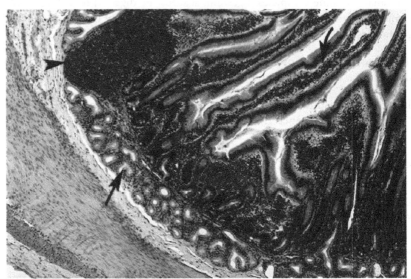

Copyright McGraw-Hill Companies. Used with permission.

Figure II-3-19. Duodenum with villi (curved arrow) and submucosal Brunner glands (arrow)

Patches of lymphatic tissue are in the lamina propria (arrowheads).

In the **jejunum,** the digestion process continues via enterocyte-produced enzymes and absorbs food products. The plicae circulares are best developed here. In the **ileum,** a major site of immune reactivity, the mucosa is more heavily infiltrated with lymphocytes and the accompanying antigen-presenting cells than the duodenum and jejunum. Numerous primary and secondary lymphatic nodules (Peyer's patches) are always present in the ileum's mucosa, though their location is not fixed in time. In the infant, maternal IgGs that are ingested are recognized by the Fc receptors in microvilli and endocytosed to provide passive immunity. In the adult, only trace amounts of intact proteins are transferred from lumen to lamina propria, but IgAs produced in GALT in the ileum are transported in the opposite direction into the lumen.

Throughout the small intestine, the simple columnar intestinal epithelium has 5 types of differentiated cells, all derived from a common pool of stem cells.

Note

Histologically, the duodenum contains submucosal Brunner's glands, and the ileum contains Peyer's patches in the lamina propria. The jejunum can be easily recognized because it has neither Brunner's glands nor Peyer's patches.

1. **Goblet cells** secrete mucous that protects the surface of the intestine with a viscous fluid consisting of glycoproteins (20% peptides, 80% carbohydrates).

2. **Enterocytes** have 2 major functions. Enterocytes participate in the final digestion steps and they absorb the digested food (in the form of amino acids, monosaccharides, and emulsified fats) by transporting it from the lumen of the intestine to the lamina propria, where it is carried away by blood vessels and lymphatics.

3. **Paneth cells** are cells located at the base of the crypts, especially in the jejunum and ileum; they contain visible acidophilic secretory granules located in the apical region of the cells. These cells protect the body against pathogenic microorganisms by secreting lysozyme and defensins (or cryptins) that destroy bacteria. Their life span is about 20 days.

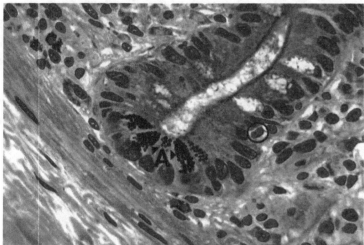

Figure II-3-20. Cells at the base of crypts of Lieberkühn include Paneth cells (A) with large apical granules of lysozyme, and an adjacent stem cell (circle) undergoing mitosis.

4. **Enteroendocrine cells** of the small and large intestine, like those of the stomach, secrete hormones that control the function of the GI tracts and associated organs. They are located in the lower half of the crypts and are detectable by silver-based stains.

5. **Stem cells** are located in the crypts, about one-third of the way up from the bottom. Their progeny differentiate into all the other cell types. **The epithelial lining of the small intestine, particularly that covering the villi, completely renews itself every 5 days (or longer, during starvation).** The newly created cells (goblet, enterocytes, and enteroendocrine cells) migrate up from the crypts, while the cells at the tips of microvilli undergo apoptosis and slough off. There is also a group of fibroblasts that accompany these epithelial cells as they move toward the tips of the villi. Other cells move to the base of the crypts, replenishing the population of Paneth and enteroendocrine cells.

Gut-associated lymphatic tissue (GALT): Throughout the intestine, the lamina propria is heavily infiltrated with macrophages and lymphocytes. Peyer's patches are patches of GALT that are prominent in the ileum. M cells in the epithelium transport luminal antigens to their base, where they are detected by B lymphocytes and taken up by antigen-presenting macrophages.

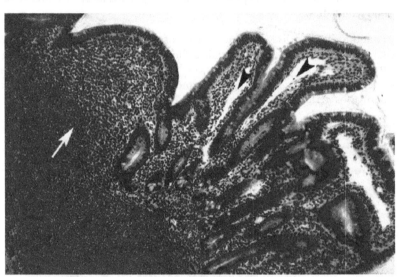

Figure II-3-21. Ileum with Payer's patches (arrow) and central lacteals (arrowheads) in the lamina propria of the villi

Large Intestine

The **large intestine** includes the cecum (with appendix), ascending, transverse, and descending colon, sigmoid colon, rectum, and anus. The large intestine has a wide lumen, strong musculature, and longitudinal muscle that is separated into 3 strands, the teniae coli. The inner surface has no plicae and no villi but consists of short crypts of Lieberkühn.

General features

- The colon is larger in diameter and shorter in length than is the small intestine. Fecal material moves from the **cecum**, through the colon (**ascending, transverse, descending,** and **sigmoid colons**), rectum, and anal canal.

- Three longitudinal bands of muscle, the **teniae coli**, constitute the outer layer. Because the colon is longer than these bands, pouching occurs, creating **haustra** between the teniae and giving the colon its characteristic "caterpillar" appearance.

- The mucosa has **no villi**, and mucus is secreted by short, inward-projecting colonic glands.

- Abundant lymphoid follicles are found in the cecum and appendix, and more sparsely elsewhere.

- The major functions of the colon are **reabsorption of fluid and electrolytes** and **temporary storage of feces**.

Defecation

Rectal distention with feces activates intrinsic and cord reflexes that cause relaxation of the internal anal sphincter (smooth muscle) and produce the urge to defecate. If the external anal sphincter (skeletal muscle innervated by the **pudendal nerve**) is then voluntarily relaxed, and intra-abdominal pressure is increased via the **Valsalva maneuver**, defecation occurs. If the external sphincter is held contracted, the urge to defecate temporarily diminishes.

Throughout the large intestine, the epithelium contains goblet, absorptive, and enteroendocrine cells. Unlike the small intestine, about half of the epithelial cells are mucus-secreting goblet cells, providing lubrication. The major function of the large intestine is fluid retrieval. Some digestion is still occurring, mainly the breakdown of cellulose by the permanent bacterial flora. Stem cells are in the lower part of the crypts.

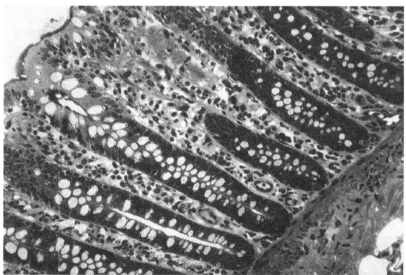

Figure II-3-22. Large intestine with crypts but no villi and many light-staining goblet cells interspersed among enterocytes

GASTROINTESTINAL GLANDS

Salivary Glands

The major salivary glands are all branched tubuloalveolar glands, with secretory **acini** that drain into **ducts**, which drain into the oral cavity. Acini contain **serous**, **mucous**, or both types of secretory cells, as well as **myoepithelial cells**, both surrounded by a basal lamina. Serous cells secrete various proteins and enzymes. Mucous cells secrete predominantly glycosylated mucins.

Table II-3-5. Gastrointestinal Glands

Salivary glands Submandibular Parotid Sublingual	• Produce approximately 1.5 L/day of saliva • Presence of food in the mouth; the taste, smell, sight, or thought of food; or the stimulation of vagal afferents at the distal end of the esophagus increase production of saliva		
Functions	• Initial triglyceride digestion (lingual lipase) • Initial starch digestion (α-amylase) • Lubrication		
Regulation	**Parasympathetic**	↑ synthesis and secretion of **watery** saliva via muscarinic receptor stimulation; (anticholinergics → dry mouth)	
	Sympathetic	↑ synthesis and secretion of **viscous** saliva via β-adrenergic receptor stimulation	

The ducts that drain the glands increase in size and are lined by an epithelium that transitions from cuboidal to columnar to pseudostratified to stratified columnar cells. The smallest ducts, **intercalated ducts**, have myoepithelial cells; the next larger ducts, **striated ducts**, have columnar cells with basal striations, caused by basal infolding of cell membranes between prominent mitochondria. These columnar cells make the saliva hypotonic by transporting Na and Cl ions out of saliva back into the blood.

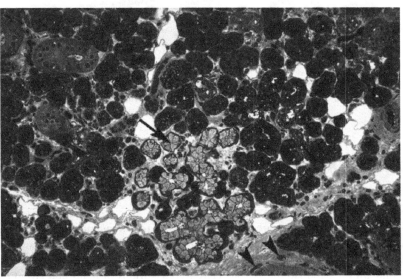

Figure II-3-23. Submandibular with a mix of light-staining mucus acini (arrow) adjacent to dark-staining serous acini

Small vessels (arrowheads)

Clinical Correlate

The parotid gland is the major site of the mumps and rabies viruses that are transmitted in saliva.

Benign tumors most frequently appear at the parotid gland; their removal is complicated by the facial nerve traversing the gland.

- The **parotid glands** lie on the surface of the masseter muscles in the lateral face, in front of each external auditory meatus. The parotids are **entirely serous** salivary glands that drain inside each cheek through **Stensen's ducts** which open above the second upper molar tooth. The parotid glands contribute 25% of the volume of saliva.

- The **submandibular glands** lie inside the lower edge of the mandible, and are mixed serous/mucous glands with a **predominance of serous** cells. They drain in the floor of the mouth near the base of the tongue through **Wharton's ducts**. The submandibular glands contribute 70% of the volume of saliva.

- The **sublingual glands** lie at the base of the tongue, and are also mixed serous/mucous glands with a **predominance of mucous** cells. They drain into the mouth through multiple small ducts, The sublingual glands contribute 5% of the volume of saliva.

Exocrine Pancreas

The pancreas is a branched tubuloacinar exocrine gland with **acini**. The acini are composed of secretory cells that produce multiple digestive enzymes including proteases, lipases, and amylases. Acinar cells are functionally polarized, with basophilic RER at their basal ends below the nucleus, and membrane-bound, enzyme-containing eosinophilic **zymogen granules** toward their apex.

The endocrine-producing cells of the **islets of Langerhans** are embedded within the exocrine pancreas.

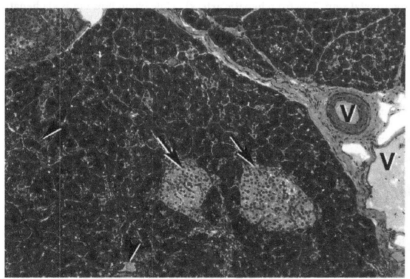

Figure II-3-24. Pancreas with light-staining islets of Langerhans (arrows) surrounded by exocrine acini with ducts (arrowheads) and adjacent blood vessels (V)

Unlike salivary glands, the **pancreas lacks myoepithelial cells** in acini and **lacks striated ducts**. Also, unlike salivary glands, the cells of the intercalated ducts extend partially into the lumen of pancreatic acini as **centroacinar cells**. The pancreas does not usually have mucinous cells in acini, but may have mucinous cells in its ducts.

Pancreatic acini drain via progressively larger ducts into the duodenum. The main pancreatic **duct (of Wirsung)** is the distal portion of the dorsal pancreatic duct that joined the ventral pancreatic duct in the head of the pancreas. The main duct typically joins with the common bile duct and enters the duodenum through the **ampulla of Vater** (controlled by the **sphincter of Oddi**). Sometimes the pancreas has a persistent accessory duct with separate drainage into the duodenum, the **accessory duct of Santorini**, and a persisting remnant of the proximal part of the dorsal pancreatic duct.

Liver

The liver is the largest visceral organ and gland (both exocrine and endocrine) in the body. **Hepatocytes**, of endodermal epithelial origin, carry out both exocrine and endocrine functions. The liver has unusual capillaries, the hepatic **sinusoids**, that facilitate exchange (uptake and secretion) between hepatocytes and blood. The liver has **Kupffer cells**, specialized cells of the mononuclear phagocyte system (blood monocyte derived) which patrol the **space of Disse** between hepatocytes and blood.

The liver has epithelial lined exocrine (excretory) ducts, the **bile ducts**, lined by **biliary epithelium**, which drain hepatocyte products (bile) into the duodenum, ultimately through the common bile duct. Blood flow into the liver is dual (75% from **portal vein**, 25% from **hepatic artery**), while blood flow out is via **hepatic veins** into the inferior vena cava.

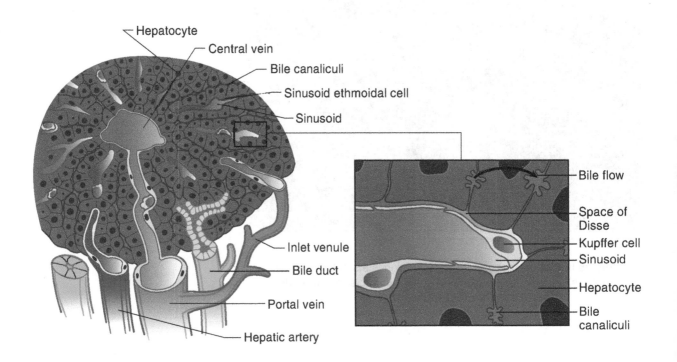

Figure II-3-25. Organization of a Liver Lobule

Hepatocytes are functionally polarized, like many other epithelial cells, but rather than being polarized along a single axis, each hepatocyte has multiple "**basal**" and "**apical**" surfaces.

- Where 2 hepatocytes abut, their "apical" surfaces form bile **canaliculi**, extracellular grooved bile channels joined by tight and occluding junctions between adjacent hepatocytes. Bile is secreted into bile canaliculi, which drains into progressively larger bile ducts and empties into the duodenum.

- Where a hepatocyte abuts a sinusoid, its membrane has microvilli, representing a "basal" or basolateral surface. Exchange between blood and hepatocytes is facilitated by the surface microvilli. This exchange occurs in the space of Disse which is between the fenestrated endothelial cells of the sinusoid and the basal surface of hepatocytes.

The hepatic artery and portal vein enter and the common hepatic duct exits the liver in the hepatic **hilum**. Within the liver, branches of the hepatic artery, portal vein, and bile duct tend to run together in thin connective tissue bands. When seen in cross section, these 3 structures and their connective tissue are called a **portal triad or portal tract**. Blood from portal vein and hepatic artery branches both flow through and mix in hepatic sinusoids that run between cords or plates of hepatocytes. After passing by hepatocytes, the sinusoidal blood flows into hepatic venules, which form progressively larger branches draining into the right and left hepatic veins which drain into the inferior vena cava.

A **classic hepatic lobule** is a hexagonal structure with a portal tract at each corner of the hexagon and a central vein in the center of the hexagon. Blood flow is from the triads into the central vein and bile flow is opposite, from the central vein to the triads.

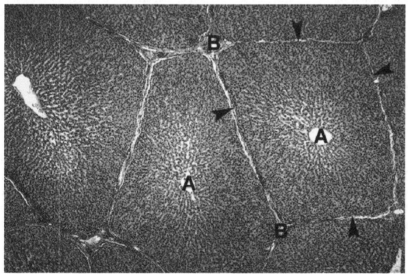

Figure II-3-26. Liver lobules with central veins (A) in the center of each lobule and connective tissue (arrowheads) separating each lobule and portal triads at each point of the lobule (B)

A **portal lobule** is a triangular structure with a central vein at each corner and a portal tract in the center. Bile flows from the periphery of the portal lobule into the central triad.

A **hepatic acinus** is based on blood flow from the hepatic artery branches to central veins. As hepatic arterial blood flow enters the sinusoids from side branches extending away from the center of the hepatic triad (rather than directly from the triad), the center of the acinus is conceived of as centered on such a branch extending out from a triad (or between 2 triads) and ending at 2 nearby central veins, resulting in a roughly elliptical structure with portal tracts at the 2 furthest poles and 2 central veins at the 2 closest edges.

In the acinus, the hepatocytes receiving the first blood flow (and the most oxygen and nutrients) are designated **zone 1**, while those receiving the last blood flow (and least oxygen and nutrients) are near the central veins and designated **zone 3**. **Zone 2** hepatocytes are in between zones 1 and 3. This model helps to explain the **differential effect on hepatocytes of changes in blood flow, oxygenation, etc**. Zone 3 is most susceptible to injury by decreased oxygenation of blood or decreased blood flow into the liver (as well as stagnation of blood drainage out of the liver due to congestive heart failure).

The metabolic activity of hepatocytes varies within the zones of the acinus. Zone 1 hepatocytes are most involved in glycogen synthesis and plasma protein synthesis (albumin, coagulation factors and complement components). Zone 3 cells are most concerned with lipid, drug, and alcohol metabolism and detoxification.

Ito cells (stellate cells) are mesenchymal cells that live in the space of Disse. They contain fat and are involved in **storage of fat-soluble vitamins, mainly vitamin A**.

Bile formation by hepatocytes serves both an exocrine and excretory function. Bile salts secreted into the duodenum aid in fat emulsification and absorption, as well as excretion of endogenous metabolites (bilirubin) and drug metabolites that cannot be excreted by the kidney.

Gallbladder

The gallbladder is lined by a simple columnar epithelium with both absorptive and mucin secretory function, with underlying lamina propria. Unlike the gut tube, the gallbladder **lacks muscularis mucosae and submucosa**, and the muscularis externa is not organized into 2 distinct layers like the gut. The surface of the gallbladder is covered by peritoneal serosa (mesothelium). The gallbladder has a wide end, the **fundus**, and a narrowing **neck**, which empties into the **cystic duct** and which has spiral valves of Heister. The cystic duct joins the **common hepatic duct** to form the **common bile duct**, which joins the pancreatic duct at or just before the ampulla of Vater.

Clinical Correlate

When stimulated during liver injury, Ito cells may release type I collagen and other matrix components into the space of Disse, **contributing to scarring** of the liver in some diseases (cirrhosis due to ethanol). This may lead to the development of portal hypertension, portacaval anastomoses, and esophageal or rectal bleeding.

Clinical Correlate

Disturbance of the balance in the components of bile can lead to precipitation of one or more of the bile components, resulting in stone (or **calculus**) formation or **lithiasis** in the gallbladder and/or bile ducts.

Note

Bile has 3 main functions:

(1) Absorption of fats from intestinal lumen

(2) Excretion

(3) Transport of IgA

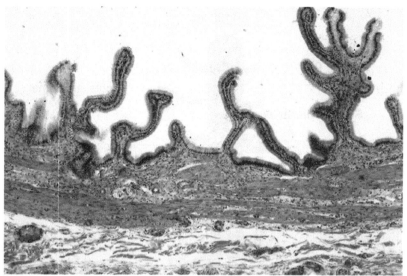

Figure II-3-27. Gallbladder with folds lined by a simple
columnar epithelium with no goblet cells

The gallbladder stores and concentrates bile by absorption of electrolytes and water. After a meal, entrance of lipid into the duodenum stimulates enteroendocrine cells of the duodenum to secrete cholecystokinin, which stimulates contraction and emptying of the gallbladder. At the same time, it relaxes the sphincter of Oddi in the ampulla of Vater. This delivers a bolus of bile into the duodenum.

ARTERIAL SUPPLY TO ABDOMINAL VISCERA

The blood supply to the abdominal viscera and the body wall is provided by branches of the abdominal aorta. The aorta enters the abdomen by passing through the aortic hiatus of the diaphragm at the **T12 vertebra** (Figure II-3-28). It descends on the lumbar vertebra just to the left of the midline and bifurcates at the **L4 vertebral** level. During its short course in the abdomen, the aorta gives origin to 3 groups of branches: (a) **3 unpaired visceral branches**, (b) **3 paired visceral branches**, and (c) several **parietal branches** to the body wall.

Note

Abdominal Aorta Branches

Visceral branches

Unpaired

- Celiac (foregut)
- Superior mesentric (midgut)
- Inferior mesentric (hindgut)

Paired

- Middle suprarenals
- Renals
- Gonadals

Parietal branches

Unpaired

- Medial sacral

Paired

- Inferior phrenics
- Lumbars
- Common iliac

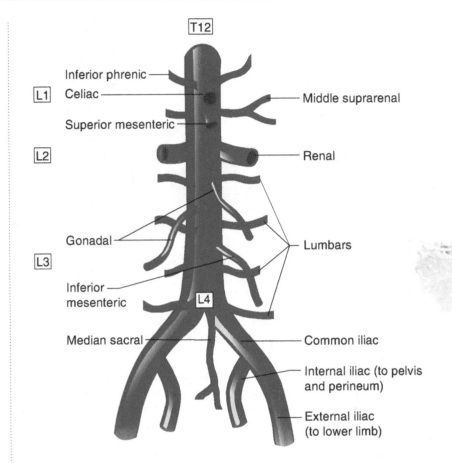

Figure II-3-28. Visceral and Parietal Branches of the Abdominal Aorta

Clinical Correlate

The most common site for an abdominal aneurysm is in the area between the renal arteries and the bifurcation of the abdominal aorta. Signs include decreased circulation to the lower limbs and pain radiating down the back of the lower limbs. The most common site of atherosclerotic plaques is at the bifurcation of the abdominal aorta.

Three Unpaired Visceral Arteries

Celiac Artery (Trunk)

The **celiac artery** (Figure II-3-29) is the blood supply to the structures derived from the foregut. The artery arises from the anterior surface of the aorta just inferior to the aortic hiatus at the level of T12–L1 vertebra. The celiac artery passes above the superior border of the pancreas and then divides into 3 retroperitoneal branches.

The **left gastric artery** courses superiorly and upward to the left to reach the **lesser curvature** of the stomach. The artery enters the lesser omentum and follows the lesser curvature distally to the pylorus. The distribution of the left gastric includes the following:

- **Esophageal branch** to the distal one inch of the esophagus in the abdomen
- **Most of the lesser curvature**

The **splenic artery** is the longest branch of the celiac trunk and runs a very tortuous course along the superior border of the pancreas. The artery is retroperitoneal until it reaches the tail of the pancreas, where it enters the splenorenal ligament to enter the hilum of the spleen. The distributions of the splenic artery include:

- Direct branches to the spleen
- Direct branches to the **neck, body, and tail of pancreas**
- **Left gastroepiploic artery** that supplies the left side of the **greater curvature** of the stomach
- **Short gastric** branches that supply to the **fundus** of the stomach

The **common hepatic artery** passes to the right to reach the superior surface of the first part of the duodenum, where it divides into its 2 terminal branches:

- **Proper hepatic artery** ascends within the hepatoduodenal ligament of the lesser omentum to reach the porta hepatis, where it divides into the **right and left hepatic arteries**. The right and left arteries enter the 2 lobes of the liver, with the right hepatic artery first giving rise to the **cystic artery** to the gallbladder.
- **Gastroduodenal artery** descends posterior to the first part of the duodenum and divides into the **right gastroepiploic artery** (supplies the pyloric end of the greater curvature of the stomach) and the **superior pancreaticoduodenal arteries** (supplies the head of the pancreas, where it anastomoses the inferior pancreaticoduodenal branches of the superior mesenteric artery).

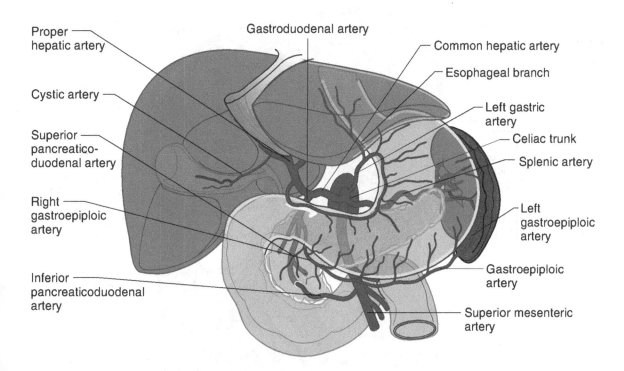

Figure II-3-29. Celiac Artery

Superior Mesenteric Artery

The **superior mesenteric artery** (SMA) (Figure II-3-30) supplies the viscera of the midgut. The SMA arises from the aorta deep to the neck of the pancreas just below the origin of the celiac artery at the L1 vertebral level. It then descends anterior to the uncinate process of the pancreas and the third part of the duodenum to enter the mesentery proper. The superior mesenteric vein is to the right of the artery. Branches of the SMA include:

1. **Inferior pancreaticoduodenal arteries** which anastomose with the superior pancreaticoduodenal branches of the gastroduodenal artery in the head of the pancreas

2. **Intestinal arteries** arise as 12–15 branches from the left side of the SMA and segmentally supply the jejunum and ileum. Distally, they form vascular arcades and vasa recta arteries at the wall of the gut.

3. **Ileocolic artery** is the most inferior branch which descends to the lower right quadrant to supply the distal ileum and cecum.

4. **Right colic artery** passes to the right to supply the ascending colon.

5. **Middle colic artery** ascends and enters the transverse mesocolon to supply the proximal two-thirds of the transverse colon.

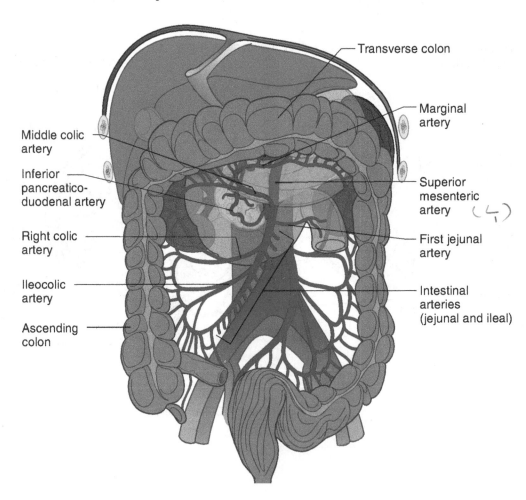

Transverse colon

Marginal artery

Middle colic artery

Inferior pancreatico-duodenal artery

Right colic artery

Ileocolic artery

Ascending colon

Superior mesenteric artery

First jejunal artery

Intestinal arteries (jejunal and ileal)

Figure II-3-30. Distribution of Superior Mesenteric Artery

Inferior Mesenteric Artery

The inferior mesenteric artery (IMA) (Figure II-3-31) is the third unpaired visceral branch of the aorta that supplies the hindgut (distal third of the transverse colon to the pectinate line). The IMA arises from the aorta just above its bifurcation at the level of the L3 vertebra. It descends retroperitoneally and inferiorly to the left and gives rise to 3 branches:

1. **Left colic artery** supplies the distal third of the transverse colon and the descending colon

2. **Sigmoid arteries** to the sigmoid colon

3. **Superior rectal artery** descends into the pelvis and supplies the superior aspect of the rectum and anal canal.

The branches of the SMA and IMA to the ascending, transverse and descending parts of the large intestines are interconnected by a continual arterial arch called the **marginal artery**. The marginal artery provides a collateral circulation between the parts of the large intestines if there is a vascular obstruction in some part of the SMA and IMA.

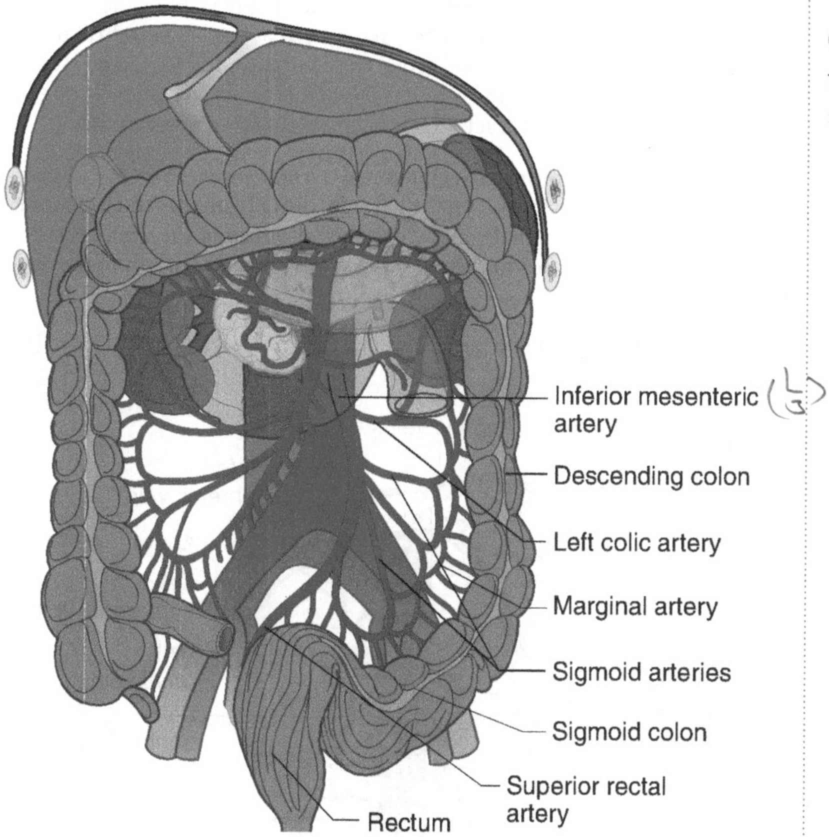

Clinical Correlate

Branches of the **celiac** and **superior mesenteric arteries** form a collateral circulation within the head of the pancreas (Figure II-3-29).

Clinical Correlate

The **splenic flexure** is the most common site of bowel ischemia.

- Inferior mesenteric artery
- Descending colon
- Left colic artery
- Marginal artery
- Sigmoid arteries
- Sigmoid colon
- Superior rectal artery
- Rectum

Figure II-3-31. Distribution of Inferior Mesenteric Artery

Three Paired Visceral Arteries

- **Middle suprarenal arteries** branch from the aorta above the renal arteries and supply the medial parts of the suprarenal gland.
- **Renal arteries** are large paired vessels that arise from the aorta at the upper border of the L2 vertebra. They course horizontally to the hila of the kidneys. The right renal artery is the longer than the left and passes posterior to the inferior vena cava.
- **Gonadal arteries** arise from the anterior surface of the aorta just inferior to the renal arteries. They descend retroperitoneally on the ventral surface of the psoas major muscle.

VENOUS DRAINAGE OF ABDOMINAL VISCERA

Inferior Vena Cava

The **inferior vena cava** forms to the right of the lumbar vertebrae and the abdominal aorta by the union of the 2 common iliac veins at the **L5 vertebral level** (Figure II-3-32). The inferior vena cava ascends to the right of the midline and passes through the caval hiatus of the diaphragm at the **T8 vertebral level**. The inferior vena cava receives blood from the lower limbs, pelvis and perineum, paired abdominal viscera, and body wall. Note that the vena cava does not receive blood directly from the GI tract, except the lower rectum and anal canal.

Note that the **right tributaries** (right gonadal, right suprarenal) drain separately into the inferior vena cava. But on the left side, the left gonadal and left suprarenal veins drain into the left renal vein, which then drains into the vena cava. The left renal vein crosses anterior to the aorta, just inferior to the origin of the superior mesenteric artery.

The drainage of the inferior vena cava and its tributaries is shown in Figure II-3-32.

Clinical Correlate

The **left renal vein may be compressed** by an **aneurysm of the superior mesenteric artery** as the vein crosses anterior to the aorta. Patients with compression of the left renal vein may have renal and adrenal hypertension on the left, and, in males, a varicocele on the left.

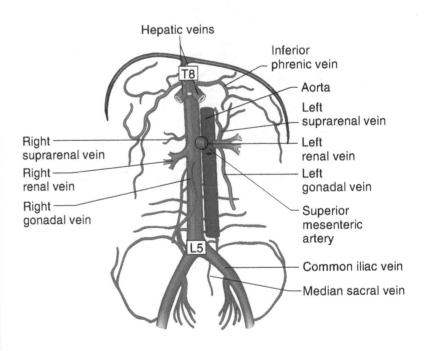

Figure II-3-32. Inferior Vena Cava and Tributaries

Hepatic veins
Inferior phrenic vein
Aorta
Left suprarenal vein
Left renal vein
Left gonadal vein
Superior mesenteric artery
Common iliac vein
Median sacral vein
Right suprarenal vein
Right renal vein
Right gonadal vein
T8
L5

Hepatic Portal System

The **hepatic portal system** is an extensive network of veins that receives the blood flow from the GI tract above the pectinate line. The venous flow is carried to the liver via the **hepatic portal vein** where it enters the liver sinusoids, which drain to the hepatic veins, which then drain into the inferior vena cava and ultimately into the right atrium.

The hepatic portal vein is formed by the union of the **superior mesenteric** (drains midgut) and **splenic** (drains foregut) veins posterior to the **neck of the pancreas**. The **inferior mesenteric vein** (drains hindgut) usually drains into splenic vein. (Figure II-3-33A and -33B).

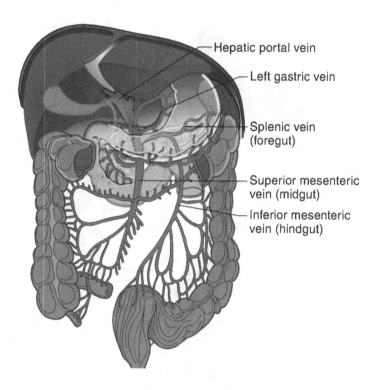

— Hepatic portal vein

— Left gastric vein

— Splenic vein (foregut)

— Superior mesenteric vein (midgut)

— Inferior mesenteric vein (hindgut)

Figure II-3-33A. Hepatic Portal System

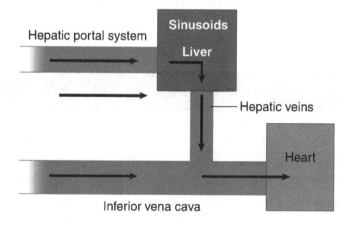

Figure II-3-33B. Comparison of Normal Caval and Portal Blood Flow

Portalcaval (Systemic) Anastomoses

If there is an obstruction to flow through the portal system (portal hypertension), blood can flow in a retrograde direction (because of the absence of valves in the portal system) and pass through anastomoses to reach the caval system. Sites for these anastomoses include the **esophageal veins, rectal veins**, and **thoracoepi-gastric veins**. Enlargement of these veins may result in esophageal varices, hemorrhoids, and a caput medusae (Figure II-3-34 and Table II-3-6).

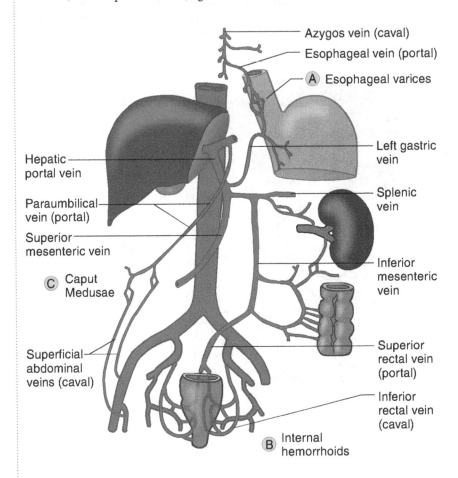

Figure II-3-34. Chief Portacaval Anastomoses

Table II-3-6. Sites of Portacaval Anastomoses

Sites of Anastomoses	Portal	Caval	Clinical Signs
Umbilicus	Paraumbilical veins ⟶	Superficial veins of the anterior abdominal wall	Caput medusa
Rectum	Superior rectal veins (inferior mesenteric vein) ⟶	Inferior rectal veins (internal iliac vein)	Internal hemorrhoids
Esophagus	Esophageal veins (left gastric veins) ⟶	Veins of the thoracic esophagus, which drain into the azygos system	Esophageal varices

POSTERIOR ABDOMINAL BODY WALL

Embryology of Kidneys and Ureter

Renal development is characterized by 3 successive, slightly overlapping kidney systems: pronephros, mesonephros, and metanephros (Figure II-3-35).

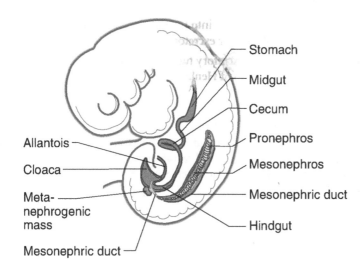

- Stomach
- Midgut
- Cecum
- Pronephros
- Mesonephros
- Mesonephric duct
- Hindgut

Allantois
Cloaca
Meta-nephrogenic mass
Mesonephric duct

Figure II-3-35. Pronephros, Mesonephros, and Metanephros

Pronephros

During week 4, segmented nephrotomes appear in the cervical intermediate mesoderm of the embryo. These structures grow laterally and canalize to form nephric tubules. The first tubules formed regress before the last ones are formed. **By the end of week 4, the pronephros disappears and does not function.**

Mesonephros

In week 5, the mesonephros appears as S-shaped tubules in the intermediate mesoderm of the thoracic and lumbar regions of the embryo.

- The medial end of each tubule enlarges to form a Bowman's capsule into which a tuft of capillaries, or glomerulus, invaginates.
- The lateral end of each tubule opens into the **mesonephric (Wolffian) duct**, an intermediate mesoderm derivative. The duct drains into the hindgut.
- Mesonephric tubules function temporarily and degenerate by the beginning of month 3. The mesonephric duct persists in the male as the ductus epididymidis, ductus deferens, and the ejaculatory duct. It disappears in the female.

Metanephros

During week 5, the metanephros, or permanent kidney, develops from 2 sources: the **ureteric bud,** a diverticulum of the mesonephric duct, and the **metanephric mass** (blastema), from intermediate mesoderm of the lumbar and sacral regions (Figure II-3-36).

The **ureteric bud** penetrates the metanephric mass, which condenses around the diverticulum to form the metanephrogenic cap. The bud dilates to form the renal pelvis, which subsequently splits into the cranial and caudal major calyces. Each major calyx buds into the metanephric tissue to form the minor calyces. One to 3 million collecting tubules develop from the minor calyces, thus forming the renal pyramids. The ureteric bud forms the **drainage components** of the urinary system (calyces, pelvis, ureter).

Penetration of collecting tubules into the **metanephric mass** induces cells of the tissue cap to form **nephrons**, or excretory units.

- Lengthening of the excretory tubule gives rise to the proximal convoluted tubule, the loop of Henle, and the distal convoluted tubule.

Positional change of the kidneys

The kidneys develop in the pelvis but appear to ascend into the abdomen as a result of fetal growth of the lumbar and sacral regions. With their ascent, the ureters elongate, and the kidneys become vascularized by arteries which arise from the abdominal aorta.

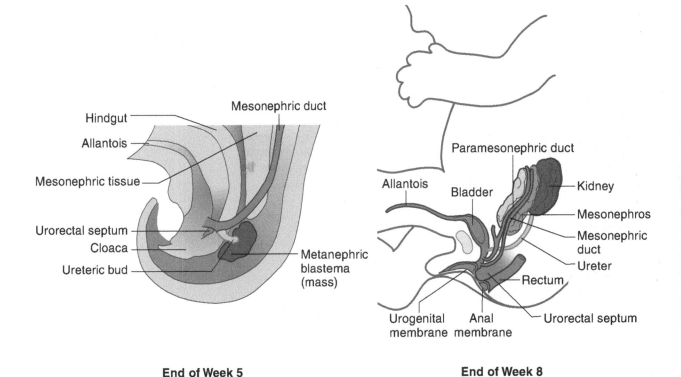

End of Week 5

End of Week 8

Figure II-3-36. Development of the Urinary System

Embryology of Bladder and Urethra

The **hindgut does not** rotate but it is divided into 2 parts by the **urorectal septum**. The urorectal septum divides the cloaca into the **anorectal canal** and the **urogenital sinus** by week 7 (Figure II-3-37).

The **urogenital sinus** is divided into 3 parts:

- The **upper** (cranial) and largest part of the urogenital sinus (endoderm) becomes the **urinary bladder**, which is initially continuous with the **allantois**.
  - The lumen of the allantois becomes obliterated to form a fibrous cord, the **urachus**. The urachus connects the apex of the bladder to the umbilicus. In the adult, this structure becomes the **median umbilical ligament**.
  - The **trigone of the bladder** is formed by the incorporation of the caudal mesonephric ducts into the dorsal bladder wall. This mesodermal tissue is eventually covered by endodermal epithelium so that the entire lining of the bladder is of **endodermal origin**. The smooth muscle of the bladder is derived from splanchnic mesoderm.
  - The mesonephric ducts also from the **ejaculatory ducts** as they enter the prostatic urethra.
- The **middle** part of the urogenital sinus (endoderm) will form all of the **urethra** of the female and the **prostatic, membranous, and proximal spongy urethra** in the male.
  - The **prostate gland** in the male is formed by an endodermal outgrowth of the prostatic urethra.
- The **inferior** part of the sinus forms the **lower vagina** and contributes to the primordia of the penis or the clitoris.

The **anorectal canal** forms the hindgut distally to the pectinate line.

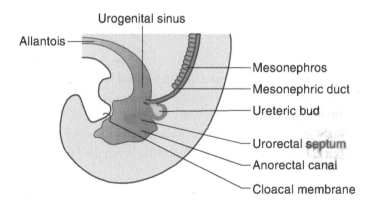

Urogenital sinus

Allantois

Mesonephros

Mesonephric duct

Ureteric bud

Urorectal septum

Anorectal canal

Cloacal membrane

Figure II-3-37. Development of Bladder and Urethra

Congenital Abnormalities of the Renal System

- **Renal agenesis**

  Renal agenesis results from failure of one or both kidneys to develop because of early degeneration of the ureteric bud. Unilateral agenesis is fairly common; bilateral agenesis is fatal (associated with oligohydramnios, and the fetus may have **Potter sequence**: clubbed feet, pulmonary hypoplasia, and craniofacial anomalies).

- **Pelvic and horseshoe kidney**

  Pelvic kidney is caused by a failure of one kidney to ascend. **Horseshoe kidney** (usually **normal renal function**, predisposition to calculi) is a fusion of both kidneys at their ends and failure of the fused kidney to ascend. The horseshoe kidney hooks under the origin of the **inferior mesenteric artery**.

- **Double ureter**

  Caused by the early splitting of the ureteric bud or the development of 2 separate buds

- **Patent urachus**

  Failure of the allantois to be obliterated results in urachal fistulas or sinuses. In male children with congenital valvular obstruction of the prostatic urethra or in older men with enlarged prostates, a patent urachus **may cause drainage of urine through the umbilicus**.

Posterior Abdominal Wall and Pelvic Viscera

Kidneys

The kidneys are a pair of bean-shaped organs approximately 12 cm long. They extend from vertebral level T12 to L3 when the body is in the erect position (Figures II-3-38A and -38B). The right kidney is positioned slightly lower than the left because of the mass of the liver.

- **Kidney's Relation to the Posterior Abdominal Wall**

  Both kidneys are in contact with the diaphragm, psoas major, and quadratus lumborum (Figures II-3-38A and -38B).

  - **Right** kidney—contacts the above structures and the 12th rib
  - **Left** kidney—contacts the above structures and the 11th and 12th ribs

Ureters

Ureters are fibromuscular tubes that connect the kidneys to the urinary bladder in the pelvis. They run posterior to the ductus deferens in males and posterior to the uterine artery in females. They begin as continuations of the renal pelves and run retroperitoneally, crossing the external iliac arteries as they pass over the pelvic brim.

Ureter's Relation to the Posterior Abdominal Wall

The ureter lies on the **anterior surface** of the **psoas major muscle**.

Clinical Correlate

Blockage by Renal Calculi

The most common sites of ureteral constriction susceptible to blockage by renal calculi are:

- Where the renal pelvis joins the ureter

- Where the ureter crosses the pelvic inlet

- Where the ureter enters the wall of the urinary bladder

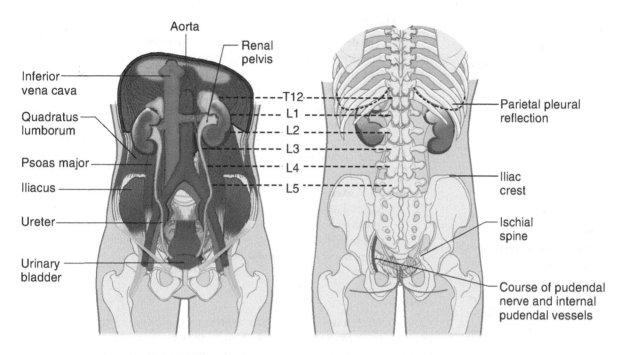

Figure II-3-38A. Muscles of the Posterior Abdominal Wall

Figure II-3-38B. Bony Landmarks of the Posterior Abdominal Wall

Labels (Figure II-3-38A): Aorta · Renal pelvis · Inferior vena cava · Quadratus lumborum · Psoas major · Iliacus · Ureter · Urinary bladder · T12 · L1 · L2 · L3 · L4 · L5

Labels (Figure II-3-38B): Parietal pleural reflection · Iliac crest · Ischial spine · Course of pudendal nerve and internal pudendal vessels

Urinary Bladder

- **Structure**
  - The urinary bladder is covered superiorly by peritoneum.
  - The body is a hollow muscular cavity.
  - The neck is continuous with the urethra (Figures II-3-47 and -48).
  - The trigone is a smooth, triangular area of mucosa located internally at the base of the bladder.
  - The base of the triangle is superior and bounded by the 2 openings of the ureters. The apex of the trigone points inferiorly and is the opening for the urethra.

- **Blood Supply**
  - The bladder is supplied by vesicular branches of the internal iliac arteries and umbilical arteries.
  - The vesicular venous plexus drains to internal iliac veins.

- **Lymphatics**
  - Drain to the external and internal iliac nodes

- **Innervation**
  - Parasympathetic innervation is from sacral segments S2, S3, and S4. The preganglionic parasympathetic fibers travel in **pelvic splanchnic nerves** to reach the **detrusor muscle**.
  - Sympathetic innervation is through fibers derived from L1 through L2 (**lumbar splanchnics**). These fibers supply the **trigone muscle** and the **internal urethral sphincter**.

In A Nutshell

Parasympathetic fibers facilitate micturition and sympathetic fibers inhibit micturition.

Clinical Correlate

Spastic bladder results from lesions of the spinal cord **above the sacral spinal cord levels**. There is a loss of inhibition of the parasympathetic nerve fibers that innervate the detrusor muscle during the filling stage. Thus, the detrusor muscle responds to a minimum amount of stretch, causing urge incontinence.

Clinical Correlate

Atonic bladder results from lesions **to the sacral spinal cord segments** or the sacral spinal nerve roots. Loss of pelvic splanchnic motor innervation with loss of contraction of the detrusor muscle results in a full bladder with a continuous dribble of urine from the bladder.

Clinical Correlate

Weakness of the **puborectalis** part of the levator ani muscle may result in **rectal incontinence.**

Weakness of the **sphincter urethrae** part of the urogenital diaphragm may result in **urinary incontinence.**

- **Muscles**
  - The **detrusor muscle** forms most of the smooth-muscle walls of the bladder and contracts during emptying of the bladder (micturition). The contraction of these muscles is under control of the parasympathetic fibers of the **pelvic splanchnics** (S2, 3, 4)
  - The **internal urethral sphincter** (sphincter vesicae) is smooth-muscle fibers that enclose the origin of the urethra at the **neck of the bladder**. These muscles are under control of the sympathetic fibers of the lower thoracic and **lumbar splanchnics** (T11-L2) and are activated during the filling phase of the bladder to prevent urinary leakage.
  - The **external urethral sphincter** (sphincter urethrae) is the voluntary skeletal muscle component of the urogenital diaphragm that encloses the urethra and is **relaxed** during micturition (voluntary muscle of micturition). The external sphincter is innervated by perineal branches of the **pudendal nerve**.

Urethra

The male urethra is a muscular tube approximately 20 cm in length. The urethra in men extends from the neck of the bladder through the prostate gland (prostatic urethra) to the urogenital diaphragm of the perineum (membranous urethra), and then to the external opening of the glans (penile or spongy urethra) (Figure II-3-47).

The male urethra is anatomically divided into 3 portions: prostatic, membranous, and spongy (penile).

- The **distal spongy urethra** of the male is derived from the ectodermal cells of the glans penis.

The female urethra is approximately 4 cm in length and extends from the neck of the bladder to the external urethral orifice of the vulva (Figure II-3-48).

URINARY HISTOLOGY AND FUNCTION

The urinary system consists of 2 kidneys, 2 ureters, the bladder, and the urethra.

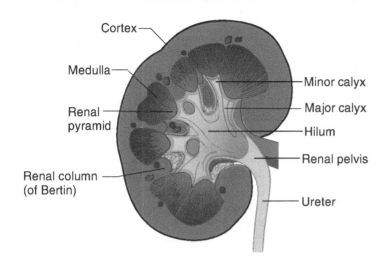

Figure II-3-39. Organization of the Kidney

Urinary Functions

The urinary system functions in the removal of waste products from blood. The kidney also functions in fluid balance, salt balance, and acid-base balance. The kidney functions as an endocrine gland; it produces and releases renin, which leads to an increase in extracellular fluid volume; erythropoietin, which stimulates erythropoiesis; and prostaglandins, which act as vasodilators.

A sagittal section through the center of a kidney shows a capsule (connective tissue) surrounding and protecting the organ, a wide band of cortex showing radial striations and the presence of glomeruli, and a medulla in the shape of an inverted pyramid. The medulla in turn shows an outer and inner zone. The blunted tip of the pyramid, called the **papilla**, borders a space that is surrounded by calices of the ureter. The collecting ducts are invaginations of the papilla's epithelium and the urine drains from their open ends into the calices.

Table II-3-7. Basic Functions of the Kidneys

Fluid balance	Maintain normal extracellular fluid (ECF) and intracellular fluid (ICF) volumes
Electrolytes	Balance excretion with intake to maintain normal plasma concentrations
Wastes	Excrete metabolic wastes (nitrogenous products, acids, toxins, etc.)
Fuels	Reabsorb metabolic fuels (glucose, lactate, amino acids, etc.)
Blood pressure	Regulate ECF volume for the long-term control of blood pressure
Acid–base	Regulate absorption and excretion of H^+ and HCO_3^- to control acid–base balance

Organization of the Kidney

The cortex is divided into lobules, and contains nephron elements mixed with vascular elements and stroma (a small amount of connective tissue). At the center of each lobule is a medullary ray, containing tubules that are parallel to each other and oriented radially in the cortex. The tubules in the medullary rays are continuous with those in the medulla. Along the 2 edges of each lobule are glomeruli, located along one or 2 rows. Radially oriented arterioles and venules with a large lumen are located at the edges of the lobules.

The medulla is comprised of radially arranged straight tubules which run from cortex to papilla, vascular elements, and stroma (a small amount of connective tissue). The medulla is divided into 2 zones. A wide strip in proximity to the cortex, the outer medulla contains profiles of tubules with different appearances. The inner medulla has fewer profiles of similar tubes.

Blood Circulation

The renal artery enters the kidney at the hilum, near the ureter. The artery branches into interlobar arteries, which travel to the medulla–cortex border remaining outside the medullary pyramids, The vessels branch into arcuate arteries (and veins) that follow the edge of the cortex. The arcuate arteries branch into interlobular arterioles that travel tangentially in the cortex at the edges of the lobules. Intralobular arterioles, feeding the glomeruli, branch off the interlobular arterioles at each renal corpuscle.

The kidneys receive 25% of total cardiac output, 1,700 liters in 24 hours. Each intralobular arteriole enters a renal corpuscle at the vascular pole as afferent arteriole and forms a convoluted tuft of capillaries (the glomerulus). A second arteriole (the efferent arteriole) exits the corpuscle. This is a unique situation due to the fact that the pressure remains high in the glomerulus in order to allow filtration.

The efferent arterioles carrying blood out of the glomeruli make a second capillary bed. This second capillary bed has lower blood pressure than the glomerulus and it connects to venules at its distal end. The arteriole-capillary-arteriole-capillary-vein sequence in the kidney is unique in the body. The efferent arterioles from glomeruli in the upper cortex divide into a complex capillary system in the cortex.

NEPHRON

The functional unit within the kidney is the nephron. Each kidney contains 1–1.3 million nephrons. Nephrons connect to collecting ducts, and collecting ducts receive urine from several nephrons and converge with each other before opening to and letting the urine flow out of the kidney. The nephron and the collecting duct form the uriniferous tubule.

The nephron is a tube about 55 mm in length in the human kidney. It starts at one end with Bowman's capsule, which is the enlarged end of the nephron. Bowman's capsule has been invaginated by a tuft of capillaries of the glomerulus so that it has 2 layers: the visceral layer is in direct contact with the capillary endothelium, and the parietal layer surrounds an approximately spherical urinary space. Bowman's capsule and glomerulus of capillaries form a renal corpuscle.

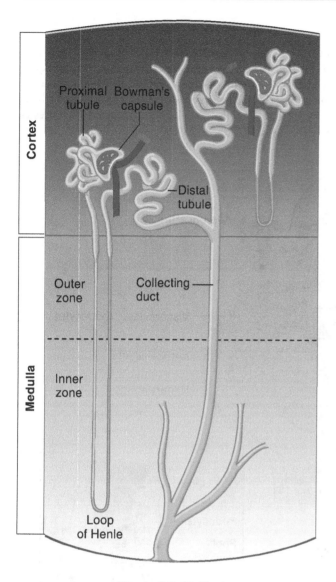

Figure II-3-40. Nephron

Renal Corpuscle

The parietal layer of Bowman's capsule is continuous with the walls of the proximal convoluted tubule (PCT). The visceral layer cells are called podocytes and have a complex shape; the cell body has extensive primary and secondary foot processes which surround the blood vessels. The foot processes of the podocytes lie a basal lamina that is shared by capillary endothelial cells. The podocyte foot processes almost completely cover the capillary surfaces, leaving small slits in between.

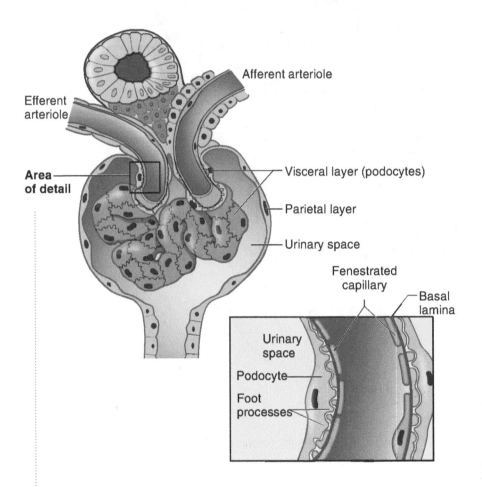

Figure II-3-41. Renal Corpuscle and Bowman's Capsule

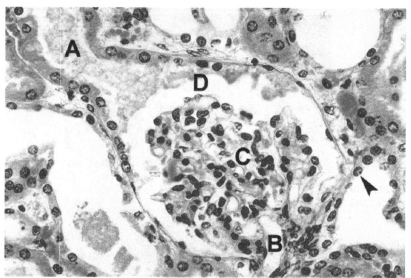

Figure II-3-42. Renal corpuscle proximal tubule (A), vascular pole (B), glomerulus (C), and urinary space (D)

Simple cuboidal epithelium of the distal tubule (arrowhead)

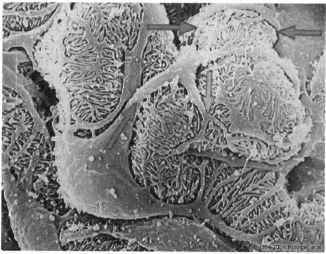

Figure II-3-43. Scanning electron micrograph demonstrating podocytes with their processes (arrows)

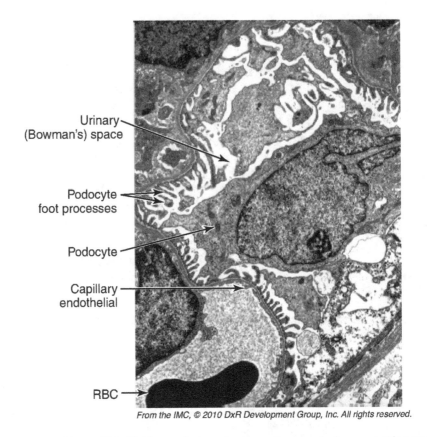

Figure II-3-44. Transmission electron micrograph demonstrating podocytes

Blood plasma is filtered from the lumen of the capillary to the urinary space across the combined capillary endothelium-podocyte complex. Fenestrations in the endothelium are large (50–100 nm) and occupy 20% of the capillary surface. Fenestrations block the exit of cells, but allow free flow of plasma. The shared basal lamina of podocytes and endothelium constitutes the first, coarser filtration barrier; it blocks the passage of molecules larger than 70 kD.

The thin diaphragms covering the slit openings between the podocyte foot processes constitutes a more selective filter. The slits are composed of elongated proteins which arise from the surface of the adjacent foot process cell membranes and join in the center of the slit, in a zipper-like configuration. The width of the junction between 2 adjacent podocytes varies between 20 and 50 nm, possibly as a function of perfusion pressures of the glomerulus.

Podocyte foot processes are motile (they contain actin and myosin). They are connected to each other by the slit diaphragm and to the basal lamina. The slit diaphragm molecular complex is associated with the actin cytoskeleton. Alterations in composition and/or arrangement of these complexes are found in many forms of human and experimental diseases.

Proximal Convoluted Tubule

The proximal convoluted tubule (PCT) opens at the urinary pole of Bowman's capsule. The PCT follows a circuitous path and ends with a straight segment that connects to the loop of Henle. PCT cells are tall, and they have a pink cytoplasm, long apical microvilli, and extensive basal invaginations. Numerous large mitochondria are located between the basal invaginations. The lateral borders of adjacent cells are extensively interdigitated. These characteristics are typical of cells involved in active transport. The lumen of the PCT is frequently clouded by microvilli which do not preserve well during the histologic preparation process.

Loop of Henle

The loop of Henle has a smaller diameter than the PCT and has descending and ascending limbs which go in opposite directions. Some loops of Henle have a wider segment before the distal tubule. The straight and convoluted segments of the distal convoluted tubule (DCT) follow. The straight portions of the PCT and DCT have traditionally been assigned to the loop of Henle (constituting the thick ascending and descending limbs) but they are now thought to be part of the PCT and DCT to which they are more similar. The special disposition of the loops of Henle descending and ascending branches, coupled with their specific transport and permeability properties, allow them to operate as "countercurrent multipliers," creating a gradient of extracellular fluid tonicity in the medulla. This is used to modulate urine tonicity and final volume.

Distal Convoluted Tubule

The DCT comes back to make contact with its own glomerulus, and then connects to the collecting tubule, which receives urine from several nephrons and is open at its far end. The epithelium of DCT, loops of Henle, and collecting ducts have variable thicknesses and more or less well-defined cell borders. Some have limited surface microvilli. In general, these tubes either do much less active transport than the PCT or are involved only in passive water movements.

Collecting Ducts

Collecting ducts are lined by principal cells and intercalated cells. The cell outline of these cells is more distinct than that of the PCT or the DCT. Principal cells respond to aldosterone.

Mesangial Cells

Mesangial cells (also known as Polkissen or Lacis cells) are located between capillaries, under the basal lamina but outside the capillary lumen. There is no basal lamina between mesangial and endothelial cells. Mesangial cells are phagocytic and may be involved in the maintenance of the basal lamina. Abnormalities of mesangial cells are detected in several diseases resulting in clogged and/or distorted glomeruli.

Note

Renal cortex and medullary fibroblasts (interstitial cells) produce erythropoetin.

Note

Diuretics act by inhibiting Na^+ resorption, leading to an increase in Na^+ and water excretion.

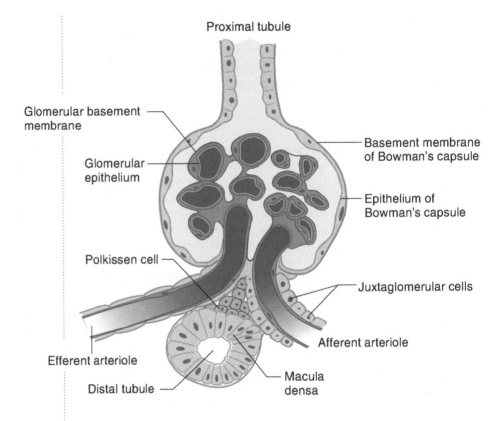

Figure II-3-45. Renal Corpuscle and Juxtaglomerular Apparatus

Juxtaglomerular Complex

The juxtaglomerular (JG) complex is a complex comprising JG apparatus (in the wall of the afferent arteriole), the macula densa (a special domain of the DCT), and a group of mesangial cells. The JG cells are modified smooth-muscle cells which secrete renin.

The macula densa is formed by tall cuboidal cells in the wall of the DCT which detect sodium levels in the tubular fluid.

PELVIS

Embryology of the Reproductive System

Table II-3-8. Embryology of Reproductive System

Male and Female Development		
Adult Female and Male Reproductive Structures Derived From Precursors of the Indifferent Embryo		
Adult Female	**Indifferent Embryo**	**Adult Male**
Ovary, follicles, rete ovarii	Gonads — TDF $\xrightarrow{+}$	Testes, seminiferous tubules, rete testes
Uterine tubes, uterus, cervix, and upper part of vagina	Paramesonephric ducts — MIF $\xrightarrow{-}$	Appendix of testes
Duct of Gartner	Mesonephric ducts — Testosterone $\xrightarrow{+}$	Epididymis, ductus deferens, seminal vesicle, ejaculatory duct
Clitoris	Genital tubercle	Glans and body of penis
Labia minora	Urogenital folds	Ventral aspect of penis	DHT
Labia majora	Labioscrotal swellings	Scrotum

Abbreviations: DHT, dihydrotestosterone; MIF, Müllerian-inhibiting factors; TDF, testes-determining factor

Congenital Reproductive Anomalies

Female Pseudointersexuality

- 46,XX genotype
- Have ovarian (but no testicular) tissue and masculinization of the female external genitalia
- Most common cause is **congenital adrenal hyperplasia**, a condition in which the fetus produces excess androgens

Male Pseudointersexuality

- 46,XY genotype
- Testicular (but no ovarian) tissue and stunted development of male external genitalia
- Most common cause is inadequate production of dihydrotestosterone due to a 5α-reductase deficiency

5α-reductase 2 deficiency

- Caused by a mutation in the **5α-reductase 2 gene** that renders 5α-reductase 2 enzyme underactive in catalyzing the conversion of testosterone to dihydrotestosterone
- *Clinical findings:* underdevelopment of the penis and emission of sperm (microphallus, hypospadias, and bifid scrotum) and prostate. The epididymis, ductus deferens, seminal vesicle, and ejaculatory duct are normal
- At puberty, these patients undergo virilization due to an increased **T:DHT ratio**.

Complete androgen insensitivity (CAIS, or testicular feminization syndrome)

- Occurs when a fetus with a 46,XY genotype develops testes and female external genitalia with a rudimentary vagina; the uterus and uterine tubes are generally absent
- Testes may be found in the labia majora and are surgically removed to circumvent malignant tumor formation.
- Individuals present as normal-appearing females, and their psychosocial orientation is female despite their genotype.
- Most common cause is a mutation in the **androgen receptor (AR) gene** that renders the AR inactive.

Abnormalities of the Penis and Testis

Hypospadias

- Occurs when the urethral folds fail to fuse completely, resulting in the external urethral orifice opening onto the **ventral** surface of the penis.
- Generally associated with a poorly developed penis that curves ventrally, known as **chordee.**

Epispadias

- Occurs when the external urethral orifice opens onto the **dorsal** surface of the penis.
- Generally associated with exstrophy of the bladder.

Undescended testes (cryptorchidism)

Occurs when the testes fail to descend into the scrotum. Normally occurs within 3 months after birth.

- Bilateral cryptorchidism results in sterility.
- The undescended testes may be found in the abdominal cavity or in the inguinal canal.

Hydrocele of the testes

Occurs when a small patency of the processus vaginalis remains so that peritoneal fluid can flow into the processus vaginalis. Results in a fluid-filled cyst near the testes.

Pelvic and Urogenital Diaphragms

The **pelvic and urogenital diaphragms** (Figure II-3-46) are 2 important skeletal muscle diaphragms that provide support of the pelvic and perineal structures. They are each innervated by branches of the pudendal nerve.

- The **pelvic diaphragm** forms the muscular floor of the pelvis and separates the pelvic cavity from the perineum. The pelvic diaphragm is a strong support for the pelvic organs and transmits the distal parts of the genitourinary system and GI tract from the pelvis to the perineum.

- The diaphragm is formed by 2 layers of fascia and the 2 muscles: the **levator ani** and coccygeus.
  - The **puborectalis** component of the levator ani muscle forms a muscular sling around the anorectal junction, marks the boundary between the rectum and anal canal and is important in fecal continence.
- The muscular **urogenital diaphragm** (Figure II-3-46) is located in the perineum inferior to the pelvic diaphragm. It is formed by 2 muscles (**sphincter urethrae** and deep transverse perineus muscles) which extend horizontally between the 2 ischiopubic rami.
  - The diaphragm is penetrated by the urethra in the male and the urethra and vagina in the female.
  - The sphincter urethrae muscle serves as an **external urethral sphincter** (voluntary muscle of micturition) which surrounds the membranous urethra and maintains urinary continence.

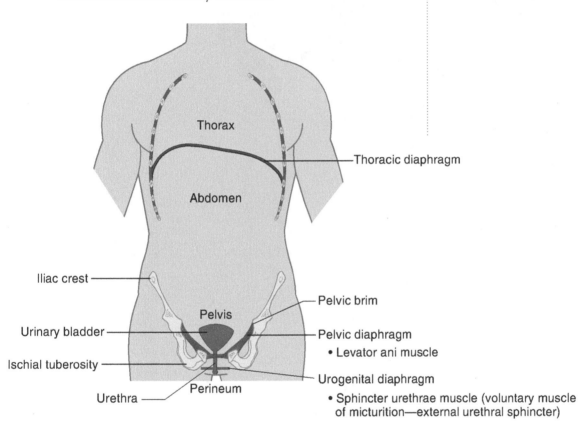

Figure II-3-46. Pelvic Diaphragm

Male Pelvic Viscera

The position of organs and peritoneum in the male pelvis is illustrated in Figure II-3-47.

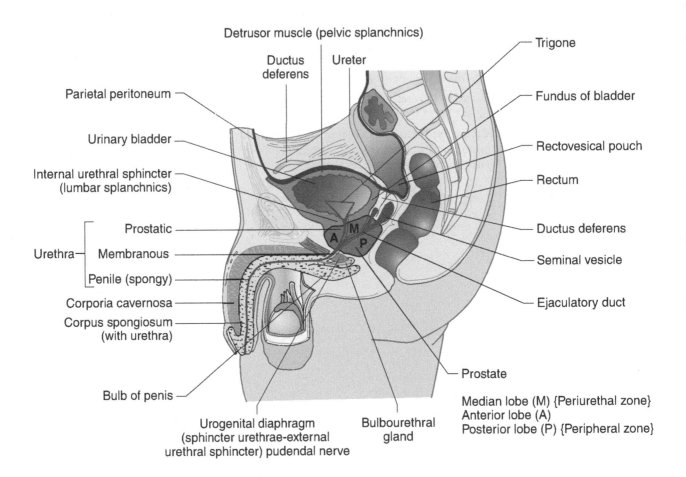

Detrusor muscle (pelvic splanchnics)

Ductus deferens

Ureter

Trigone

Parietal peritoneum

Fundus of bladder

Urinary bladder

Rectovesical pouch

Internal urethral sphincter (lumbar splanchnics)

Rectum

Urethra — Prostatic

Membranous

Penile (spongy)

A M P

Ductus deferens

Seminal vesicle

Corporia cavernosa

Corpus spongiosum (with urethra)

Ejaculatory duct

Bulb of penis

Prostate

Urogenital diaphragm (sphincter urethrae-external urethral sphincter) pudendal nerve

Bulbourethral gland

Median lobe (M) {Periurethal zone}
Anterior lobe (A)
Posterior lobe (P) {Peripheral zone}

Figure II-3-47. Male Pelvis

Clinical Correlate

Hyperplasia of the Prostate

An enlarged prostate gland will compress the urethra. The patient will complain of the urge to urinate often and has difficulty with starting urination.

Because the prostate gland is enclosed in a dense connective tissue capsule, hypertrophy will compress the prostatic portion of the urethra.

Female Pelvic Viscera

The position of organs and peritoneum in the female pelvis is illustrated in Figure II-3-48.

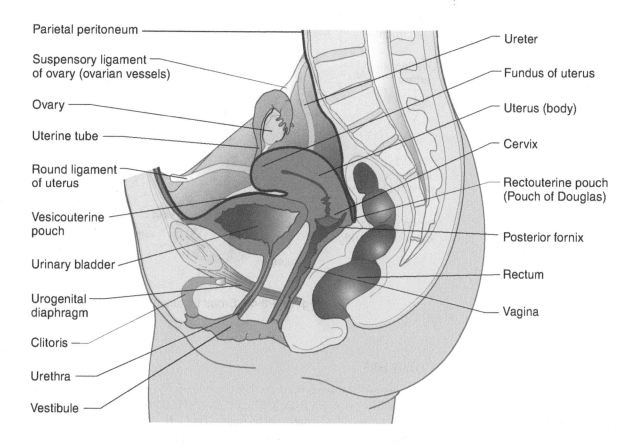

Parietal peritoneum

Suspensory ligament of ovary (ovarian vessels)

Ovary

Uterine tube

Round ligament of uterus

Vesicouterine pouch

Urinary bladder

Urogenital diaphragm

Clitoris

Urethra

Vestibule

Ureter

Fundus of uterus

Uterus (body)

Cervix

Rectouterine pouch (Pouch of Douglas)

Posterior fornix

Rectum

Vagina

Figure II-3-48. Female Pelvis

Clinical Correlate

The ureter courses just medial to the suspensory ligament of the ovary and must be protected when ligating the ovarian vessels.

Clinical Correlate

Support for pelvic viscera is provided by the pelvic and urogenital diaphragms, perineal membrane, perineal body, and the transverse (cardinal) cervical and uterosacral ligaments. Weakness of support structures may result in **prolapse** of the uterus into the vagina or **herniation** of the bladder or rectum into the vagina.

Clinical Correlate

The ureter passes **inferior** to the uterine artery 1 to 2 centimeters from the cervix ("water under the bridge") and must be avoided during surgical procedures.

Clinical Correlate

A **pudendal nerve block** to anesthetize the perineum is performed as the pudendal nerve crosses posterior to the **ischial spine** (Figure II-3-24B).

Uterus and Broad Ligament

Figure II-3-28 illustrates **a posterior view** of the female reproductive tract.

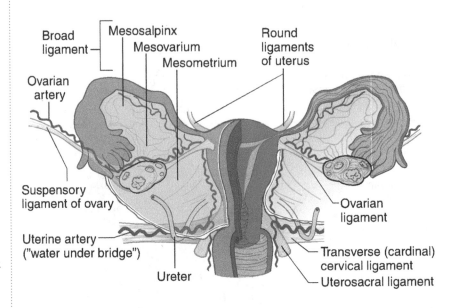

Figure II-3-49. Broad Ligament

PERINEUM

The **perineum** is the diamond-shaped outlet of the pelvis located below the pelvic diaphragm. The perineum is divided by a transverse line between the ischial tuberosities into the **anal** and **urogenital triangles** (Figure II-3-52).

- The sensory and motor innervation to the perineum is provided by the **pudendal nerve** (S2, 3, 4) of the sacral plexus.
- The blood supply is provided by the **internal pudendal artery,** a branch of the internal iliac artery.
- The pudendal nerve and vessels cross the ischial spine posteriorly to enter the perineum (Figure II-3-38B).

Anal Triangle

The **anal triangle** is posterior and contains the **anal canal** surrounded by the fat-filled **ischioanal fossa**.

- The anal canal is guarded by a smooth-muscle **internal anal sphincter** innervated by the ANS and an **external anal sphincter** of skeletal muscle innervated by the pudendal nerve.
- The pudendal canal transmitting the pudendal nerve and internal pudendal vessels is found on the lateral aspect of the ischioanal fossa (Figure II-3-52).

Urogenital Triangle

The **urogenital triangle** forms the anterior aspect of the perineum and contains the superficial and root structures of the external genitalia. The urogenital triangle is divided into **superficial** and **deep perineal spaces (pouches)** (Figure II-3-50).

Superficial Perineal Pouch (Space)

The superficial perineal pouch is located between the **perineal membrane** of the urogenital diaphragm and the **superficial perineal (Colles') fascia**.

It contains:

- Crura of penis or clitoris: erectile tissue
- Bulb of penis (in the male): erectile tissue; contains urethra
- Bulbs of vestibule (in the female): erectile tissue in lateral walls of vestibule
- Ischiocavernosus muscle: skeletal muscle that covers crura of penis or clitoris
- Bulbospongiosus muscle: skeletal muscle that covers bulb of penis or bulb of vestibule
- Greater vestibular (Bartholin) gland (in female only): homologous to Cowper gland

Deep Perineal Pouch (Space)

The deep perineal pouch is formed by the fasciae and muscles of the **urogenital diaphragm**. It contains:

- Sphincter urethrae muscle—serves as voluntary external sphincter of the urethra
- Deep transverse perineal muscle
- Bulbourethral (Cowper) gland (in the male only)—duct enters bulbar urethra

In A Nutshell

The **bulbourethral (Cowper) glands** are located in the **deep perineal pouch** of the male.

The **greater vestibular (Bartholin) glands** are located in the **superficial perineal pouch** of the female.

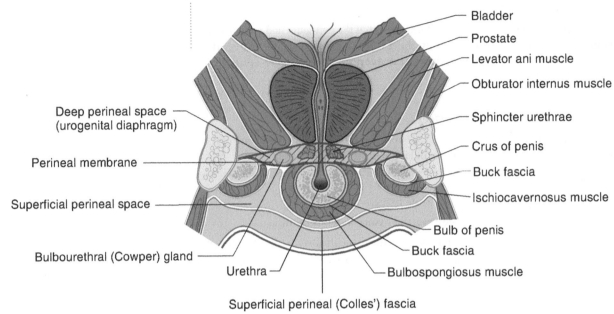

Figure II-3-50. Superficial and Deep Perineal Pouches of Male

External Genitalia

Male

Crura of penis are continuous with the corpora cavernosa of the penis.
Bulb of penis is continuous with corpus spongiosus of the penis (contains urethra).

Corpora cavernosa and corpus spongiosus form the shaft of the penis.

Clinical Correlate

In the male, injury to the bulb of the penis may result in extravasation of urine from the urethra into the superficial perineal space. From this space, urine may pass into the scrotum, into the penis, and onto the anterior abdominal wall in the plane deep to Scarpa fascia (green arrows).

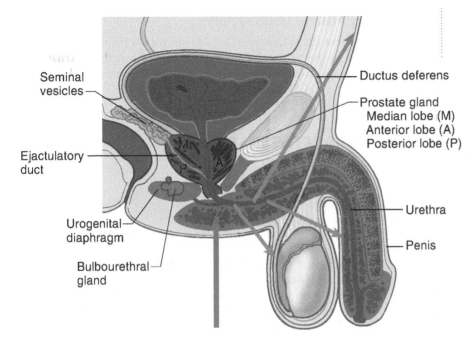

Figure II-3-51. Male Reproductive System

Female

Crura of the clitoris are continuous with the corpora cavernosa of the clitoris.

Bulbs of vestibule are separated from the vestibule by the labia minora.

Urethra and vagina empty into the vestibule.

Duct of greater vestibular glands enters the vestibule.

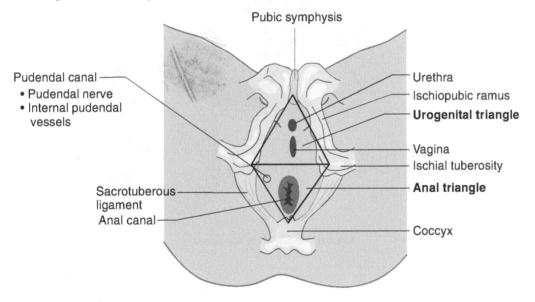

Figure II-3-52. Perineum of Female

Pelvic and Perineal Innervation

The **pudendal nerve (S2, S3, S4 ventral rami) and its branches** innervate the skeletal muscles in the pelvic and urogenital diaphragms, the external anal sphincter and the sphincter urethrae, skeletal muscles in both perineal pouches, and the skin that overlies the perineum.

MALE REPRODUCTIVE HISTOLOGY

Testis

The testis is surrounded by a dense fibrous capsule called the **tunica albuginea**. The tunica albuginea is continuous with many of the interlobular septa that divide the testis into approximately 250 pyramidal compartments (testicular lobules).

Within each lobule are 1-4 tubes, **seminiferous tubules,** where spermatozoa are produced. Each tubule is a coiled, non-branching closed loop that is 150–200 μm in diameter and 30–70 cm in length. Both ends of each tubule converge on the rete testes. The seminiferous tubules contain spermatogenic cells, Sertoli cells, and a well-defined basal lamina.

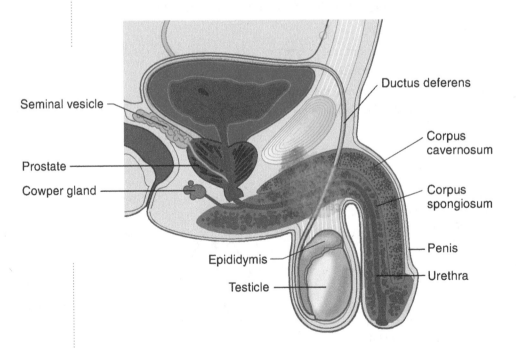

Seminal vesicle

Prostate

Cowper gland

Ductus deferens

Corpus cavernosum

Corpus spongiosum

Penis

Urethra

Epididymis

Testicle

Figure II-3-53. Male reproductive system

Note

The blood–testis barrier is formed by tight junctions between Sertoli cells and protects primary spermatocytes and their progeny.

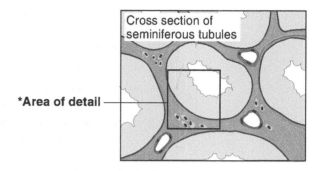

Cross section of seminiferous tubules

*Area of detail

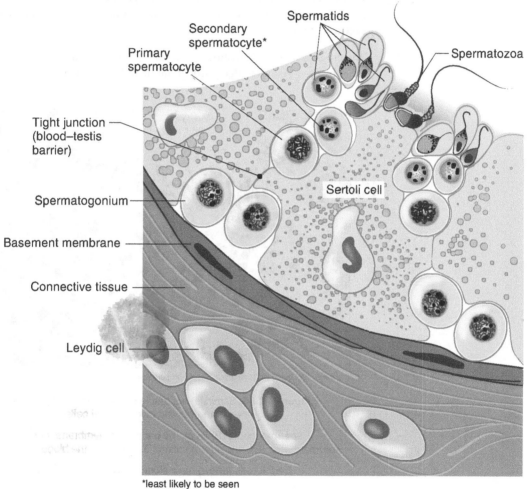

*least likely to be seen

Figure II-3-54. Seminiferous tubule diagram

Spermatogenesis

The spermatogenic cells (germinal epithelium) are stacked in 4 to 8 layers that occupy the space between the basement membrane and the lumen of the seminiferous tubule. The stem cells (**spermatogonia**) are adjacent to the basement membrane. As the cells develop, they move from the basal to the luminal side of the tubule.

At puberty the stem cells resume mitosis, producing more stem cells as well as differentiated spermatogonia (type A and B) that are committed to meiosis. **Type B spermatogonia** differentiate into primary spermatocytes that enter meiosis. **Primary spermatocytes** (4n, diploid) pass through a long prophase (10 days to 2 weeks) and after the first meiotic division form 2 secondary spermatocytes (2n, haploid). The **secondary spermatocytes** rapidly undergo the second meiotic division in a matter of minutes **(and are rarely seen in histologic sections)** to produce the **spermatids** (1n, haploid).

The progeny of a single maturing spermatogonium remain connected to one another by cytoplasmic bridges throughout their differentiation into mature sperm.

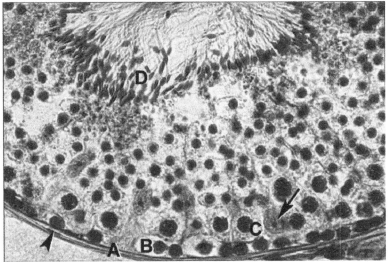

Figure II-3-55. Seminiferous tubule surrounded by a basement membrane (A) and myoepithelial cells

Spermatogonia (B) lie on the basement membrane, primary spermatocytes (C), and spermatozoa (D) are inside the blood testis barrier.

Sertoli cells (arrow) have elongate, pale-staining nuclei.

Spermiogenesis

Spermiogenesis transforms haploid spermatids into spermatozoa. This process of differentiation involves formation of the acrosome, condensation, and elongation of the nucleus; development of the flagellum; and loss of much of the cytoplasm.

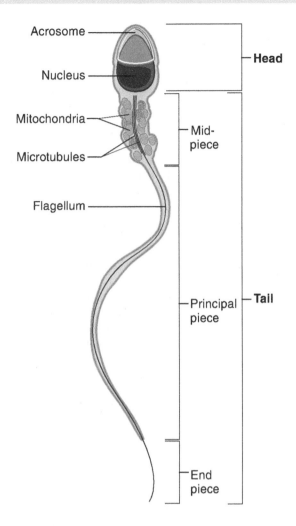

Figure II-3-56. Spermatozoan

The **acrosome**, which is located over the anterior half of the nucleus, is derived from the Golgi complex of the spermatid and contains several hydrolytic enzymes such as hyaluronidase, neuraminidase, and acid phosphatase; these enzymes dissociate cells of the corona radiata and digest the zona pellucida of the recently produced secondary oocyte.

The basic structure of a flagellum is similar to that of a cilium. Movement is a result of the interaction among microtubules, ATP, and dynein.

Sertoli Cells and the Blood–Testis Barrier

Sertoli cells are tall columnar epithelial cells. These multifunctional cells are the predominant cells in the seminiferous tubule prior to puberty and in elderly men but comprise only 10% of the cells during times of maximal spermatogenesis.

- Irregular in shape; the base adheres to the basal lamina and the apical end extends to the lumen. The nucleus tends to be oval with the long axis oriented perpendicular to the basement membrane.
- The cytoplasmic extensions make contact with neighboring Sertoli cells via tight junctions, forming the **blood–testis barrier** by separating the seminiferous tubule into a basal and an adlumenal compartment.
- Do not divide during the reproductive period.
- Support, protect, and provide nutrition to the developing spermatozoa. During spermiogenesis, the excess spermatid cytoplasm is shed as residual bodies that are phagocytized by Sertoli cells. They also phagocytize germ cells that fail to mature.
- Secrete **androgen-binding protein** that binds testosterone and dihydrotestosterone. High concentrations of these hormones are essential for normal germ-cell maturation. The production of androgen-binding protein is stimulated by **follicle-stimulating hormone** (FSH receptors are on Sertoli cells).
- Secrete **inhibin**, which suppresses FSH synthesis.
- Produce anti-Müllerian hormone during fetal life that suppresses the development of female internal reproductive structures.

The blood–testis barrier is a network of Sertoli cells which divides the seminiferous tubule into a basal compartment (containing the spermatogonia and the earliest primary spermatocytes) and an adlumenal compartment (containing the remaining spermatocytes and spermatids). The basal compartment has free access to material found in blood, while the more advanced stages of spermatogenesis are protected from blood-borne products by the **barrier** formed by the tight junctions between the Sertoli cells. The primary spermatocytes traverse this barrier by a mechanism not yet understood.

Interstitial Tissues of the Testis

The interstitial tissue lying between the seminiferous tubules is a loose network of connective tissue composed of fibroblasts, collagen, blood and lymphatic vessels, and **Leydig cells** (also called interstitial cells). The Leydig cells synthesize testosterone.

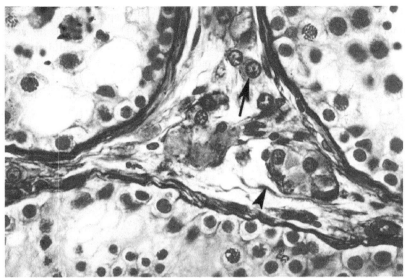

Figure II-3-57. Interstitium between seminiferous tubules contains Leydig cells (arrow) and fibroblasts (arrowhead)

Genital Ducts

The seminiferous tubules empty into the **rete testis** and then into 10–20 **ductuli efferentes**. The ductuli are lined by a single layer of epithelial cells, some of which are ciliated. The ciliary action propels the nonmotile spermatozoa. The non-ciliated cells reabsorb some of the fluid produced by the testis. A thin band of smooth muscle surrounds each ductus.

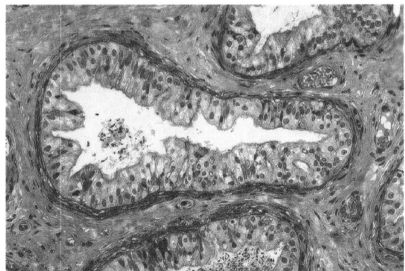

Figure II-3-58. Efferent ductules with ciliated cuboidal and columnar cells

The spermatozoa pass from the ducti efferentes to the **epididymis**. The major function of this highly convoluted duct (approximately 5 m long) is the accumulation, storage, and maturation of spermatozoa. It is in the **epididymis** that the spermatozoa become motile. The epididymis is lined with a pseudostratified columnar epithelium which contains stereocilia (tall microvilli) on the luminal surface. This epithelium resorbs testicular fluid, phagocytizes residual bodies and poorly formed spermatozoa, and secretes substances thought to play a role in the maturation of spermatozoa.

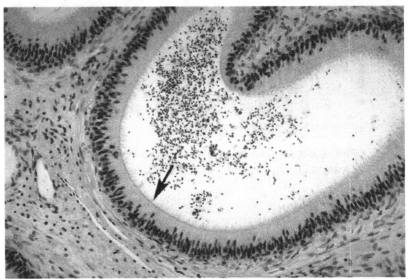

Copyright McGraw-Hill Companies. Used with permission.

Figure II-3-59. Epididymis lined by pseudostratified columnar epithelium with stereocilia (arrow)

The **ductus (vas) deferens** conducts spermatozoa from the epididymis to the ejaculatory duct and then into the prostatic **urethra**. The ductus (vas) deferens is a thick walled muscular tube consisting of an inner and outer layer of longitudinal smooth muscle and an intermediate circular layer. Vasectomy or the bilateral ligation of the vas deferens prevents movement of spermatozoa from the epididymis to the urethra.

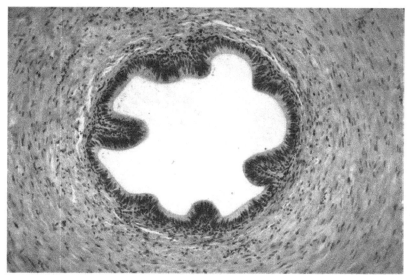

Figure II-3-60. Ductus deferens with thick layers of smooth muscle

Accessory Glands

Seminal Vesicles

The **seminal vesicles** are a pair of glands situated on the posterior and inferior surfaces of the bladder. These highly convoluted glands have a folded mucosa lined with pseudostratified columnar epithelium. The columnar epithelium is rich in secretory granules that displace the nuclei to the cell base.

The seminal vesicles produce a secretion that constitutes approximately 70% of human ejaculate and is rich in spermatozoa-activating substances such as fructose, citrate, prostaglandins, and several proteins. Fructose, which is a major nutrient for sperm, provides the energy for motility. The duct of each seminal vesicle joins a ductus deferens to form an ejaculatory duct. The ejaculatory duct traverses the prostate to empty into the prostatic urethra.

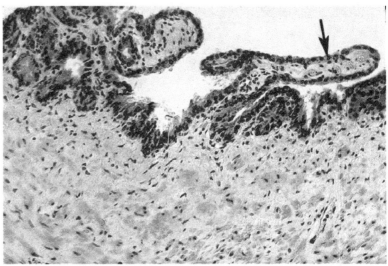

Figure II-3-61. Seminal vesicle showing mucosal folds lined with
pseudostratified columnar epithelium (arrow)

Prostate

The **prostate** is a collection of 30–50 branched tubuloalveolar glands whose
ducts empty into the urethra. The prostate is surrounded by a fibroelastic capsule that is rich in smooth muscle. There are 2 types of glands in the prostate,
periurethral submucosal glands and the main prostatic glands in the periphery.
Glandular epithelium is pseudostratified columnar with pale, foamy cytoplasm
and numerous secretory granules. The products of the secretory granules include acid phosphatase, citric acid, fibrinolysin, and other proteins.

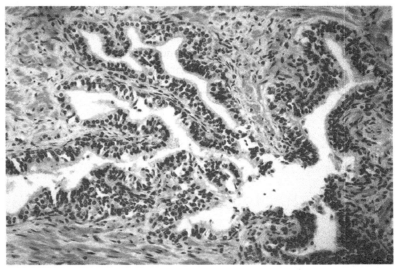

Figure II-3-62. Prostate with tubuloalveolar glands lined by
pseudostratified columnar epithelium

Table II-3-9. Male Reproductive Physiology

Penile Erection
Erection occurs in response to **parasympathetic** stimulation (pelvic splanchnic nerves). **Nitric oxide** is released, causing relaxation of the corpus cavernosum and corpus spongiosum, which allows blood to accumulate in the trabeculae of erectile tissue.

Ejaculation
• **Sympathetic** nervous system stimulation (lumbar splanchnic nerves) mediates movement of mature spermatozoa from the epididymis and vas deferens into the ejaculatory duct.
• Accessory glands such as the bulbourethral (Cowper) glands, prostate, and seminal vesicles secrete fluids that aid in sperm survival and fertility.
• **Somatic motor efferents** (pudendal nerve) that innervate the bulbospongiosus and ischiocavernous muscles at the base of the penis stimulate the rapid ejection of semen out the urethra during ejaculation. Peristaltic waves in the vas deferens aid in a more complete ejection of semen through the urethra.

Clinical Correlate
• Injury to the bulb of the penis may result in extravasation of urine from the urethra into the superficial perineal space. From this space, urine may pass into the scrotum, into the penis, and onto the anterior abdominal wall.
• Accumulation of fluid in the scrotum, penis, and anterolateral abdominal wall is indicative of a laceration of either the membranous or penile urethra (deep to Scarpa fascia). This can be caused by trauma to the perineal region (saddle injury) or laceration of the urethra during catheterization.

FEMALE REPRODUCTIVE HISTOLOGY

Ovary

The paired **ovaries** have 2 major functions: to produce the female gametes and to produce the steroid hormones which prepare the endometrium for conception and maintain pregnancy should fertilization occur. The ovaries are 3 cm long, 1.5 cm wide, and 1 cm thick. They consist of a **medullary region**, which contains a rich vascular bed with a cellular loose connective tissue, and a **cortical region** where the ovarian follicles reside.

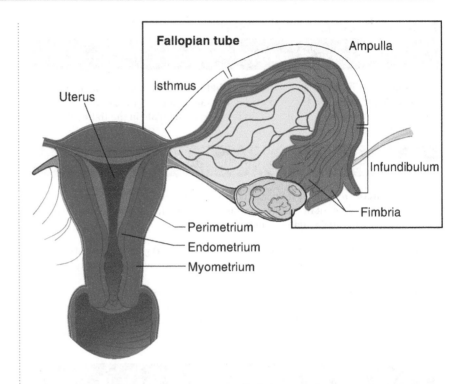

Figure II-3-63. Female Reproductive System

Folliculogenesis and Ovulation

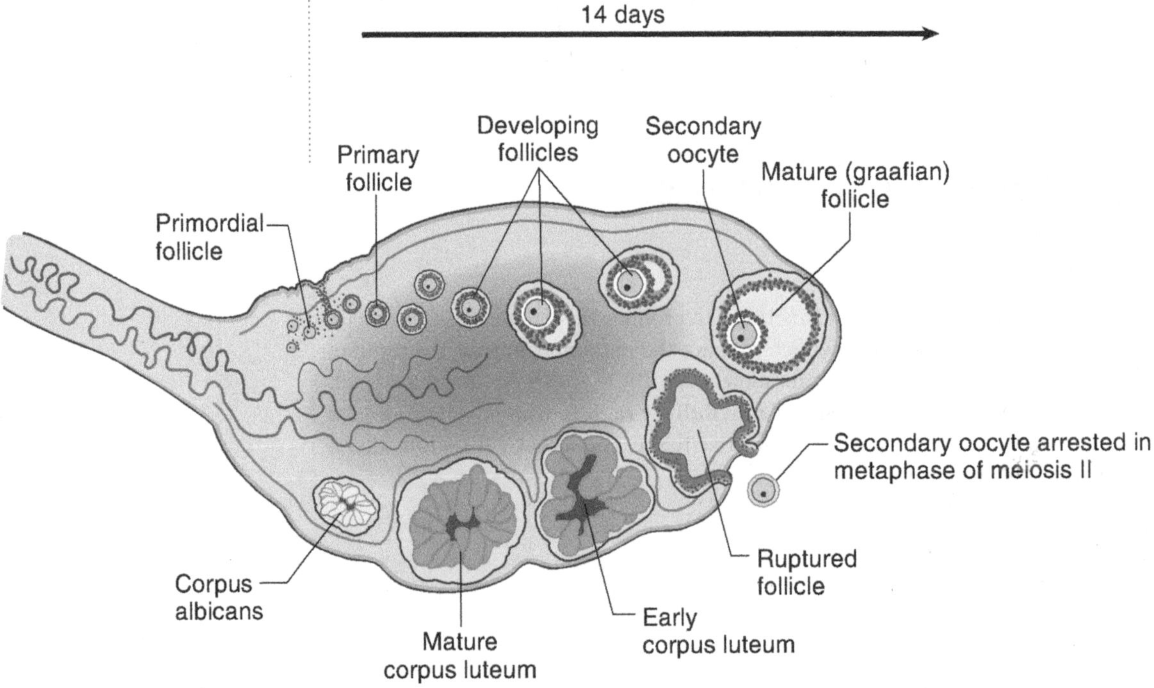

Figure II-3-64. Follicular Development

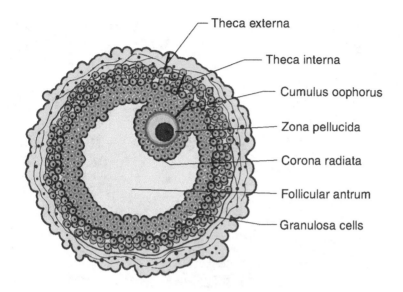

Figure II-3-65. Graafian Follicle

Ovarian Follicles

An ovarian follicle consists of an oocyte surrounded by one or more layers of follicular cells, the **granulosa cells**. In utero, each ovary initially contains 3 million primordial germ cells. Many undergo atresia as the number of follicles in a normal young adult woman is estimated to be 400,000. A typical woman will ovulate only around 450 ova during her reproductive years. All other follicles (with their oocytes) will fail to mature and will undergo atresia.

Before birth, primordial germ cells differentiate into oogonia that proliferate by mitotic division until they number in the millions. They all enter prophase of the first meiotic division in utero and become arrested (they are now designated as **primordial follicles**). The primordial follicles consist of a primary oocyte surrounded by a single layer of squamous follicular cells, which are joined to one another by desmosomes.

Around the time of sexual maturity, the primordial follicles undergo further growth to become **primary follicles** in which the oocyte is surrounded by 2 or more layers of cuboidal cells. In each menstrual cycle after puberty, several primary follicles enter a phase of rapid growth. The oocyte enlarges and the surrounding follicular cells (now called granulosa cells) proliferate. Gap junctions form between the granulosa cells. A thick layer of glycoprotein called the **zona pellucida** is secreted (probably by both the oocyte and granulosa cells) in the space between the oocyte and granulosa cells. Cellular processes of the granulosa cells and microvilli of the oocyte penetrate the zona pellucida and make contact with one another via gap junctions. Around this time the stroma surrounding the follicle differentiates into a cellular layer called the **theca folliculi**. These cells are separated from the granulosa cells by a thick basement membrane. As development proceeds, 2 zones are apparent in the theca: the **theca interna** (richly vascularized) and the **theca externa** (mostly connective tissue). Cells of the theca interna synthesize androgenic steroids that diffuse into the follicle and are converted to estradiol by the granulosa cells.

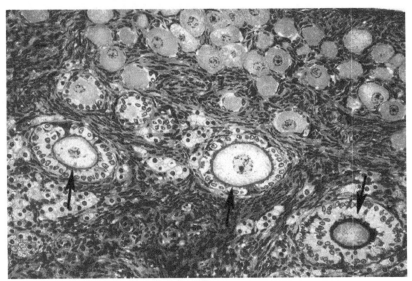

Figure II-3-66. Ovary

Small primordial follicles are at top and 3 primary follicles (arrows)
with cuboidal granulosa cells and a thin zona pellucida are below.

As the follicle grows, follicular fluid, which contains mainly plasma, glycosaminoglycans and steroids accumulates between the cells. The cavities containing the fluid coalesce and form a larger cavity, the **antrum**. At this point, when the antrum is present, the follicles are called **secondary follicles**. The oocyte is at its full size and it is situated in a thickened area of the granulosa called the **cumulus oophorus**.

The mature follicle (**graafian follicle**) completes the first meiotic division (haploid, 2N amount of DNA) just prior to ovulation. The first polar body contains little cytoplasm and remains within the zona pellucida. The Graafian follicle rapidly commences the second meiotic division where it arrests in metaphase awaiting ovulation and fertilization. The second meiotic division is not completed unless fertilization occurs. The fluid filled antrum has greatly enlarged in the Graafian follicle and the cumulus oophorus diminishes leaving the oocyte surrounded by the corona radiata. After ovulation, the corona radiata remains around the ovum where it persists throughout fertilization and for some time during the passage of the ovum through the oviduct.

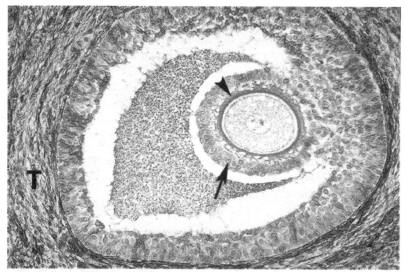

Figure II-3-67. Secondary follicle with an antrum

Follicle is surrounded by a corona radiata of
granulosa cells (arrow) and by a zona pellucida.

Ovulation

Ovulation occurs approximately mid-cycle and is stimulated by a surge of luteinizing hormone secreted by the anterior pituitary. Ovulation consists of rupture of the mature follicle and liberation of the secondary oocyte (ovum) that will be caught by the infundibulum, the dilated distal end of the oviduct. The ovum remains viable for a maximum of 24 hours. Fertilization most commonly occurs in the ampulla of the oviduct. If not fertilized, the ovum undergoes autolysis in the oviduct.

Corpus Luteum

After ovulation, the wall of the follicle collapses and becomes extensively infolded, forming a temporary endocrine gland called the **corpus luteum**. During this process the blood vessels and stromal cells invade the previously avascular layer of granulosa cells and the granulosa cells and those of the theca interna hypertrophy and form lutein cells (granulosa lutein cells and theca lutein cells). The granulosa lutein cells now secrete progesterone and estrogen and the theca lutein cells secrete androstenedione and progesterone. Progesterone prevents the development of new follicles, thereby preventing ovulation.

In the absence of pregnancy the corpus luteum lasts only 10–14 days. The lutein cells undergo apoptosis and are phagocytized by invading macrophages. The site of the corpus luteum is subsequently occupied by a scar of dense connective tissue, the **corpus albicans**.

When pregnancy does occur, human chorionic gonadotropin produced by the placenta will stimulate the corpus luteum for about 6 months and then decline. It continues to secrete progesterone until the end of pregnancy. The corpus luteum of pregnancy is large, sometimes reaching 5 cm in diameter.

Oviducts

The **oviduct** (Fallopian tube) is a muscular tube of about 12 cm in length. One end extends laterally into the wall of the uterus and the other end opens into the peritoneal cavity next to the ovary. The oviduct receives the ovum from the ovary, provides an appropriate environment for its fertilization, and transports it to the uterus. The **infundibulum** opens into the peritoneal cavity to receive the ovum. Finger-like projections (fimbriae) extend from the end of the tube and envelop the ovulation site to direct the ovum to the tube.

Adjacent to the infundibulum is the **ampulla**, where fertilization usually takes place. A slender portion of the oviduct called the **isthmus** is next to the ampulla. The **intramural segment** penetrates the wall of the uterus.

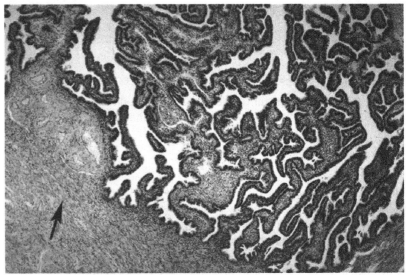

Figure II-3-68. Oviduct with simple columnar epithelium and underlying layer of smooth muscle (arrow)

The wall of the oviduct has 3 layers: a mucosa, a muscularis, and a serosa composed of visceral peritoneum. The mucosa has longitudinal folds that are most numerous in the ampulla. The epithelium lining the mucosa is simple columnar. Some cells are ciliated and the other are secretory. The cilia beat toward the uterus, causing movement of the viscous liquid film (derived predominantly from the secretory cells) that covers the surface of the cells. The secretion has nutrient and protective functions for the ovum and promotes activation of spermatozoa. Movement of the liquid together with contraction of the muscle layer transports the ovum or fertilized egg (zygote) to the uterus.

Ciliary action is not essential, so women with **immotile cilia syndrome (Kartagener's syndrome)** will have a normal tubal transport of the ovum. The muscularis consists of smooth-muscle fibers in a inner circular layer and an outer longitudinal layer.

An **ectopic pregnancy** occurs when the fertilized ovum implants, most commonly in the wall of the ampulla of the oviduct. Partial development proceeds for a time but the tube is too thin and the embryo cannot survive. The vascular placental tissues that have penetrated the thin wall cause brisk bleeding into the lumen of the tube and peritoneal cavity when the tube bursts.

Uterus

The **uterus** is a pear-shaped organ that consists of a fundus which lies above the entrance sties of the oviducts; a **body** (**corpus**) which lies below the entry point of the oviducts and the internal os; a narrowing of the uterine cavity; and a lower cylindrical structure, the **cervix**, which lies below the internal os. The wall of the uterus is relatively thick and has 3 layers. Depending upon the part of the uterus, there is either an outer serosa (connective tissue and mesothelium) or adventitia (connective tissue). The 2 other layers are the **myometrium** (smooth muscle) and the **endometrium** (the mucosa of the uterus).

The myometrium is composed of bundles of smooth-muscle fibers separated by connective tissue. During pregnancy, the myometrium goes through a period of growth as a result of hyperplasia and hypertrophy. The endometrium consists of epithelium and lamina propria containing simple tubular glands that occasionally branch in their deeper portions. The epithelial cells are a mixture of ciliated and secretory simple columnar cells.

The endometrial layer can be divided into 2 zones. The **functionalis** is the part that is sloughed off at menstruation and replaced during each menstrual cycle, and the **basalis** is the portion retained after menstruation that subsequently proliferates and provides a new epithelium and lamina propria. The bases of the uterine glands, which lie deep in the basalis, are the source of the stem cells that divide and migrate to form the new epithelial lining.

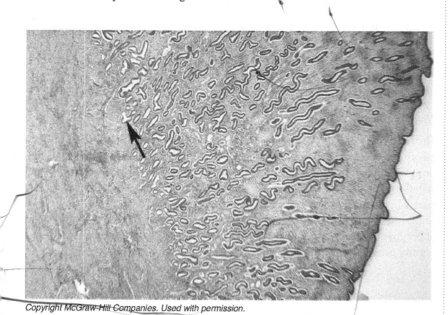

Figure II-3-69. Uterine wall with endometrium

Simple tubular glands to the right of arrow
and myometrium to the left of arrow

Vagina

The wall of the **vagina** has no glands and consists of 3 layers: the mucosa, a muscular layer, and an adventitia. The mucus found in the vagina comes from the glands of the uterine cervix. The epithelium of the mucosa is stratified squamous. This thick layer of cells contains glycogen granules and may contain some keratohyalin. The muscular layer of the vagina is composed of longitudinal bundles of smooth muscle.

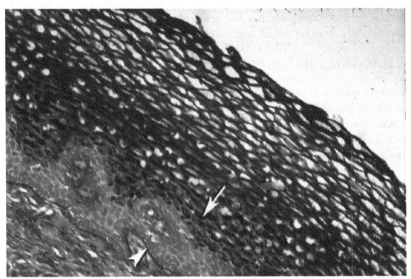

Copyright McGraw-Hill Companies. Used with permission.

Figure II-3-70. Vaginal epithelium with vacuolated stratified squamous epithelial cells that contain glycogen, which is removed during histological processing

Mammary Glands

The mammary glands enlarge significantly during pregnancy as a result of proliferation of alveoli at the ends of the terminal ducts. Alveoli are spherical collections of epithelial cells that become the active milk-secreting structures during lactation. The milk accumulates in the lumen of the alveoli and in the lactiferous ducts. Lymphocytes and plasma cells are located in the connective tissue surrounding the alveoli. The plasma cell population increases significantly at the end of pregnancy and is responsible for the secretion of IgA that confers passive immunity on the newborn.

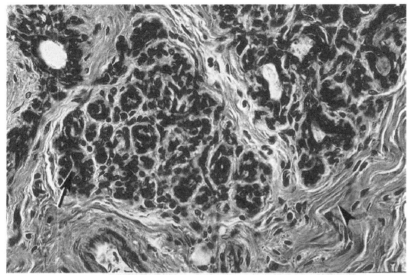

Figure II-3-71. Breast tissue containing modified mammary gland tissue (arrow) surrounded by dense regular connective tissue (arrowhead)

RADIOLOGY OF THE ABDOMEN AND PELVIS

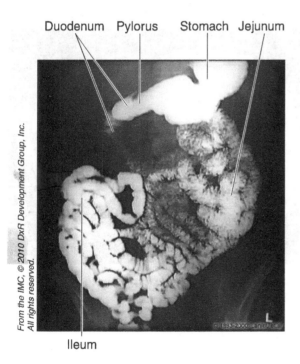

Figure II-3-72. Abdomen: Upper GI, Small Bowel

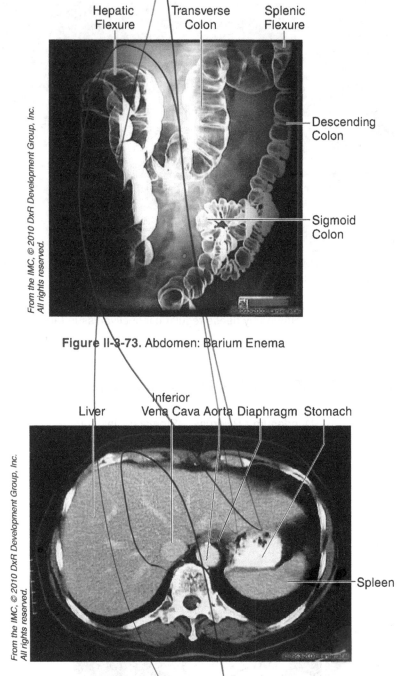

Hepatic Flexure

Transverse Colon

Splenic Flexure

Descending Colon

Sigmoid Colon

Figure II-3-73. Abdomen: Barium Enema

Liver

Inferior Vena Cava Aorta Diaphragm Stomach

Spleen

Figure II-3-74. Abdomen: CT, T11

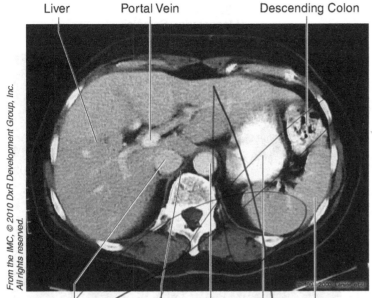

Liver Portal Vein Descending Colon

Inferior Vena Cava Diaphragm Aorta Stomach Spleen

Figure II-3-75. Abdomen: CT, T12

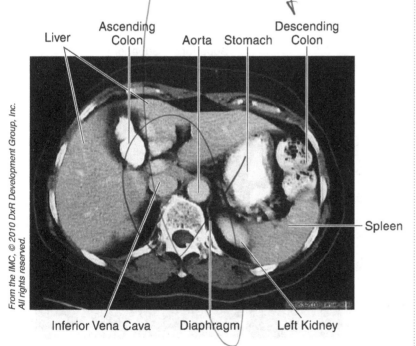

Liver Ascending Colon Aorta Stomach Descending Colon

Spleen

Inferior Vena Cava Diaphragm Left Kidney

Figure II-3-76. Abdomen: CT, T12

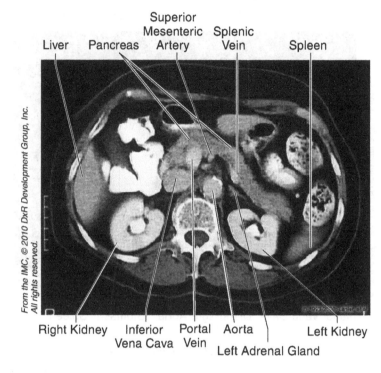

Figure II-3-77. Abdomen: CT, L1

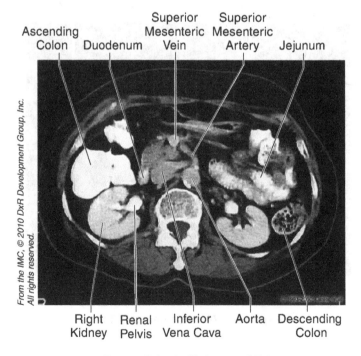

Figure II-3-78. Abdomen: CT, L2

Duodenum
Inferior
Vena Cava
Superior
Mesenteric
Artery
Aorta

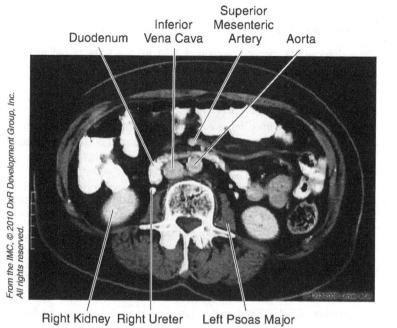

Right Kidney Right Ureter Left Psoas Major

Figure II-3-79. Abdomen: CT, L3

Ureter
Inferior
Vena Cava
Left Common
Iliac Artery

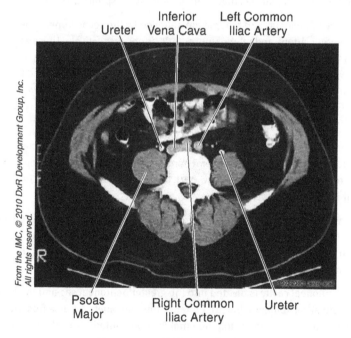

Psoas
Major
Right Common
Iliac Artery
Ureter

Figure II-3-80. Abdomen: CT, L4

Chapter Summary

- The abdominal wall consists primarily of 3 flat muscles (external oblique, internal oblique, and transversus abdominis muscles), rectus abdominis muscle, and the transversalis fascia.

- The inguinal canal contains the round ligament in the female and the spermatic cord in the male. It is an oblique canal through the lower abdominal wall beginning with the deep inguinal ring laterally and the superficial inguinal ring medially. Weakness of the walls of the canal can result in 2 types of inguinal hernias: direct and indirect.

- A direct hernia emerges through the posterior wall of the inguinal canal medial to the inferior epigastric vessels. An indirect hernia passes through the deep inguinal ring lateral to the inferior epigastria vessels and courses through the inguinal canal to reach the superficial inguinal ring.

- A persistent processus vaginalis often results in a congenital indirect inguinal hernia.

- The gastrointestinal (GI) system develops from the primitive gut tube formed by the incorporation of the yolk sac into the embryo during body foldings. The gut tube is divided in the foregut, midgut, and hindgut.

- Defects in the development of the GI tract include annular pancreas, duodenal atresia, Meckel diverticulum, and Hirschsprung disease.

- The foregut, midgut, and hindgut are supplied by the celiac trunk, superior mesenteric artery, and inferior mesenteric artery, respectively. These arteries and their branches reach the viscera mainly by coursing in different parts of the visceral peritoneum. Venous return from the abdomen is provided by the tributaries of the inferior vena cava, except for the GI tract. Blood flow from the GI tract is carried by the hepatic portal system to the liver before returning to the inferior vena cava by the hepatic veins.

- Diseases of the liver result in obstruction of flow in the portal system and portal hypertension. Four collateral portal-caval anastomoses develop to provide retrograde venous flow back to the heart: esophageal, rectal, umbilical, and retroperitoneal.

- The viscera of the GI system are covered by the peritoneum, which is divided into the parietal layer lining the body wall and the visceral layer extending from the body wall and covering the surface of the viscera. Between these layers is the potential space called the peritoneal cavity.

- The peritoneal cavity is divided into the greater peritoneal sac and the lesser peritoneal sac (omental bursa). Entrance into the omental bursa from the greater sac is the epiploic foramen that is bound anteriorly by the lesser omentum and posteriorly by the inferior vena cava.

- The **GI system** includes the **digestive tract** and its associated **glands**. The associated **glands** are **salivary glands, pancreas, liver, and the gallbladder**.

(Continued)

Chapter Summary (*Cont'd*)

- The **pancreas** has an *exocrine* portion and an *endocrine* portion. The exocrine portion is composed of *acini* and *duct cells*. **Acini** secrete enzymes that cleave proteins, carbohydrates, and nucleic acids. **Duct cells** secrete water, electrolytes, and bicarbonate.

- The **liver** is the largest gland in the body. The parenchyma is made up of hepatocytes arranged in cords within lobules.

  - Hepatocytes produce proteins, secrete bile, store lipids and carbohydrates, and convert lipids and amino acids into glucose. They detoxify drugs by oxidation, methylation, or conjugation, and they are capable of regeneration.

Liver **sinusoids**, found between hepatic cords, are lined with endothelial cells and scattered **Kupffer cells**, which phagocytose red blood cells.

- The **biliary system** is composed of bile caliculi, hepatic ducts, the cystic duct, and the common bile duct. The **gallbladder** is lined by simple tall columnar cells and has a glycoprotein surface coat. It concentrates bile by removing water through active transport of sodium and chloride ions (especially the former).

  - Gallbladder contraction is mediated via cholecystokinin, a hormone produced by enteroendocrine cells in the mucosa of the small intestine.

- The kidneys develop from intermediate mesoderm by 3 successive renal systems: pronephros, mesonephros, and metanephros. The mesonephric kidney is the first functional kidney that develops during the first trimester. The final or metanephric kidney develops from 2 sources: the ureteric bud that forms the drainage part of the kidney and the metanephric mass that forms the nephron of the adult kidney.

- The urinary bladder develops from the urogenital sinus, which is formed after division of the cloaca by the urorectal septum.

- The kidneys are located against the posterior abdominal wall between the T12 and L3 vertebrae. Posterior to the kidneys lie the diaphragm and the psoas major and quadratus lumborum muscles. The superior pole of the kidney lies against the parietal pleura posteriorly. The ureters descend the posterior abdominal wall on the ventral surface of the psoas major muscle and cross the pelvic brim to enter the pelvic cavity.

- The **kidney** has 3 major regions: the hilum, cortex, and medulla.

  - The **hilum** is the point of entrance and exit for the renal vessels and ureter. The upper expanded portion of the ureter is called **the renal pelvis**, and divides into 2 or 3 **major calyces** and several **minor calyces**.

  - The **cortex** has several renal columns that penetrate the entire depth of the kidney.

(Continued)

Chapter Summary (*Cont'd*)

- The **medulla** forms a series of pyramids that direct the urinary stream into a minor calyx.

● The **uriniferous tubule** is composed of the **nephron** and **collecting tubule**.

- The **nephron** contains the **glomerulus** (a tuft of capillaries interposed between an afferent and efferent arteriole). Plasma filtration occurs here. **Bowman's capsule** has an inner visceral and outer parietal layer. The space between is the urinary space. The **visceral layer** is composed of podocytes resting on a basal lamina, which is fused with the capillary endothelium. The **parietal layer** is composed of simple squamous epithelium that is continuous with the proximal tubule epithelial lining. The **proximal convoluted tubule** is the longest and most convoluted segment of the nephron. Most of the glomerular filtrate is reabsorbed here. The **loop of Henle** extends into the medulla and has a thick and thin segment. It helps to create an osmotic gradient important for concentration of the tubular filtrate. The **distal convoluted tubule** reabsorbs sodium and chloride from the tubular filtrate.

- The **collecting tubules** have a range of cells from cuboidal to columnar. Water removal and urine concentration occur here with the help of the antidiuretic hormone. The blood supply is via renal artery and vein.

● The **vasa rectae** supply the medulla. They play an important role in maintaining the **osmotic gradient**. The **juxtaglomerular apparatus (JGA)** is composed of **juxtaglomerular cells**, which are myoepithelial cells in the afferent arteriole. They secrete **renin**. The JGA also contains **Polkissen cells** (function unknown), located between afferent and efferent arterioles, and the **macula densa**. Macula densa cells are located in the wall of the distal tubule, located near the afferent arteriole. They sense sodium concentration in tubular fluid.

Pelvis

● The pelvic cavity contains the inferior portions of the GI and urinary systems along with the reproductive viscera. The pelvic viscera and their relationships are shown for the male and female pelvis in Figures II-3-26 and II-3-27, respectively.

● There are 2 important muscular diaphragms related to the floor of the pelvis and the perineum: the pelvic diaphragm and the urogenital diaphragm, respectively. Both of these consist of 2 skeletal muscle components under voluntary control and are innervated by somatic fibers of the lumbosacral plexus.

● The pelvic diaphragm forms the floor of the pelvis where it supports the weight of the pelvic viscera and forms a sphincter for the anal canal. The urogenital diaphragm is located in the perineum (deep perineal space) and forms a sphincter for the urethra. Both diaphragms are affected by an epidural injection.

(Continued)

Chapter Summary (*Cont'd*)

- The broad ligament of the female is formed by 3 parts: the mesosalpinx, which is attached to the uterine tube; the mesovarium attached to the ovary; and the largest component, the mesometrium, attached to the lateral surface of the uterus. In the base of the broad ligament, the ureter passes inferior to the uterine artery just lateral to the cervix.

- The suspensory ligament of the ovary is a lateral extension of the broad ligament extending upward to the lateral pelvic wall. This ligament contains the ovarian vessels, lymphatics, and autonomic nerves.

Perineum

- The perineum is the area between the thighs bounded by the pubic symphysis, ischial tuberosity, and coccyx. The area is divided into 2 triangles. Posteriorly, the anal triangle contains the anal canal, external anal sphincter, and the pudendal canal that contains the pudendal nerve and internal pudendal vessels. Anteriorly is the urogenital triangle, containing the external and deep structures of the external genitalia.

- The urogenital triangle is divided into 2 spaces. The superficial perineal space contains the root structures of the penis and clitoris, associated muscles, and the greater vestibular gland in the female. The deep perineal space is formed by the urogenital diaphragm and contains the bulbourethral gland in the male.

Male Reproductive System

- The **testes** contain seminiferous tubules and connective tissue stroma. **Seminiferous tubules** are the site of spermatogenesis. The epithelium contains Sertoli cells and spermatogenic cells.

  - **Sertoli cells** synthesize **androgen-binding protein** and provide the **blood–testis barrier**.

  - **Spermatogenic cells** are germ cells located between Sertoli cells. They include spermatogonia, primary and secondary spermatocytes, spermatids, and spermatozoa.

  Spermatozoa number about 60,000 per mm^3 of seminal fluid. Each one has a **head**, which contains chromatin. At the apex of the nucleus is the **acrosome**. The tail contains **microtubules**.

- **Interstitial cells of Leydig** are located between the seminiferous tubules in the interstitial connective tissue. They synthesize **testosterone** and are activated by **luteinizing hormone** from the anterior pituitary.

- The **genital ducts** are composed of tubuli recti, rete testis, efferent ductules, ductus epididymis, ductus deferens, and ejaculatory ducts.

  - Spermatozoa undergo maturation and increased motility within the ductus (vas) epididymis.

  - Spermatozoa are stored in the efferent ductules, epididymis, and proximal ductus deferens.

(Continued)

Clinical Correlate

Breast cancer affects about 9% of women born in the United States. Most of the cancers (carcinomas) arise from epithelial cells of the lactiferous ducts.

Chapter Summary (*Cont'd*)

- The **urethra** extends from the urinary bladder to the tip of the penis. The prostatic urethra is composed of transitional epithelium and the distal urethra of stratified epithelium.

- **Seminal vesicles** secrete alkaline, viscous fluid rich in fructose. They do not store spermatozoa.

- Secretions from the **prostate gland** are rich in citric acid, lipids, zinc, and acid phosphatase.

- **Bulbourethral gland** secretes mucous fluid into the urethra for lubrication prior to ejaculation.

- The **penis** is composed of 3 cylindrical bodies of erectile tissue: **corpora cavernosa, corpus spongiosum, and trabeculae of erectile tissue**. The corpora cavernosa is surrounded by the **tunica albuginea**.

Female Reproductive System

- The female reproductive system is composed of ovaries, fallopian tubes, uterus, cervix, vagina, external genitalia, and mammary glands. The **ovaries** have 2 regions, the **cortex** and **medulla**. The former contain **follicles** and the latter vascular and neural elements. There are approximately 400,000 follicles at birth, of which approximately 450 reach maturity in the adult. The remaining follicles undergo atresia.

- Maturation involves the formation of the primary, secondary, and finally, the **Graafian follicle**. During ovulation, a rise in antral fluid causes the follicle to rupture. The ovum will degenerate in 24 hours unless fertilized by the spermatozoan. Following ovulation, the **follicle changes** in the following manner: **theca interna cells** become theca lutein cells and secrete **estrogen**; while follicular cells become **granulosa lutein cells**, producing **progesterone**. If the ovum is fertilized, the **corpus luteum** persists for 3 months, producing progesterone. Its survival is dependent upon **human chorionic gonadotropin** secreted by the developing embryo. Thereafter, the placenta produces progesterone, required to maintain pregnancy.

- The **fallopian tube** is divided into the infundibulum, ampulla, isthmus, and interstitial segment. Fallopian tubes are lined by a mucosa containing cilia that beat toward the uterus, except in the infundibulum, where they beat toward the fimbria. Fertilization occurs in the ampulla, which is also the most frequent site of ectopic pregnancies.

- The **uterus** has 3 coats in its wall:

  - The **endometrium** is a basal layer and superficial functional layer. The latter is shed during menstruation.

  - The **myometrium** is composed of smooth muscle.

  - The **perimetrium** consists of the peritoneal layer of the broad ligament.

(Continued)

Chapter Summary (*Cont'd*)

The **menstrual cycle** results in cyclical endometrial changes. The first 3–5 days are characterized by menstrual flow. Thereafter, the **proliferative stage** commences. During this time, lasting 14 days, the endometrium regrows. This phase is estrogen-dependent. During the **secretory phase**, the endometrium continues to hypertrophy, and there is increased vascularity. This phase is progesterone-dependent. The **premenstrual phase** is marked by constriction of spiral arteries leading to breakdown of the functional layer. Failure of fertilization leads to a drop in progesterone and estrogen levels, and degeneration of the corpus luteum about 2 weeks after ovulation.

- The **placenta** permits exchange of nutrients and removal of waste products between maternal and fetal circulations. The fetal component consists of the **chorionic plate** and **villi**. The maternal component is **decidua basalis**. Maternal blood is separated from fetal blood by the cytotrophoblast and syncytiotrophoblast.

- The **vagina** contains no glands. It is lined by stratified, squamous epithelium, rich in glycogen. During the **estrogenic phase**, its pH is acidic. During the **postestrogenic phase**, the pH is alkaline and vaginal infections could occur.

Upper Limb 4

Learning Objectives

❏ Solve problems concerning brachial plexus

❏ Answer questions about muscle innervation

❏ Solve problems concerning sensory innervation

❏ Solve problems concerning nerve injuries

❏ Solve problems concerning upper and lower brachial plexus lesions

❏ Use knowledge of lesions of branches of the brachial plexus

❏ Use knowledge of arterial supply and major anastomoses

❏ Solve problems concerning carpal tunnel

❏ Interpret scenarios on rotator cuff

❏ Use knowledge of radiology

BRACHIAL PLEXUS

The **brachial plexus** provides the motor and sensory innervation to the upper limb and is formed by the ventral rami of C5 through T1 spinal nerves (Figure II-4-1).

Five major nerves arise from the brachial plexus:

- The **musculocutaneous, median,** and **ulnar** nerves contain **anterior division fibers** and innervate muscles in the anterior arm, anterior forearm, and palmer compartments that function mainly as flexors.

- The **axillary** and **radial** nerves contain **posterior division fibers** and innervate muscles in the posterior arm and posterior forearm compartments that function mainly as extensors.

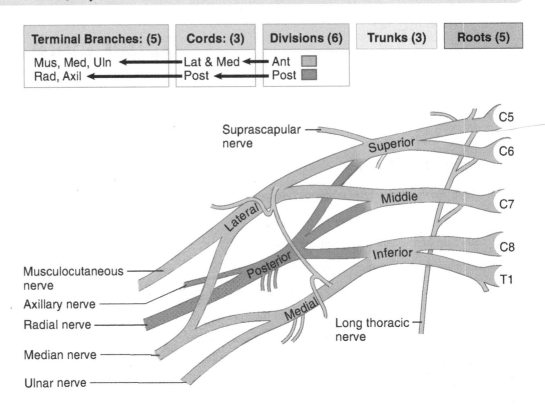

Terminal Branches: (5)	Cords: (3)	Divisions (6)	Trunks (3)	Roots (5)
Mus, Med, Uln ◄────	──Lat & Med ◄──	─ Ant ▢		
Rad, Axil ◄────	──Post ◄──	─ Post ▢		

Suprascapular nerve

Superior

C5

C6

Middle

C7

Lateral

Inferior

C8

Posterior

T1

Musculocutaneous nerve

Axillary nerve

Medial

Radial nerve

Long thoracic nerve

Median nerve

Ulnar nerve

Figure II-4-1. Brachial Plexus

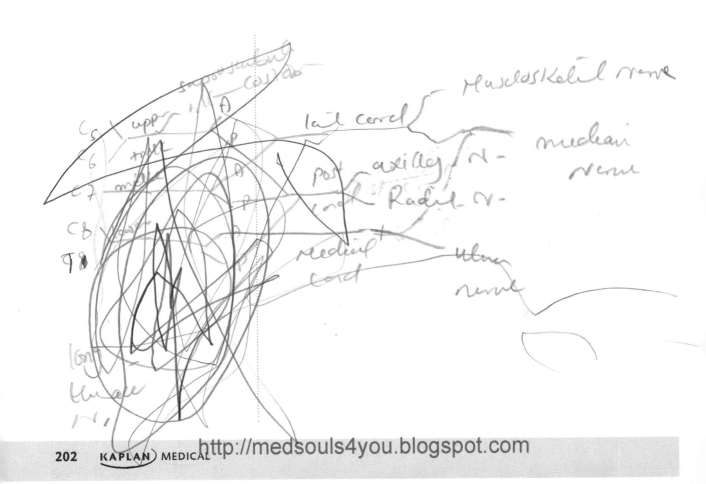

MUSCLE INNERVATION

Terminal Nerves of Upper Limbs

The motor innervation by the 5 terminal nerves of the arm muscles is summarized in Table II-4-1.

Table II-4-1. Major Motor Innervations by the 5 Terminal Nerves

Terminal Nerve	Muscles Innervated	Primary Actions
Musculocutaneous nerve C5–6	All the muscles of the **anterior compartment** of the arm	Flex elbow Supination (biceps brachii)
Median nerve C5–T1	**A. Forearm** • **Anterior compartment** except 1.5 muscles by ulnar nerve (flexor carpi ulnaris and the ulnar half of the flexor digitorum profundus) **B. Hand** • **Thenar compartment** • **Central compartment** Lumbricals: Digits 2 and 3	Flex wrist and all digits Pronation Opposition of thumb Flex metacarpophalangeal (MP) and extend interphalangeal (PIP and DIP) joints of digits 2 and 3
Ulnar nerve C8–T1	**A. Forearm** Anterior Compartment: 1 [1/2] muscles not innervated by the median nerve **B. Hand** • Hypothenar compartment • **Central compartment** – Interossei muscles: Palmar and Dorsal • Lumbricals: Digits 4 & 5 • Adductor pollicis	Flex wrist (weak) and digits 4 and 5 Dorsal – Abduct digits 2-5 (DAB) Palmar – Adduct digits 2-5 (PAD) Assist Lumbricals in MP flexion and IP extension digits 2–5 Flex MP and extend PIP & DIP joints of digits 4 and 5 Adduct the thumb
Axillary nerve C5–6	Deltoid Teres minor	Abduct shoulder—15°–110° Lateral rotation of shoulder
Radial nerve C5–T1	**Posterior compartment** muscles of the arm and forearm	Extend MP, wrist, and elbow Supination (supinator muscle)

Collateral Nerves

In addition to the 5 terminal nerves, there are several collateral nerves that arise from the brachial plexus proximal to the terminal nerves (i.e., from the rami, trunks, or cords). These nerves innervate proximal limb muscles (shoulder girdle muscles). Table II-4-2 summarizes the collateral nerves.

Table II-4-2. The Collateral Nerves of the Brachial Plexus

Collateral Nerve	Muscles or Skin Innervated
Dorsal scapular nerve	Rhomboids
Long thoracic nerve	Serratus anterior—protracts and rotates scapula superiorly
Suprascapular nerve C5–6	Supraspinatus—abduct shoulder 0–15° Infraspinatus—laterally rotate shoulder
Lateral pectoral nerve	Pectoralis major
Medial pectoral nerve	Pectoralis major and minor
Upper subscapular nerve	Subscapularis
Middle subscapular (thoracodorsal) nerve	Latissimus dorsi
Lower subscapular nerve	Subscapularis and teres major
Medial brachial cutaneous nerve	Skin of medial arm
Medial antebrachial cutaneous nerve	Skin of medial forearm

Segmental Innervation to Muscles of Upper Limbs

The **segmental innervation** to the muscles of the upper limbs has a **proximal–distal gradient**, i.e., the more proximal muscles are innervated by the higher segments (C5 and C6) and the more distal muscles are innervated by the lower segments (C8 and T1). Therefore, the intrinsic shoulder muscles are innervated by C5 and C6, the intrinsic hand muscles are innervated by C8 and T1, the distal arm and proximal forearm muscles are innervated by C6 and C7, and the more distal forearm muscles are innervated by C7 and C8.

SENSORY INNERVATION

The skin of the palm is supplied by the median and ulnar nerves. The **median** supplies the lateral 3½ digits and the adjacent area of the lateral palm and the thenar eminence. The **ulnar** supplies the medial 1½ digits and skin of the hypothenar eminence. The **radial** nerve supplies skin of the dorsum of the hand in the area of the first dorsal web space, including the skin over the anatomic snuffbox.

The sensory innervation of the hand is summarized in Figure II-4-2.

Note: Palm sensation is not affected by carpal tunnel syndrome; the superficial palmar cutaneous branch of median nerve passes superficial to the carpal tunnel.

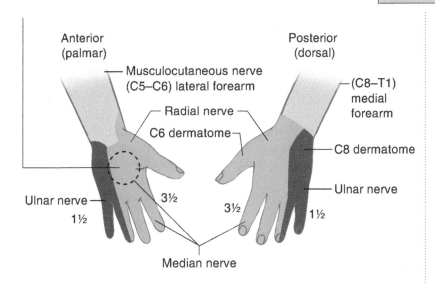

Figure II-4-2. Sensory Innervation of the Hand and Forearm

NERVE INJURIES

Remember: Follow clues in the questions as to the location of the injury. An injury will manifest in symptoms distal to the site of injury.

Thoughts on Muscle–Nerve Lesions

- Without specifically naming all the muscles, assign a function to the various compartments of the limbs.

    Example: posterior arm = extension of the forearm and shoulder

- List the nerve(s) that innervate those muscles or that area.

    Example: posterior arm = radial nerve

- You have an area of the limb, a function of the muscles within that area, and a nerve responsible for that function.

Now you can damage a nerve and note what function(s) is lost or weakened.

UPPER AND LOWER BRACHIAL PLEXUS LESIONS

Upper (C5 and C6) Brachial Plexus Lesion: Erb-Duchenne Palsy (Waiter's Tip Syndrome)

- Usually occurs when the head and shoulder are forcibly separated (e.g., accident or birth injury or herniation of disk)
- Trauma will damage **C5** and **C6** spinal nerves (roots) of the upper trunk.
- Primarily affects the **axillary, suprascapular, and musculocutaneous nerves** with the loss of intrinsic muscles of the shoulder and muscles of the anterior arm (Figure II-4-1).
- Arm is medially rotated and adducted at the shoulder: Loss of **axillary** and **suprascapular** nerves. The unopposed latissimus dorsi and pectoralis major muscles pull the limb into adduction and medial rotation at the shoulder.
- The forearm is extended and pronated: loss of **musculocutaneous** nerve.
- **Sign is "waiter's tip."**
- Sensory loss on lateral forearm to base of thumb: loss of musculocutaneous nerve

Lower (C8 and T1) Brachial Plexus Lesion: Klumpke's Paralysis

- Usually occurs when the upper limb is forcefully abducted above the head (e.g., grabbing an object when falling, thoracic outlet syndrome or birth injury)
- Trauma will injure the **C8 and T1** spinal nerve roots of inferior trunk.
- Primarily affects the ulnar nerve and the intrinsic muscles of the hand with a weakness of the median innervated muscles of the hand (Figure II-4-1)
- Sign is combination of **"claw hand"** and "ape hand" (median nerve).
- May include a Horner syndrome.
- Sensory loss on medial forearm and medial 1½ digits

Table II-4-3. Lesions of Roots of Brachial Plexus

Lesioned Root	C5	C6	C8	T1
Dermatome paresthesia	Lateral border of upper arm	Lateral forearm to thumb	Medial forearm to little finger	Medial arm to elbow
Muscles affected	Deltoid Rotator cuff Serratus anterior Biceps Brachioradialis	Biceps Brachioradialis Brachialis Supinator	Finger flexors Wrist flexors Hand muscles	Hand muscles
Reflex test	—	Biceps tendon	—	—
Causes of lesions	Upper trunk compression	Upper trunk compression	Lower trunk compression	Lower trunk compression

LESIONS OF BRANCHES OF THE BRACHIAL PLEXUS

- Sensory deficits precede motor weakness
- Proximal lesions: more signs

Radial Nerve

Axilla: (Saturday night palsy or using crutches)

- Loss of extension at the elbow, wrist and MP joints
- Weakened supination
- Sensory loss on posterior arm, forearm, and dorsum of thumb
- Distal sign is **"wrist drop."**

Mid-shaft of humerus at radial groove or lateral elbow (lateral epicondyle or radial head dislocation)

- Loss of forearm extensors of the wrist and MP joints
- Weakened supination
- Sensory loss on the posterior forearm and dorsum of thumb
- Distal sign is **"wrist drop."**

Note: Lesions of radial nerve distal to axilla, elbow extension are spared.

Wrist: laceration

- No **motor loss**
- Sensory loss only on dorsal aspect of thumb (first dorsal web space)

Median Nerve

Elbow: (Supracondylar fracture of humerus)

- Weakened wrist flexion (with ulnar deviation)
- Loss of pronation
- Loss of digital flexion of lateral 3 digits resulting in the inability to make a complete fist; sign is **"hand of benediction"**
- Loss of thumb opposition (opponens pollicis muscle); sign is **ape (simian) hand**
- Loss of first 2 lumbricals
- Thenar atrophy (flattening of thenar eminence)
- Sensory loss on palmar surface of the lateral hand and the palmar surfaces of the lateral 3½ digits

Note: A lesion of median nerve at elbow results in the "hand of benediction" and "ape hand."

Wrist: carpal tunnel or laceration

- Loss of thumb opposition (opponens pollicis muscle); sign is **ape or simian hand**
- Loss of first 2 lumbricals

- Thenar atrophy (flattening of thenar eminence)
- Sensory loss on the palmar surfaces of lateral 3½ digits. Note sensory loss on lateral palm may be spared (Figure II-4-2).

Note: Lesions of median nerve at the wrist present without benediction hand and with normal wrist flexion, digital flexion, and pronation.

Ulnar Nerve

Elbow (medial epicondyle), wrist (lacerations), or fracture of hook of hamate

- Loss of hypothenar muscles, third and fourth lumbricals, all interossei and adductor pollicis
- With elbow lesion there is minimal weakening of wrist flexion with radial deviation
- Loss of **abduction** and **adduction of digits 2–5** (interossei muscles)
- Weakened interphalangeal (IP) extension of digits 2–5 (more pronounced in digits 4 and 5)
- Loss of thumb adduction
- Atrophy of the hypothenar eminence
- Sign is **"claw hand."** Note that clawing is greater with a wrist lesion.
- Sensory loss on medial 1½ digits

Axillary Nerve

Fracture of the surgical neck of the humerus or inferior dislocation of the shoulder

- Loss of abduction of the arm to the horizon
- Sensory lost over the deltoid muscle

Musculocutaneous Nerve

- Loss of elbow flexion and weakness in supination
- Loss of sensation on lateral aspect of the forearm

Long Thoracic Nerve

- Often damaged during a radical mastectomy or a stab wound to the lateral chest (nerve lies on superficial surface of serratus anterior muscle).
- Loss of abduction of the arm above the horizon to above the head
- Sign of **"winged scapula"**; patient unable to hold the scapula against the posterior thoracic wall

Suprascapular Nerve

- Loss of shoulder abduction between 0 and 15 degrees (supraspinatus muscle)
- Weakness of lateral rotation of shoulder (infraspinatus muscle)

Table II-4-4. Effects of Lesions to Branches of the Brachial Plexus

Lesioned Nerve	Axillary (C5, C6)	Musculo-cutaneous (C5, C6, C7)	Radial (C5, C6, C7, C8)	Median (C6, C7, C8, T1)	Ulnar (C8, T1)
Altered sensation	Lateral arm	Lateral forearm	Dorsum of hand over first dorsal interosseous and anatomic snuffbox	Lateral 3½ digits; lateral palm	Medial 1½ digits; medial palm
Motor weakness	Abduction at shoulder	Flexion of forearm Supination	Wrist extension Metacarpo-phalangeal extension Supination	Wrist flexion Finger flexion Pronation Thumb opposition	Wrist flexion Finger spreading Thumb adduction Finger extension
Common sign of lesion	—	—	Wrist drop	Ape hand Hand of benediction Ulnar deviation at wrist	Claw hand Radial deviation at wrist
Causes of lesions	Surgical neck fracture of humerus Dislocated humerus	Rarely lesioned	Saturday night palsy Midshaft fracture of humerus Subluxation of radius Dislocated humerus	Carpal tunnel compression Supracondylar fracture of humerus Pronator teres syndrome	Fracture of medial epicondyle of humerus Fracture of hook of hamate Fracture of clavicle

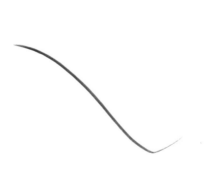

ARTERIAL SUPPLY AND MAJOR ANASTOMOSES

Arterial Supply to the Upper Limb (Figure II-4-3)

Subclavian artery

Branch of brachiocephalic trunk on the right and aortic arch on the left.

Axillary artery

- From the first rib to the posterior edge of the teres major muscle
- Three major branches:
  - Lateral thoracic artery—supplies mammary gland; runs with long thoracic nerve
  - Subscapular artery—collateral to shoulder with suprascapular branch of subclavian artery
  - Posterior humeral circumflex artery—at surgical neck with axillary nerve

Brachial artery

Profunda brachii artery with radial nerve in radial groove—at midshaft of humerus

Radial artery

Deep palmar arch

Ulnar artery

- Common interosseus artery
- Superficial palmar arch

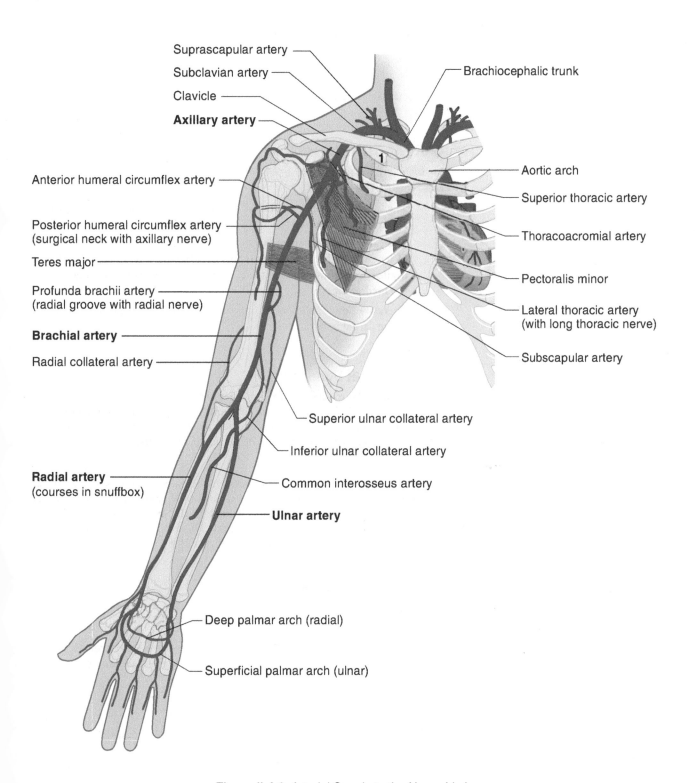

Figure II-4-3. Arterial Supply to the Upper Limb

Collateral Circulation

Shoulder

Subscapular branch of axillary and suprascapular branch of subclavian arteries

Hand

Superficial and deep palmar arches

CARPAL TUNNEL

The carpal tunnel is the fibro-osseous tunnel located on the ventral aspect of the wrist (Figure II-4-4).

- The tunnel is bounded **anteriorly** by the **flexor retinaculum** and **posteriorly** by the proximal row of **carpal bones (lunate)**.
- The carpal tunnel transmits 9 tendons and the radial and ulnar bursae (4 tendons of **the flexor digitorum superficialis**, 4 tendons of the **flexor digitorum profundus**, and the tendon of the **flexor pollicis longus**) and the **median nerve**.
- There are **no** blood vessels or any branches of the radial or ulnar nerves in the carpal tunnel.

Carpal Tunnel Syndrome

Entrapment of the median nerve and other structures in the carpal tunnel due to any condition that reduces the space results in **carpal tunnel syndrome**. The median nerve is the only nerve affected and the patient will present with atrophy of the thenar compartment muscles and weakness of the thenar muscles (opposition of the thumb—**ape hand**).

There is also **sensory loss** and numbness on the palmar surfaces of the **lateral 3½ digits**. Note that the skin on the lateral side of the palm (thenar eminence) is spared because the **palmar cutaneous branch of the median nerve** which supplies the lateral palm enters the hand **superficial** to the flexor retinaculum and does not course through the carpal tunnel (Figure II-4-2).

Clinical Correlate

Carpal tunnel syndrome compresses the median nerve.

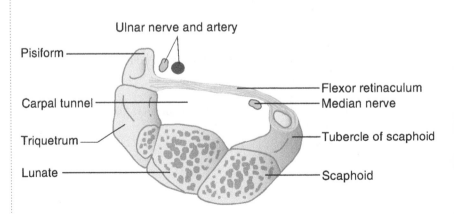

Figure II-4-4. Carpal Tunnel at Proximal Row of Carpal Bones

ROTATOR CUFF

The tendons of rotator cuff muscles strengthen the glenohumeral joint and include the **supraspinatus**, **infraspinatus**, **teres minor**, and **subscapularis** (the **SITS**) muscles. The tendons of the muscles of the rotator cuff may become torn or inflamed.

The tendon of the **supraspinatus** is most commonly affected. Patients with rotator cuff tears experience pain anteriorly and superiorly to the glenohumeral joint during abduction.

Clinical Correlate

Humeral Head Dislocation

Dislocation of the humeral head from the glenohumeral joint typically occurs through the inferior portion of the joint capsule where the capsule is the slackest and is not reinforced by a rotator cuff tendon (Figure II-4-5). After inferior dislocation, the humeral head is pulled superiorly and comes to lie anterior to the glenohumeral joint.

Dislocation may injure the **axillary** or **radial** nerve.

Clinical Correlate

A rupture or tear of the rotator cuff follows chronic use of the shoulder or a fall with an abducted upper limb. The **supraspinatus muscle** is the most frequently damaged muscle of the rotator cuff.

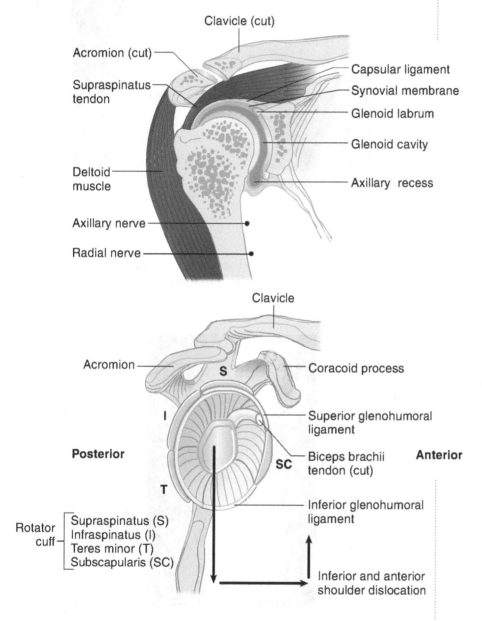

Figure II-4-5. Rotator Cuff

Clinical Correlate

Humeral Surgical Neck Fracture

The axillary nerve accompanies the posterior humeral circumflex artery as it passes around the surgical neck of the humerus.

A fracture in this area could lacerate both the artery and nerve.

Mid-Shaft (Radial Groove) Humeral Fracture

The radial nerve accompanies the profunda brachii artery.

Both could be damaged as a result of a mid-shaft humeral fracture.

What deficits would result from laceration of the radial nerve?

RADIOLOGY

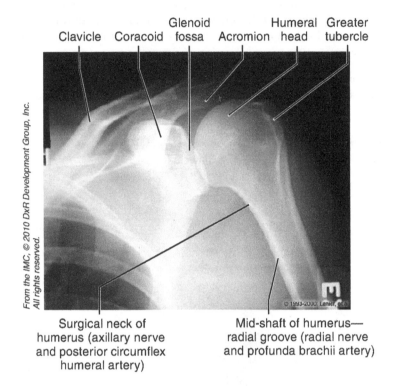

Surgical neck of humerus (axillary nerve and posterior circumflex humeral artery)

Mid-shaft of humerus— radial groove (radial nerve and profunda brachii artery)

Figure II-4-6. Upper Extremities: Anteroposterior View of Shoulder (External Rotation)

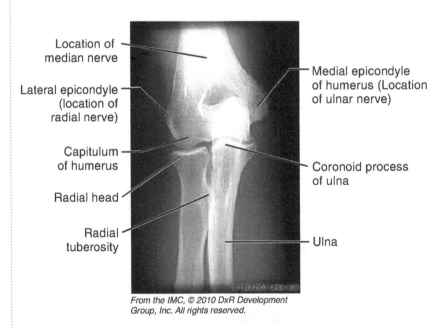

Figure II-4-7. Upper Extremities: Anteroposterior View of Elbow

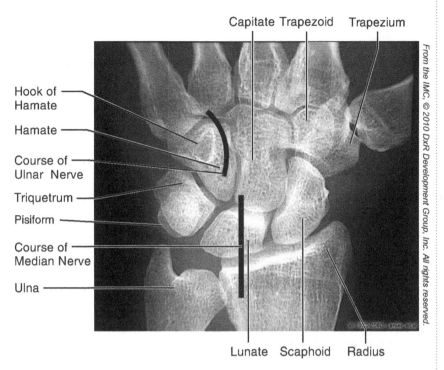

Capitate   Trapezoid   Trapezium

Hook of Hamate

Hamate

Course of Ulnar Nerve

Triquetrum

Pisiform

Course of Median Nerve

Ulna

Lunate   Scaphoid   Radius

Figure II-4-8. Upper Extremities: Posteroanterior View of Wrist

Clinical Correlate

The **scaphoid** is the most frequently fractured of the carpal bones. This fracture may separate the proximal head of the scaphoid from its blood supply (which enters the bone at the distal head) and may result in **avascular necrosis** of the proximal head.

The **lunate** is the most commonly dislocated carpal bone (it dislocates anteriorly into the carpal tunnel and may compress the median nerve).

Clinical Correlate

- **Carpal tunnel syndrome** results from compression of the median nerve within the tunnel.

- A fall on the outstretched hand may **fracture the hook of the hamate,** which may damage the ulnar nerve as it passes into the hand.

Chapter Summary

- The motor and sensory supply of the upper limb is provided by the brachial plexus. The plexus is formed by the ventral rami of spinal nerves C5–T1. These rami form superior, middle, and inferior trunks in the posterior triangle of the neck. Anterior and posterior division fibers from each of the 3 trunks enter the axilla and establish the innervation of the muscles in the anterior and posterior compartment of the limb. The compartments of the limb and their innervations are given in Table II-4-1.

- In the axilla, cords of the brachial plexus are formed and give rise to many of the named branches of the brachial plexus including the 5 terminal branches: musculocutaneous, median, ulnar, radial, and axillary nerves.

- Damage to the upper trunk (C5 and C6) of the brachial plexus (Erb paralysis) results in the arm being medially rotated and adducted with the forearm extended and pronated due to loss of the axillary, suprascapular, and musculocutaneous nerves. A lower trunk (C8 and T1) lesion causes a combined claw and ape hand.

- Other major lesions of branches of the brachial plexus include wrist drop (radial nerve), ape hand (median nerve), claw hand (ulnar nerve), loss of elbow flexion (musculocutaneous nerve), and loss of shoulder abduction (suprascapular and axillary nerves).

- Sensory supply from the palmar surface of the hand is supplied by the median nerve (laterally) and the ulnar nerve (medially) and on the dorsal surface of the hand by the radial nerve (laterally) and the ulnar nerve (medially).

- The shoulder joint is supported by the rotator cuff muscles: supraspinatus, infraspinatus, teres minor, and subscapularis muscles. These muscles hold the head of the humerus in the glenoid fossa.

- At the wrist, the carpal tunnel is the space deep to the flexor retinaculum and ventral to the carpal bones. The median nerve passes through the canal with the tendons of the flexor digitorum superficialis and flexor digitorum profundus and the tendon of the flexor pollicis longus muscle. There are no vessels in the carpal tunnel.

- The arteries that supply blood to the upper limb are a continuation of the subclavian artery. The axillary, brachial, radial, ulnar, and the superficial and deep palmar arch arteries give rise to a number of branches to the limb (Figure II-4-3).

Lower Limb 5

Learning Objectives

❏ Explain information related to lumbosacral plexus

❏ Solve problems concerning nerve injuries and abnormalities of gait

❏ Demonstrate understanding of arterial supply and major anastomoses

❏ Use knowledge of femoral triangle

❏ Demonstrate understanding of hip

❏ Explain information related to knee joint

❏ Use knowledge of ankle joint

❏ Solve problems concerning radiology

LUMBOSACRAL PLEXUS

The **lumbosacral plexus** provides the motor and sensory innervation to the lower limb and is formed by ventral rami of the L2 through S3 spinal nerves.

- The major nerves of the plexus are the:
    - **Femoral nerve**—posterior divisions of L2 through L4
    - **Obturator nerve**—anterior divisions of L2 through L4
    - **Tibial nerve**—anterior divisions of L4 through S3
    - **Common fibular nerve**—posterior divisions of L4 through S2
    - **Superior gluteal nerve**—posterior divisions of L4 through S1
    - **Inferior gluteal nerve**—posterior divisions of L5 through S2

- The tibial nerve and common fibular nerve travel together through the gluteal region and thigh in a common connective tissue sheath and together are called the **sciatic nerve.**

- The common fibular nerve divides in the proximal leg into the **superficial and deep fibular nerves.**

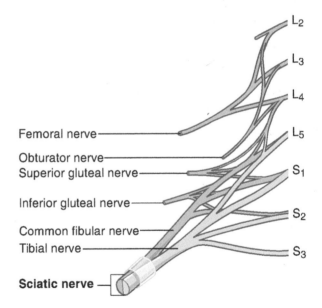

Figure II-5-1. Lumbosacral Plexus

Terminal Nerves of Lumbosacral Plexus

The terminal nerves of the lumbosacral plexus are described in Table II-5-1.

Table II-5-1. Terminal Nerves of Lumbosacral Plexus

Terminal Nerve	Origin	Muscles Innervated	Primary Actions
Femoral nerve	L2 through L4 posterior divisions	Anterior compartment of thigh (quadriceps femoris, sartorius, pectineus)	Extend knee Flex hip
Obturator nerve	L2 through L4 anterior divisions	Medial compartment of thigh (gracilis, adductor longus, adductor brevis, anterior portion of adductor magnus)	Adduct thigh Medially rotate thigh
Tibial nerve	L4 through S3 anterior divisions	Posterior compartment of thigh (semimembranosus, semitendinosus, long head of biceps femoris, posterior portion of adductor magnus)	Flex knee Extend thigh
		Posterior compartment of leg (gastrocnemius, soleus, flexor digitorum longus, flexor hallucis longus, tibialis posterior)	Plantar flex foot (S1–2) Flex digits Inversion
		Plantar muscles of foot	
Common fibular nerve	L4 through S2 posterior divisions	Short head of biceps femoris	Flex knee
Superficial fibular nerve		Lateral compartment of leg (fibularis longus, fibularis brevis)	Eversion
Deep fibular nerve		Anterior compartment of leg (tibialis anterior, extensor hallucis, extensor digitorum, fibularis tertius)	Dorsiflex foot (L4–5) Extend digits Inversion

Collateral Nerves of Lumbosacral Plexus

The collateral nerves of the lumbosacral plexus (to the lower limb) are summarized in Table II-5-2.

Table II-5-2. Collateral Nerves of Lumbosacral Plexus

Collateral Nerve	Origin	Muscles or Skin Innervated	Primary Actions
Superior gluteal nerve	L4 through S1 posterior divisions	Gluteus medius, gluteus minimus, tensor fasciae latae	Stabilize pelvis / Abduct hip
Inferior gluteal nerve	L5 through S2 posterior divisions	Gluteus maximus	Extension of hip / Lateral rotation of thigh
Nerve to superior gemellus and obturator internus	L5 through S2 posterior divisions	Superior gemellus, obturator internus	Lateral rotation of thigh
Nerve to inferior gemellus and quadratus femoris	L4 through S1 posterior divisions	Inferior gemellus, quadratus femoris	Lateral rotation of thigh
Lateral femoral cutaneous nerve	L2 through L3 posterior divisions	Skin of anterolateral thigh	—
Posterior femoral cutaneous nerve	S1 through S2 posterior divisions and S2 through S3 anterior divisions	Skin of posterior thigh	—

Segmental Innervation to Muscles of Lower Limb

The **segmental innervation** to the muscles of the lower limb has a **proximal–distal gradient**, i.e., the more proximal muscles are innervated by the higher segments and the more distal muscles are innervated by the lower segments.

- The muscles that cross the **anterior side of the hip** are innervated by **L2 and L3.**
- The muscles that cross the **anterior side of the knee** are innervated by **L3 and L4.**
- The muscles that cross the **anterior side of the ankle** are innervated by **L4 and L5 (dorsiflexion).**
- The muscles that cross the **posterior side of the hip** are innervated by **L4 and L5.**
- The muscles that cross the **posterior side of the knee** are innervated by **L5 and S1.**
- The muscles that cross the **posterior side of the ankle** are innervated by **S1 and S2** (plantar flexion).

NERVE INJURIES AND ABNORMALITIES OF GAIT

Superior Gluteal Nerve
- Weakness in abduction of the hip
- Impairment of gait; patient cannot keep pelvis level when standing on one leg.
- Sign is "Trendelenburg gait."

Inferior Gluteal Nerve
- Weakened hip extension
- Difficulty rising from a sitting position or climbing stairs

Femoral Nerve
- Weakened hip flexion
- Weakened extension of the knee
- Sensory loss on the anterior thigh, medial leg, and foot

Obturator Nerve
- Loss of adduction of the thigh as well as sensory loss on medial thigh

Sciatic Nerve
- Weakened extension of the thigh
- Loss of flexion of the knee
- Loss of all functions below the knee
- Sensory loss on the posterior thigh, leg (except medial side), and foot

Tibial nerve only
- Weakness in flexion of the knee
- Weakness in plantar flexion
- Weakened inversion
- Sensory loss on the leg (except medial) and plantar foot

Common fibular nerve (neck of fibula)
Produces a combination of deficits of lesions of the deep and superficial fibular nerves

Deep fibular nerve
- Weakened inversion
- Loss of extension of the digits
- Loss of dorsiflexion ("foot drop")
- Sensory loss limited to skin of the first web space between the great and second toes

Clinical Correlate
The **common fibular nerve** crosses the lateral aspect of the knee at the neck of the fibula, where it is the most frequently damaged nerve of the lower limb. Patients will present with loss of dorsiflexion at the ankle (**foot drop**), loss of **eversion**, and sensory loss on the lateral surface of the leg and the dorsum of the foot.

Clinical Correlate
The **common fibular nerve** may be compressed by the **piriformis muscle** when the nerve passes through the piriformis instead of inferior to the muscle with the tibial nerve. **Piriformis syndrome** results in motor and sensory loss to the lateral and anterior compartments of the leg.

Clinical Correlate
The **sciatic nerve** is often damaged following posterior hip dislocation. A complete sciatic nerve lesion results in sensory and motor deficits in the posterior compartment of the thigh and all functions below the knee.

Superficial fibular nerve

- Loss of eversion of the foot
- Sensory loss on anterolateral leg and dorsum of the foot, except for the first web space

Sensory Innervation of the Lower Leg and Foot

- The lateral leg and the dorsum of the foot are supplied mainly by the **superficial fibular nerve**, with the exception of the first dorsal web space, which is supplied by the **deep fibular nerve** (Figure II-5-2).
- The sole of the foot is supplied by the **lateral** and **medial plantar branches** of the **tibial nerve**.
- The sural nerve (a combination of both peroneal and tibial branches) supplies the posterior leg and lateral side of the foot.
- The **saphenous nerve** (a branch of the femoral nerve) supplies the medial leg and medial foot.

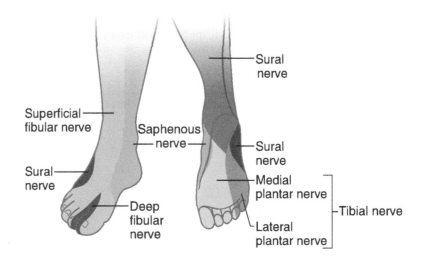

Figure II-5-2. Sensory Innervation of the Lower Leg and Foot

Clinical Correlate

Most of the blood supply to the head of the femur (arising mostly from the medial femoral circumflex artery) ascends along the neck of the femur. Fracture of the femoral neck can compromise this blood supply and lead to **avascular necrosis of the head of the femur.**

ARTERIAL SUPPLY AND MAJOR ANASTOMOSES

Figure II-5-3 illustrates the arterial supply to the legs.

Obturator artery—supplies medial compartment of thigh

External iliac artery

Femoral artery

Profunda femoris artery

- Medial circumflex femoral artery—supplies head of femur (avascular necrosis)
- Lateral circumflex femoral artery
- Perforating arteries—supplies posterior compartment of thigh

Popliteal artery—supplies knee joint

Anterior tibial artery—courses with deep fibular nerve in anterior compartment of leg

- Dorsalis pedis artery—pulse on dorsum of foot lateral to extensor hallucis longus tendon; used to note quality of blood supply to foot

Posterior tibial artery—courses with tibial nerve in posterior compartment of leg and passes posterior to the medial malleolus

- Fibular artery—supplies lateral compartment of leg
- Plantar arterial arch
- Lateral plantar artery
- Medial plantar artery

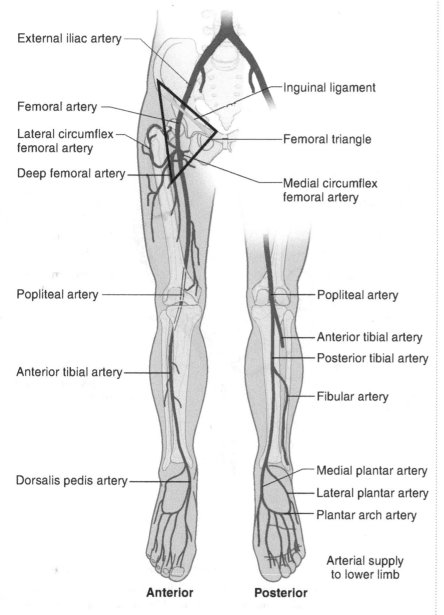

External iliac artery

Femoral artery

Lateral circumflex femoral artery

Deep femoral artery

Inguinal ligament

Femoral triangle

Medial circumflex femoral artery

Popliteal artery — — Popliteal artery

Anterior tibial artery

Posterior tibial artery

Fibular artery

Anterior tibial artery

Medial plantar artery

Lateral plantar artery

Plantar arch artery

Dorsalis pedis artery

Arterial supply to lower limb

Anterior **Posterior**

Figure II-5-3. Arterial Supply to Lower Limb

Clinical Correlate

Tibial shaft fractures can cause lacerations of the anterior or posterior tibial arteries, producing either anterior or posterior **compartment syndromes**.

FEMORAL TRIANGLE

- The femoral triangle is bounded by the inguinal ligament, and the sartorius and adductor longus muscles (Figure II-5-3).
- Within the triangle are the femoral sheath (containing the femoral artery and vein and canal) and the femoral nerve (which is outside of the femoral sheath).
- Passing under the inguinal ligament (from lateral to medial) are the femoral nerve, femoral artery, femoral vein, an empty space within the femoral sheath called the femoral canal, and inguinal lymph nodes within the femoral canal (NAVEL). The femoral canal is the site of **femoral hernias**.

HIP

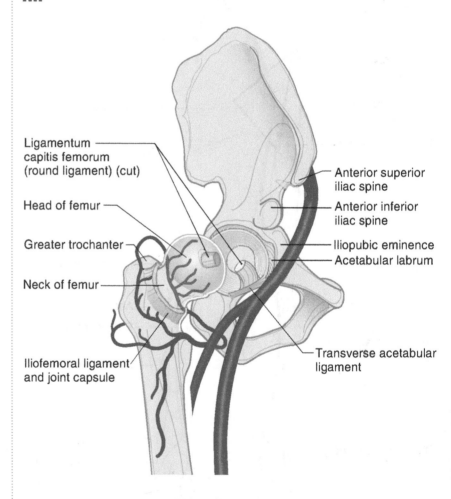

Figure II-5-4. Hip

- The hip joint is formed by the **head of the femur** and the **acetabulum**.
- The fibrous capsule of the hip joint is reinforced by 3 ligamentous thickenings: **iliofemoral ligament, ischiofemoral ligament,** and **pubofemoral ligament**.

- Most of the blood supply to the head of the femur (arising mostly from the medial femoral circumflex artery) ascends along the neck of the femur. Fracture of the femoral neck can compromise this blood supply and lead to **avascular necrosis of the head of the femur.**

KNEE JOINT

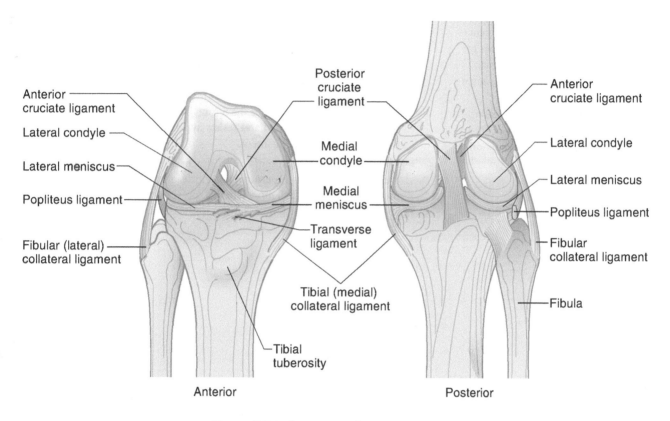

Figure II-5-5. Structures of the Knee

The knee joint is a synovial joint formed by the articulations of the **medial and lateral femoral condyles**, the **medial and lateral tibial condyles**, and the **patella** (Figure II-5-5). The primary movement at the knee joint is flexion and extension of the leg.

The knee joint is a weight-bearing joint and the stability of the joint depends on the muscles (quadriceps and hamstring muscles) that cross the joint. The knee is strengthened by several sets of ligaments.

Tibial (Medial) and Fibular (Lateral) Collateral Ligaments

Tibial collateral ligament extends from the medial epicondyle of the femur inferiorly to attach to the medial aspect of the tibia. It is firmly attached to the capsule and medial meniscus. The tibial ligament prevents **lateral displacement** (abduction) of the tibia under the femur.

Clinical Correlate

The tibial collateral ligament is the most frequently torn ligament at the knee, commonly seen following lateral trauma to the knee.

Fibular collateral ligament extends from the lateral condyle of the femur inferiorly to attach to the head of the fibula and is not attached to the lateral meniscus. The fibular ligament prevents **medial displacement** (adduction) of the tibia under the femur.

The collateral ligaments are taut with knee extension.

Anterior and Posterior Cruciate Ligaments

These are intracapsular ligaments but are located outside the synovial membrane (Figures II-5-5 and -6).

- **Anterior cruciate ligament** (ACL) attaches to the anterior aspect of the tibia and courses superiorly, posteriorly, and laterally to attach to the lateral condyle of the femur. The anterior ligament prevents **anterior displacement** of the tibia under the femur. Tension on the ACL is greatest when the knee is extended and resists hyperextension. It is weaker than the posterior cruciate ligament.
- **Posterior cruciate ligament** (PCL) attaches to the posterior aspect of the tibia and courses superiorly, anteriorly, and medially to attach to the medial condyle of the femur. The PCL prevents **posterior displacement** of the tibia under the femur. Tension on the PCL is greatest when the knee is flexed.

Clinical Correlate

The tests for the integrity of the anterior and posterior cruciate ligaments are the **anterior and posterior drawer signs.** Tearing of the anterior cruciate ligaments allows the tibia to be easily pulled **forward** (anterior drawer sign). Tearing of the posterior cruciate ligament allows the tibial to be easily pulled **posteriorly** (posterior drawer sign).

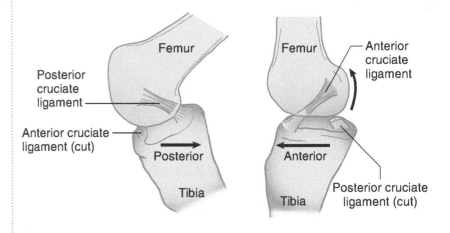

Figure II-5-6. Anterior and Posterior Cruciate Ligaments

Medial and Lateral Menisci

These are intracapsular wedges of fibrocartilage located between the articulating condyles that help make the articulating surfaces more congruent and also serve as shock absorbers.

- **Medial meniscus** is C-shaped and is firmly attached to the tibial collateral ligament. Therefore, it is less mobile and is more frequently injured than the lateral meniscus.
- **Lateral meniscus** is circular and more mobile. It is not attached to the fibular collateral ligament.

Common Knee Injuries

The 3 **most commonly injured structures at the knee** are the tibial collateral ligament, the medial meniscus, and the ACL (**the terrible or unhappy triad**)—usually results from a blow to the lateral aspect of the knee with the foot on the ground.

Patients with a **medial meniscus tear** have pain when the leg is medially rotated at the knee.

ANKLE JOINT

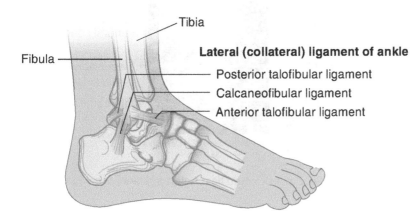

Tibia

Fibula

Lateral (collateral) ligament of ankle

Posterior talofibular ligament
Calcaneofibular ligament
Anterior talofibular ligament

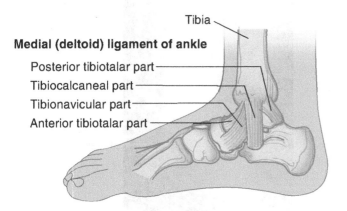

Tibia

Medial (deltoid) ligament of ankle

Posterior tibiotalar part
Tibiocalcaneal part
Tibionavicular part
Anterior tibiotalar part

Figure II-5-7. Structures of the Ankle

Clinical Correlate

– Inversion sprains are most common.
– Anterior talofibular ligament is frequently damaged.

RADIOLOGY

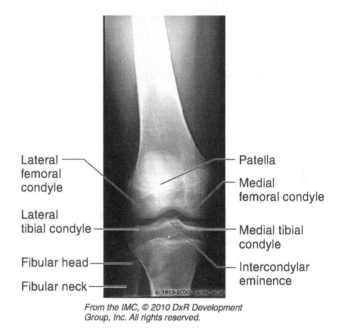

Lateral femoral condyle

Lateral tibial condyle

Fibular head

Fibular neck

Patella

Medial femoral condyle

Medial tibial condyle

Intercondylar eminence

Figure II-5-8. Lower Extremities: Anteroposterior View of Knee

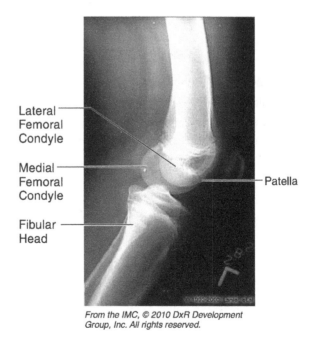

Lateral Femoral Condyle

Medial Femoral Condyle

Fibular Head

Patella

Figure II-5-9. Lower Extremities: Lateral Knee

Chapter Summary

- The lumbosacral plexus is formed by the ventral rami of spinal nerves L1–S4, which provide the major motor and sensory innervation for the lower limb. The primary named nerves are the femoral, obturator, tibial, and common fibular (superior and deep) nerves. The nerves supply the major muscular compartments of the lower limb.

- The major nerve lesions of the lower limb include Trendelenburg gait (superior gluteal nerve), difficulty standing or climbing (inferior gluteal nerve), loss of knee extension (femoral nerve), loss of hip adduction (obturator nerve), loss of knee flexion and plantar flexion (tibial nerve), foot drop (common or deep fibular nerves), loss of eversion (common or superficial fibular nerves), and loss of inversion (deep fibular and tibial nerves).

- The sensory supply from most of the dorsal surface of the foot is provided by the superficial fibular nerve, except between the great and second toes, which is supplied by the deep fibular nerve.

- On the sole of the foot, sensory supply is provided by the medial plantar nerve from the medial toes and the lateral plantar nerve from the lateral toes.

- Blood supply to the lower limb is mostly derived from the femoral artery, a continuation of the external iliac artery. The named arterial branches to the limb include the obturator, femoral, popliteal, anterior and posterior tibial arteries, and the plantar arterial arch.

- The articulation of the knee joint is formed by the condyles of the femur and tibia. This joint is strengthened by the medial and lateral collateral ligaments, the anterior and posterior cruciate ligaments, and the medial and lateral menisci.

Head and Neck 6

Learning Objectives

❏ Explain information related to neck

❏ Answer questions about carotid and subclavian arteries

❏ Demonstrate understanding of embryology of the head and neck

❏ Solve problems concerning cranium

❏ Answer questions about cranial meninges and dural venous sinuses

❏ Use knowledge of intracranial hemorrhage

❏ Interpret scenarios on orbital muscles and their innervation

NECK

Thoracic Outlet

The thoracic outlet is the space bounded by the manubrium, the first rib, and T1 vertebra. The interval between the anterior and middle scalene muscles and the first rib (**scalene triangle**) transmits the structures coursing between the thorax, upper limb and lower neck.

- The triangle contains the **trunks of the brachial plexus** and the **subclavian artery** (Figure II-6-1).

- Note that the subclavian vein and the phrenic nerve (C 3, 4, and 5) are on the anterior surface of the anterior scalene muscle and are not in the scalene triangle.

Thoracic Outlet Syndrome

Thoracic outlet syndrome results from the compression of the **trunks of the brachial plexus and the subclavian artery** within the scalene triangle. Compression of these structures can result from tumors of the neck (Pancoast on apex of lung), a cervical rib or hypertrophy of the scalene muscles. The lower trunk of the brachial plexus (C8, T1) is usually the first to be affected. Clinical symptoms include the following:

- Numbness and pain on the medial aspect of the forearm and hand
- Weakness of the muscles supplied by the ulnar nerve in the hand (claw hand)
- Decreased blood flow into the upper limb, indicated by a weakened radial pulse
- Compression can also affect the cervical sympathetic trunk (Horner's syndrome) and the recurrent laryngeal nerves (hoarseness).

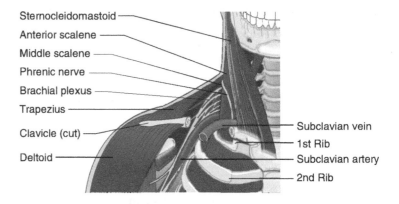

Figure II-6-1. Scalene Triangle of the Neck

CAROTID AND SUBCLAVIAN ARTERIES

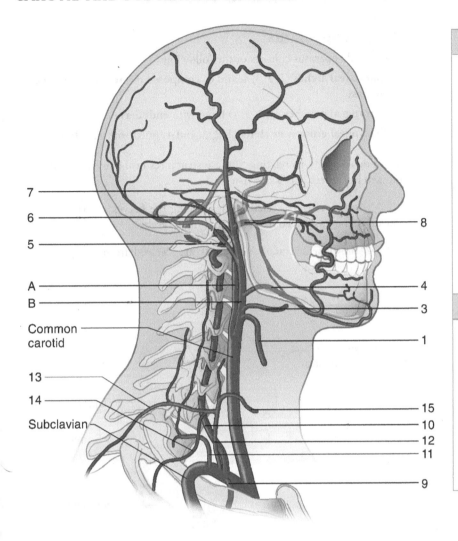

Figure II-6-2. Arteries to the Head and Neck

Common Carotid Artery
A. Internal carotid artery—opthalmic artery and brain
B. External carotid artery
1. Superior thyroid
2. Ascending pharyngeal (not shown)
3. Lingual
4. Facial
5. Occipital
6. Posterior auricular
7. Superficial temporal
8. Maxillary—deep face; middle meningeal artery

Subclavian Artery
9. Internal thoracic—cardiac bypass
10. Vertebral—brain
11. Costocervical
12. Thyrocervical
13. Transverse cervical
14. Suprascapular—collaterals to shoulder
15. Inferior thyroid

Clinical Correlate

The most significant artery of the external carotid system is the middle meningeal artery. It arises from the maxillary artery in the infratemporal fossa and enters the skull through the foramen spinosum to supply skull and dura. Lacerations of this vessel result in an epidural hematoma.

EMBRYOLOGY OF THE HEAD AND NECK

Pharyngeal Apparatus

The pharyngeal apparatus consists of the following:

- **Pharyngeal arches** (1, 2, 3, 4, and 6) composed of **mesoderm and neural crest**
- **Pharyngeal pouches** (1, 2, 3, 4) lined with **endoderm**
- **Pharyngeal grooves or clefts** (1, 2, 3, and 4) lined with **ectoderm**

The anatomic associations relating to these structures in the fetus and adult are summarized in Figures II-6-3 and II-6-4.

Table II-6-1 summarizes the relationships among the nerves, arteries, muscles, and skeletal elements derived from the pharyngeal arches.

Table II-6-2 shows which adult structures are derived from the pharyngeal pouches.

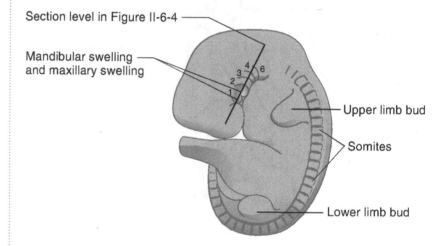

Figure II-6-3. The Fetal Pharyngeal Apparatus

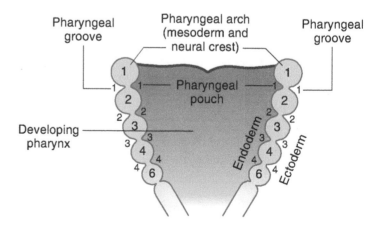

Figure II-6-4. Section through the Developing Pharynx

Pharyngeal arches

The components of the pharyngeal arches are summarized in Table II-6-1.

Table II-6-1. Components of the Pharyngeal Arches

Arch	Nerve* (Neural Ectoderm)	Artery (Aortic Arch Mesoderm)	Muscle (Mesoderm)	Skeletal/Cartilage (Neural Crest)
1	Trigeminal: mandibular nerve		Four muscles of mastication: • Masseter • Temporalis • Lateral pterygoid • Medial pterygoid Plus: • Digastric (anterior belly) • Mylohyoid • Tensor tympani • Tensor veli palatini	Maxilla Mandible Incus Malleus
2	VII		Muscles of facial expression: Plus: • Digastric (posterior belly) • Stylohyoid • Stapedius	Stapes Styloid process Lesser horn and upper body of hyoid bone
3	IX	Right and left common carotid arteries Right and left internal carotid arteries	Stylopharyngeus muscle	Greater horn and lower body of hyoid bone
4	X – Superior laryngeal nerve – Pharyngeal branches	Right subclavian artery (right arch) Arch of aorta (left arch)	Cricothyroid muscle Soft palate Pharynx (5 muscles)	Thyroid cartilage
6	X Recurrent laryngeal nerve	Right and left pulmonary arteries Ductus arteriosus (left arch)	Intrinsic muscles of larynx (except cricothyroid muscle)	All other laryngeal cartilages

*Nerves are not derived from pharyngeal arch; they grow into the arch.

Note: The **ocular muscles** (III, IV, VI) and the **tongue muscles** (XII) do not derive from pharyngeal arch mesoderm but from mesoderm of the occipital somites (somitomeres).

Pharyngeal pouches

The anatomic structures relating to the pharyngeal pouches are summarized in Figure II-6-5 and Table II-6-2.

IP: Inferior parathyroid gland
SP: Superior parathyroid gland
T: Thymus
C: C-cells of thyroid

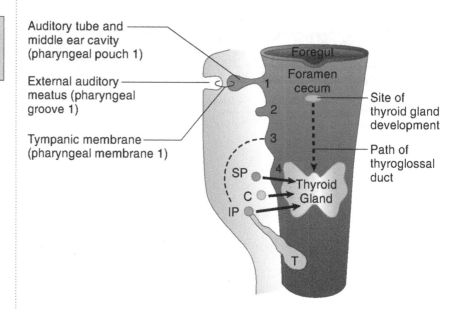

Figure II-6-5. Fetal Pharyngeal Pouches

The adult structures derived from the fetal pharyngeal pouches are summarized in Table II-6-2.

Clinical Correlate

Normally, the second, third, and fourth pharyngeal grooves are obliterated by overgrowth of the second pharyngeal arch. Failure of a cleft to be completely obliterated results in a branchial cyst or **lateral cervical cyst**.

Clinical Correlate

The **DiGeorge sequence** presents with immunologic problems and hypocalcemia, and may be combined with cardiovascular defects (persistent troncus arteriosis), abnormal ears, and micrognathia.

Table II-6-2. Adult Structures Derived From the Fetal Pharyngeal Pouches

Pouch	Adult Derivatives
1	Epithelial lining of auditory tube and middle ear cavity
2	Epithelial lining of crypts of palatine tonsil
3	Inferior parathyroid (IP) gland
	Thymus (T)
4	Superior parathyroid (SP) gland
	C-cells of thyroid

*Neural crest cells migrate to form parafollicular C-cells of the thyroid.

Pharyngeal grooves (clefts)

Pharyngeal groove 1 gives rise to the epithelial lining of **external auditory meatus.**

All other grooves are obliterated.

Thyroid Gland

The thyroid gland does not develop from a pharyngeal pouch. It develops from the **thyroid diverticulum,** which forms from the midline endoderm in the floor of the pharynx.

- The thyroid diverticulum migrates caudally to its adult anatomic position in the neck but remains connected to the foregut via the **thyroglossal duct,** which is later obliterated.
- The former site of the thyroglossal duct is indicated in the adult by the **foramen cecum** (Figures II-6-5 and II-6-6).

Tongue

The **anterior two-thirds of the tongue** is associated with **pharyngeal arches 1 and 2.** General sensation is carried by the lingual branch of the mandibular nerve (cranial nerve [CN] V). Taste sensation is carried by **chorda tympani of CN VII** (Figure II-6-6).

The **posterior one third of the tongue** is associated with **pharyngeal arch 3.** General sensation and taste are carried by **CN IX.**

Most of the muscles of the tongue are innervated by CN XII.

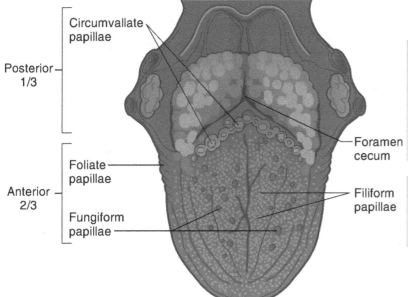

Sensory		
	General sensation	*Taste*
Post 1/3	IX	IX
Ant 2/3	V	VII
	Lingual branch of mandibular	Chorda tympani branch of VII nerve

Somatic Motor
CN XII innervates the intrinsic and extrinsic skeletal muscles of the tongue except palatoglossus muscle.

Figure II-6-6. Tongue

Development of the Face and Palate

The **face** develops from 5 primordia of mesoderm (neural crest) of the first pharyngeal arch: a single frontonasal prominence, the pair of maxillary prominences, and the pair of mandibular prominences.

- The **intermaxillary segment** forms when the 2 medial nasal prominences of the frontonasal prominences fuse together at the midline and form the **philtrum of the lip** and the **primary palate**.

- The **secondary palate** forms from palatine shelves (maxillary prominence), which fuse in the midline, posterior to the incisive foramen.

- The primary and secondary palates fuse at the **incisive foramen** to form the definitive hard palate.

Clinical Correlate

Cleft lip occurs when the maxillary prominence fails to fuse with the medial nasal prominence.

Cleft palate occurs when the palatine shelves fail to fuse with each other or the primary palate.

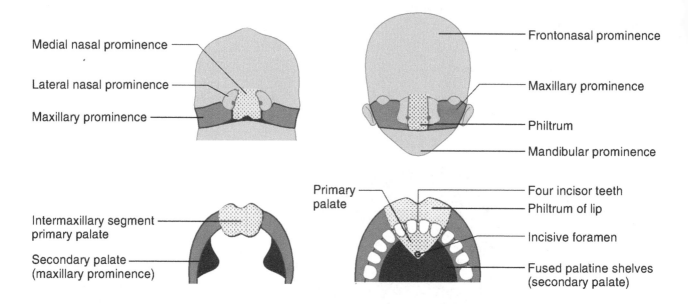

Medial nasal prominence

Lateral nasal prominence

Maxillary prominence

Frontonasal prominence

Maxillary prominence

Philtrum

Mandibular prominence

Intermaxillary segment primary palate

Secondary palate (maxillary prominence)

Primary palate

Four incisor teeth

Philtrum of lip

Incisive foramen

Fused palatine shelves (secondary palate)

Figure II-6-7. Face and Palate Development

Clinical Correlate

First arch syndrome results from abnormal formation of pharyngeal arch 1 because of faulty migration of neural crest cells, causing facial anomalies. Two well-described syndromes are Treacher Collins syndrome and Pierre Robin sequence. Both defects involve neural crest cells.

Pharyngeal fistula occurs when pouch 2 and groove 2 persist, thereby forming a fistula generally found along the anterior border of the   muscle.

Pharyngeal cyst occurs when pharyngeal grooves that are normally obliterated persist, forming a cyst usually located at the angle of the mandible.

Ectopic thyroid, parathyroid, or thymus results from abnormal migration of these glands from their embryonic position to their adult anatomic position. Ectopic thyroid tissue is found along the midline of the neck. Ectopic parathyroid or thymus tissue is generally found along the lateral aspect of the neck. May be an important issue during neck surgery.

Thyroglossal duct cyst or fistula occurs when parts of the thyroglossal duct persist, generally in the midline near the hyoid bone. The cyst may also be found at the base of the tongue (lingual cyst).

DiGeorge sequence occurs when pharyngeal pouches 3 and 4 fail to differentiate into the parathyroid glands and thymus. Neural crest cells are involved.

Clinical Correlate

Robin sequence presents with a triad of poor mandibular growth, cleft palate, and a posteriorly placed tongue.

Treacher Collins syndrome also presents with mandibular hypoplasia, zygomatic hypoplasia, down-slanted palpebral fissures, colobomas, and malformed ears.

Clinical Correlate

Cribriform plate fractures may result in dysosmia and rhinorrhea (CSF).

CRANIUM

Cranial Fossae

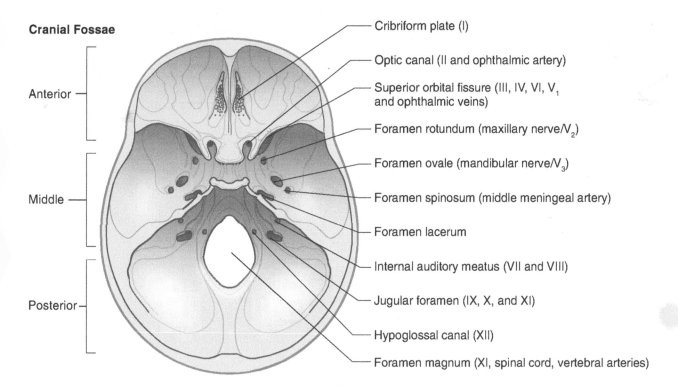

Cribriform plate (I)

Optic canal (II and ophthalmic artery)

Superior orbital fissure (III, IV, VI, V_1 and ophthalmic veins)

Foramen rotundum (maxillary nerve/V_2)

Foramen ovale (mandibular nerve/V_3)

Foramen spinosum (middle meningeal artery)

Foramen lacerum

Internal auditory meatus (VII and VIII)

Jugular foramen (IX, X, and XI)

Hypoglossal canal (XII)

Foramen magnum (XI, spinal cord, vertebral arteries)

Anterior

Middle

Posterior

Figure II-6-8. Foramina: Cranial Fossae

Clinical Correlate

Jugular foramen syndrome may be caused by a tumor pressing on CN IX, X, and XI. Patients present with hoarseness, dysphagia (CN IX and X), loss of sensation over the oropharynx and posterior third of the tongue (CN IX), and trapezius and sternocleidomastoid weakness (CN XI). The nearby CN XII may be involved producing tongue deviation to the lesioned side.

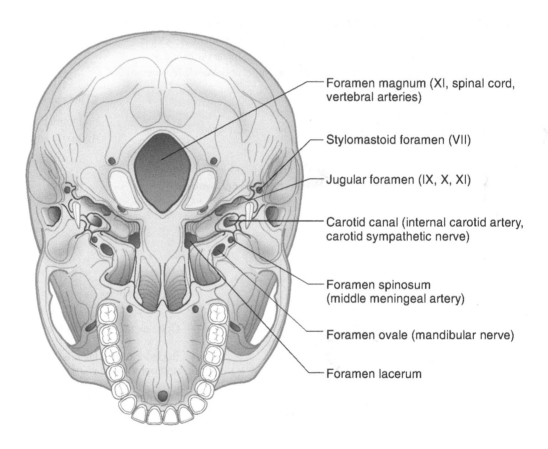

Foramen magnum (XI, spinal cord, vertebral arteries)

Stylomastoid foramen (VII)

Jugular foramen (IX, X, XI)

Carotid canal (internal carotid artery, carotid sympathetic nerve)

Foramen spinosum (middle meningeal artery)

Foramen ovale (mandibular nerve)

Foramen lacerum

Figure II-6-9. Foramina: Base of Skull

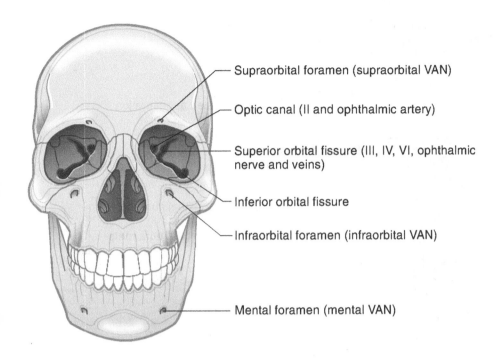

Supraorbital foramen (supraorbital VAN)

Optic canal (II and ophthalmic artery)

Superior orbital fissure (III, IV, VI, ophthalmic nerve and veins)

Inferior orbital fissure

Infraorbital foramen (infraorbital VAN)

Mental foramen (mental VAN)

Figure II-6-10. Foramina: Front of Skull

CRANIAL MENINGES AND DURAL VENOUS SINSUSES

Cranial Meninges

The brain is covered by 3 meninges that are continuous through the foramen magnum with the spinal meninges. There are several similarities and differences between spinal and cranial meninges (Figure II-6-11).

- **Pia mater** tightly invests the surfaces of the brain and cannot be dissected away, having the same relationship with the brain as spinal pia mater.

- **Dura mater** is the thickest of the 3 meninges and, unlike the spinal dura, consists of 2 layers (**periosteal and meningeal**) that are fused together during most of their course in the cranial cavity.

  - **Periosteal layer**: This outer layer lines the inner surfaces of the flat bones and serves as their periosteum. The periosteal layer can easily be peeled away from the bones.

  - **Meningeal (true dura) layer**: This is the innermost layer that is mostly fused with the periosteal dura mater throughout the cranial cavity. At certain points in the cranium, the meningeal layer separates from the periosteal layer and forms the dural venous sinuses and connective tissue foldings or duplications: **falx cerebri, diaphragma sellae and tentorium cerebelli**. These duplications separate and support different parts of the CNS.

- **Arachnoid** is the thin, delicate membrane which lines and follows the inner surface of the meningeal dura.

  - Projections of arachnoid called **arachnoid granulations** penetrate through the dura mater and extend into the superior sagittal dural venous sinus. Arachnoid granulations are where CSF returns to the systemic venous circulation.

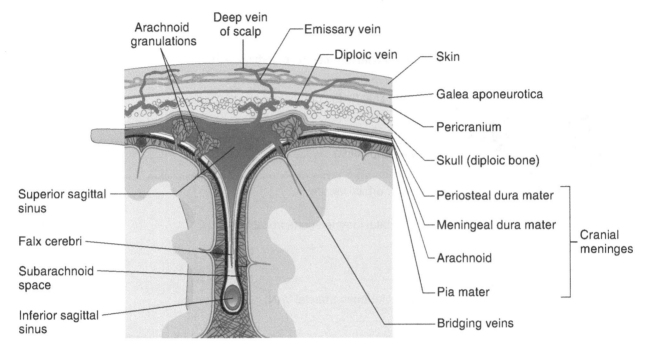

Figure II-6-11. Coronal Section of the Dural Sinuses

Spaces related to the cranial meninges

- **Epidural space** is a potential space between the periosteal dura and the bones of the skull: site of epidural hematomas (described later).
- **Subdural space** is the potential space between the meningeal dura and the arachnoid membrane: site of subdural hematomas (described later).
- **Subarachnoid space** lies between the arachnoid and pia mater containing CSF: site of subarachnoid hemorrhage (described later).

Dural Venous Sinuses

Dural venous sinuses are formed at different points in the cranial cavity where the **periosteal** and **meningeal** dural layers separate to form endothelial lined venous channels called dural venous sinuses (Figures II-6-11 and II-6-12). The sinuses provide the major venous drainage from most structures within the cranial cavity. They drain mostly into the internal jugular vein, which exits the cranial floor at the jugular foramen. Most of the dural venous sinuses are located in the 2 largest duplications of meningeal dura mater (**falx cerebri** and the **tentorium cerebelli**).

The primary tributaries that flow into the sinuses are the following:

- **Cerebral** and **cerebelli** veins that form **bridging veins** which pass across the subdural space to drain into the sinuses
- **Emissary veins** are valveless channels that course through the bones of the skull and allow dural sinuses to communicate with extracranial veins.
- **Diploic veins** drain the spongy (diploe) core of the flat bones.
- **Arachnoid granulations** are where CSF returns to the venous circulation.
- **Meningeal veins** drain the meninges.

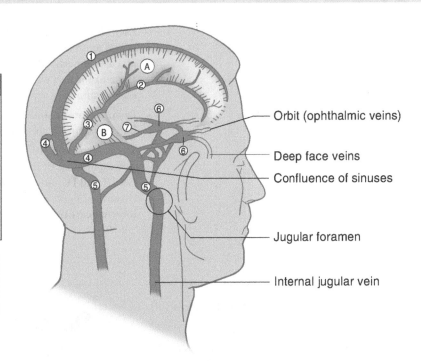

Names of the Major Dural Sinuses

1. Superior sagittal*
2. Inferior sagittal
3. Straight*
4. Transverse* (2)
5. Sigmoid (2)
6. Cavernous (2)
7. Superior petrosal (2)

* Drain into the confluence of sinuses located at the inion.

Folds (Duplications) of Dura Mater

A. Falx cerebri
B. Tentorium cerebelli

Orbit (ophthalmic veins)

Deep face veins

Confluence of sinuses

Jugular foramen

Internal jugular vein

Figure II-6-12. Dural Venous Sinuses

Major dural venous sinuses

The major dural venous sinuses are the following (Figure II-6-12):

- The **superior sagittal sinus** is located in the midsagittal plane along the superior aspect of the falx cerebri. It drains primarily into the confluence of the sinuses.

- The **inferior sagittal sinus** is located in the midsagittal plane near the inferior margin of the falx cerebri. It terminates by joining with the great cerebral vein (of Galen) to form the straight sinus at the junction of the falx cerebri and tentorium cerebelli.

- The **straight sinus** is formed by the union of the inferior sagittal sinus and the great cerebral vein. It usually terminates by draining into the confluens of sinuses (or into the transverse sinus).

- The **occipital sinus** is a small sinus found in the posterior border of the tentorium cerebelli. It drains into the confluens of sinuses.

- The **confluens of sinuses** is formed by the union of the superior sagittal, straight, and occipital sinuses posteriorly at the occipital bone. It drains laterally into the 2 transverse sinuses.

- The **transverse sinuses** are paired sinuses in the tentorium cerebelli and attached to the occipital bone that drain venous blood from the confluens of sinuses into the sigmoid sinuses.

- The **sigmoid sinuses** are paired and form a S-shaped channel in the floor of the posterior cranial fossa. The sigmoid sinus drains into the **internal jugular vein** at the **jugular foramen**.

- The paired **cavernous sinuses** are located on either side of the body of the sphenoid bone (Figure II-6-13).

– Each sinus receives blood primarily from the **orbit (ophthalmic veins)** and via emissary veins from the **deep face** (pterygoid venous plexus). Superficial veins of the maxillary face drain into the medial angle of the eye, enter the ophthalmic veins, and drain into the cavernous sinus.

– Each cavernous sinus 1 via the superior and inferior petrosal sinuses into the sigmoid sinus and internal jugular vein, respectively.

– The cavernous sinuses are the **most clinically significant** dural sinuses because of their relationship to a number of cranial nerves. **CN III** and **IV** and the **ophthalmic and maxillary** divisions of the trigeminal nerve are located in lateral wall of the sinus. **CN VI** and **internal carotid artery** are located centrally in the sinus.

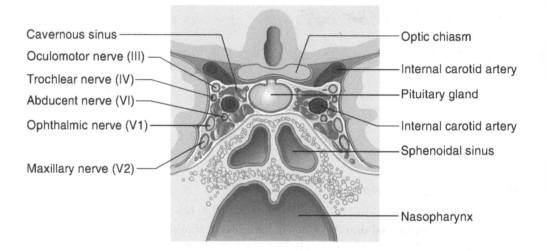

Cavernous sinus

Oculomotor nerve (III)

Trochlear nerve (IV)

Abducent nerve (VI)

Ophthalmic nerve (V1)

Maxillary nerve (V2)

Optic chiasm

Internal carotid artery

Pituitary gland

Internal carotid artery

Sphenoidal sinus

Nasopharynx

Figure II-6-13. Coronal Section Through Pituitary Gland and Cavernous Sinuses

Clinical Correlate

Cavernous Sinus Thrombosis

Infection can spread from the superficial and deep face into the cavernous sinus, producing a thrombosis that may result in swelling of sinus and damage the cranial nerves that are related to the cavernous sinus.

CN III and IV and the ophthalmic and maxillary divisions of CN V will be compressed in the lateral wall of the sinus.

CN VI and the internal carotid artery with its periarterial plexus of postganglionic sympathetic fibers will be compressed in the central part of the cavernous sinus. CN VI is typically affected first in a cavernous sinus thrombosis with the other nerves being affected later. Initially, patients have an internal strabismus (medially deviated eyeball) (CN VI lesion). Later, all eye movements are affected, along with altered sensation in the skin of the upper face and scalp.

INTRACRANIAL HEMORRHAGE

Epidural Hematoma

An **epidural hematoma** (Figure II-6-14A) results from trauma to the lateral aspect of the skull which lacerates the middle meningeal artery. Arterial hemorrhage occurs rapidly in the epidural space between the periosteal dura and the skull.

- Epidural hemorrhage forms a **lens-shaped** (biconvex) hematoma at the lateral hemisphere.
- Epidural hematoma is associated with a momentary loss of consciousness followed by a lucid (asymptomatic) period of up to 48 hours.
- Patients then develop symptoms of elevated intracranial pressure such as headache, nausea, and vomiting, combined with neurological signs such as hemiparesis.
- Herniation of the temporal lobe, coma, and death may occur rapidly if the arterial blood is not evacuated.

Subdural Hematoma

A **subdural hematoma** (Figure II-6-14B) results from head trauma that tears superficial ("bridging") cerebral veins at the point where they enter the superior sagittal sinus. A subdural hemorrhage occurs between the meningeal dura and the arachnoid.

- Subdural hemorrhage forms a **crescent-shaped** hematoma at the lateral hemisphere.
- Large subdural hematomas result in signs of elevated intracranial pressure such as headache and nausea.
- Small or chronic hematomas are often seen in elderly or chronic alcoholic patients.
- Over time, herniation of the temporal lobe, coma, and death may result if the venous blood is not evacuated.

Nolte: The Human Brain.
Copyright Mosby, an imprint of Elsevier, Inc. Used with permission.

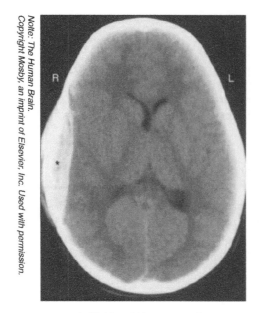

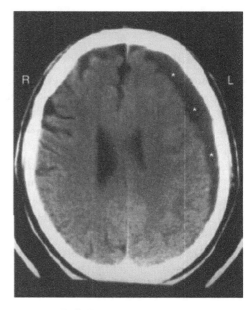

A. Epidural Hematoma* B. Subdural Hematoma*

Figure II-6-14. Intracranial Hemorrhage

Subarachnoid Hemorrhage

A **subarachnoid hemorrhage** results from a rupture of a berry aneurysm in the circle of Willis. The most common site is in the anterior part of the circle of Willis at the branch point of the anterior cerebral and anterior communicating arteries. Other common sites are in the proximal part of the middle cerebral artery or at the junction of the internal carotid and posterior communicating arteries.

- Typical presentation associated with a subarachnoid hemorrhage is the onset of a severe headache.

ORBITAL MUSCLES AND THEIR INNERVATION

In the orbit, there are 6 extraocular muscles that move the eyeball (Figure II-6-15). A seventh muscle, the levator palpebrae superioris, elevates the upper eyelid.

- Four of the 6 extraocular muscles (the superior, inferior, and medial rectus, and the inferior oblique, plus the levator palpebrae superioris) are innervated by the oculomotor nerve (CN III).

- The superior oblique muscle is the only muscle innervated by the trochlear nerve (CN IV).

- The lateral rectus is the only muscle innervated by the abducens nerve (CN VI).

- The levator palpebrae superioris is composed of skeletal muscle innervated by the oculomotor nerve (CN III) and smooth muscle (the superior tarsal muscle) innervated by sympathetic fibers.

- Sympathetic fibers reach the orbit from a plexus on the internal carotid artery of postganglionic axons that originate from cell bodies in the superior cervical ganglion.

- The orbital muscles and their actions are illustrated in Figure II-6-15.

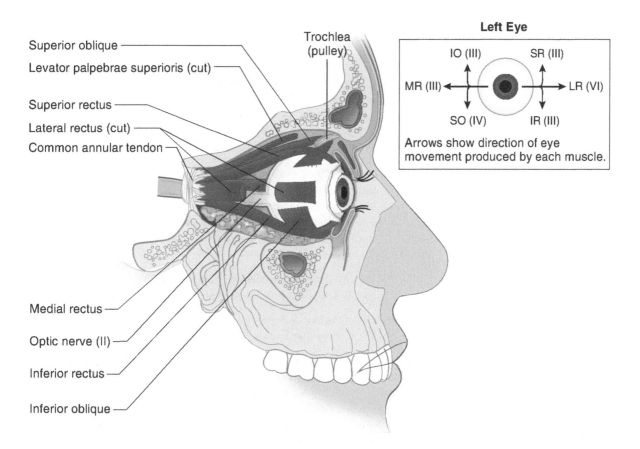

Superior oblique

Levator palpebrae superioris (cut)

Superior rectus

Lateral rectus (cut)

Common annular tendon

Trochlea (pulley)

Left Eye

IO (III)   SR (III)

MR (III) ←————→ LR (VI)

SO (IV)   IR (III)

Arrows show direction of eye movement produced by each muscle.

Medial rectus

Optic nerve (II)

Inferior rectus

Inferior oblique

Figure II-6-15. Muscles of the Eye

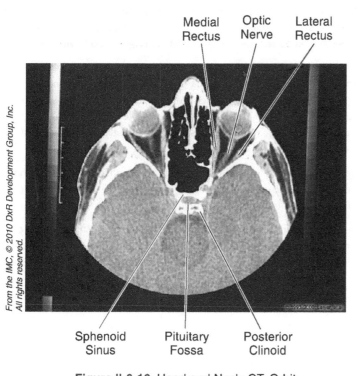

Medial Rectus   Optic Nerve   Lateral Rectus

Sphenoid Sinus   Pituitary Fossa   Posterior Clinoid

Figure II-6-16. Head and Neck: CT, Orbit

Chapter Summary

- The neck is divided by the sternocleidomastoid muscle into an anterior and posterior triangle. The **anterior triangle** contains vascular structures (carotid artery and internal jugular vein), cranial nerve (CN) X, and the respiratory (trachea and larynx) and digestive (pharynx and esophagus) visceral structures. The **posterior triangle** contains the muscles associated with the cervical vertebrae, CN XI, cervical plexus, and the origins of the brachial plexus.

- Many structures of the head and neck develop from the branchial (pharyngeal) apparatus. The apparatus consists of pharyngeal arches, pouches, and grooves. The grooves are composed of ectoderm, the pouches are composed of endoderm, and the arches are composed of mesoderm and neural crest cells. The adult derivatives of the arches and pouches are given in Tables II-6-1 and II-6-2, respectively.

- The anterior 2/3 of the tongue develops from the first pharyngeal arch, and the posterior 1/3 develops from the third pharyngeal arch.

- The muscles of the tongue derive from myoblasts that migrate into the head from the occipital somites and are innervated by CN XII.

- The face develops from 5 structures derived from the first pharyngeal arch: frontonasal prominence, a pair of maxillary prominences, and a pair of mandibular prominences. The mandibular prominences form the lower jaw, the frontonasal prominence forms the forehead, and the maxillary prominences form the cheek, lateral upper lip, and the secondary palate. The midline of the upper lip, the nasal septum, and the primary palate are formed by the medial nasal prominence. The primary and secondary palate fuse to form the definite palate.

- The floor of the cranial cavity is divided into the anterior, middle, and posterior cranial fossae. The openings in the skull provide for passage of the cranial nerves and blood vessels. These are listed in Figures II-6-8 and II-6-9.

- Venous return from the brain and other structures of the cranial vault is provided by the dural venous sinuses, which ultimately drain into the internal jugular vein at the jugular foramen. Most of these sinuses are located in the folds of the dura mater (falx cerebri and tentorium cerebelli). The major ones are the superior and inferior sagittal and the transverse, sigmoid, and cavernous sinuses.

- The cavernous sinus is significant because CN III and IV and the ophthalmic and maxillary divisions of CN V course in the lateral wall of the cavernous sinus, and the internal carotid artery and CN VI are found in the lumen.

- The orbit contains the ocular muscles, eyeball, and transmits the optic nerve and ophthalmic artery. CN VI innervates the lateral rectus muscle, CN IV innervates the superior oblique muscle, and the remaining muscles are innervated by CN III.

SECTION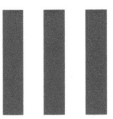

Neuroscience

Nervous System Organization and Development

1

Learning Objectives

❑ Explain information related to autonomic nervous system

❑ Use knowledge of general organization

The central nervous system consists of the brain and spinal cord, which develop from the neural tube.

The peripheral nervous system (PNS) contains cranial and spinal nerves that consist of neurons that give rise to axons, which grow out of the **neural tube**, and neurons derived from **neural crest cells**. Skeletal motor neurons and axons of preganglionic autonomic neurons are derived from the neural tube (Figures III-1-1, -2, -3, -4, -5, and -6).

Neural crest cells form sensory neurons and postganglionic autonomic neurons. The neuronal cell bodies of these neurons are found in ganglia. Therefore, all ganglia found in the PNS contain either sensory or postganglionic autonomic neurons and are derived from neural crest cells.

Chromaffin cells are neural crest cells, which migrate into the adrenal medulla to form postganglionic sympathetic neurons.

Development of the Nervous System

Neurulation

- **Neurulation** begins in the third week; both CNS and PNS derived from neuroectoderm.
- The **notochord** induces the overlying ectoderm to form the **neural plate (neuroectoderm)**.
- By end of the third week, **neural folds** grow over midline and fuse to form **neural tube**.
- During closure, **neural crest** cells also form from neuroectoderm.
- **Neural tube** 3 primary vesicles → 5 primary vesicles → brain and spinal cord
- Brain stem and spinal cord have an **alar** plate (**sensory**) and a **basal** plate (**motor**); plates are separated by the **sulcus limitans**.
- **Neural crest** → sensory and postganglionic autonomic neurons, and other non-neuronal cell types.
- **Peripheral NS (PNS):** cranial nerves (12 pairs) and spinal nerves (31 pairs)

Note

Alpha-fetoprotein (AFP) levels may also be elevated in gastroschisis and omphalocele. AFP levels are low in pregnancy of down syndrom fetus.

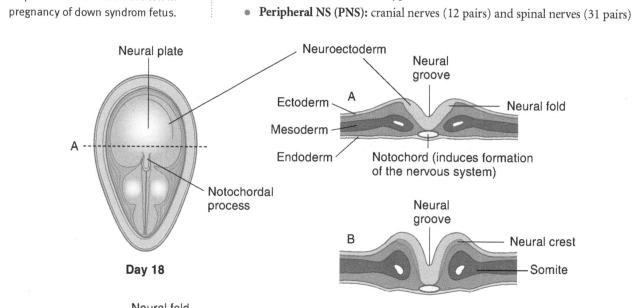

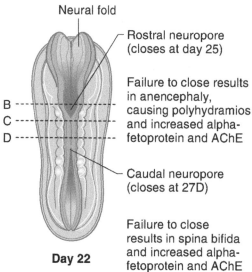

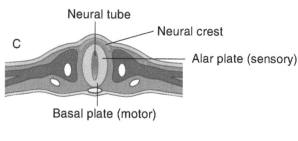

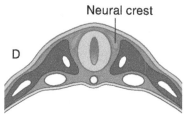

Figure III-1-1. Development of Nervous System

Central Nervous System

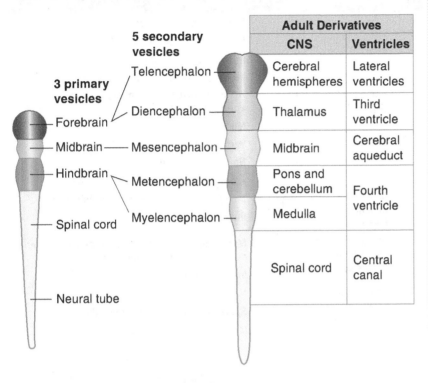

Figure III-1-2. **Adult Derivatives of Secondary Brain Vesicles**

Clinical Correlate

Axonal polyneuropathies produce distal "glove-and-stocking" weakness or sensory deficits, and are related to axonal transport failure. Diabetes mellitus patients present with sensory neuropathies.

Table III-1-1. Adult Derivatives of Secondary Brain Vesicles

	Structures	Neural Canal Remnant
Telencephalon	Cerebral hemispheres, most of basal ganglia	Lateral ventricles
Diencephalon	Thalamus, hypothalamus, subthalamus, epithalamus (pineal gland), retina and optic nerve	Third ventricle
Mesencephalon	Midbrain	Cerebral aqueduct
Metencephalon	Pons, cerebellum	Fourth ventricle
Myelencephalon	Medulla	
	Spinal cord	Central canal

Table III-1-2. Congenital Malformations of the Nervous System

Condition	Types	Description
Anencephaly	—	Failure of **anterior neuropore** to close
		Brain does not develop
		Incompatible with life
		Increased AFP during pregnancy and AChE
Spina bifida	Spina bifida occulta **(Figure A)**	Failure of **posterior neuropore** to close, or to induce bone growth around it.
		Mildest form
		Vertebrae fail to form around spinal cord
		No increase in **AFP**
		Asymptomatic; tuft of hair over defect.
	Spina bifida with meningocele **(Figure B)**	**Meninges** protrude through vertebral defect
		Increase in AFP
	Spina bifida with meningomyelocele **(Figure C)**	**Meninges** and **spinal cord** protrude through vertebral defect; seen with Arnold-Chiari Type II
		Increase in AFP
	Spina bifida with myeloschisis **(Figure D)**	Most severe
		Spinal cord can be seen **externally**
		Increase in AFP and AChE

Muscle — Skin
- Unfused laminae
- Dura and arachnoid
- Subarachnoid space
- Spinal cord
- Vertebral body

A   B   C

Condition	Types	Description
Arnold-Chiari malformation	Type I	Most common
		Mostly **asymptomatic** in children
		Downward displacement of cerebellar tonsils through foramen magnum
		Frequent association with **syringomyelia**
	Type II	More often **symptomatic**
		Downward displacement of **cerebellar vermis** and **medulla** through foramen magnum
		Compression of IV ventricle → obstructive **hydrocephaly**
		Frequent lumbar **meningomyelocele**
Dandy-Walker malformation		Failure of foramina of Luschka and Magendie to open → **dilation of IV ventricle**
		Agenesis of cerebellar vermis and splenium of the corpus callosum
Hydrocephalus		Most often caused by stenosis of cerebral aqueduct
		CSF accumulates in ventricles and subarachnoid space
		Increased head circumference
Holoprosencephaly		Incomplete separation of cerebral hemispheres
		One ventricle in telencephalon
		Seen in trisomy 13 (Patau)

Abbreviation: AFP, α-fetoprotein

Table III-1-3. Germ Layer Derivatives

Ectoderm	Mesoderm	Endoderm
Surface ectoderm	Muscle	**Forms epithelial parts of:**
Epidermis	Smooth	Tonsils
Hair	Cardiac	Thymus
Nails	Skeletal	Pharynx
Inner ear, external ear	Connective tissue	Larynx
Enamel of teeth	All serous membranes	Trachea
Lens of eye	Bone and cartilage	Bronchi
Anterior pituitary (Rathke's pouch)	Blood, lymph, cardiovascular organs	Lungs
Parotid gland	Adrenal cortex	Urinary bladder
	Gonads and internal reproductive organs	Urethra
Neuroectoderm	Spleen	Tympanic cavity
Neural tube	Kidney and ureter	Auditory tube
Central nervous system	Dura mater	GI tract
Retina and optic nerve		
Pineal gland		**Forms parenchyma of:**
Neurohypophysis		Liver
Astrocytes		Pancreas
Oligodendrocytes (CNS myelin)		Tonsils
		Thyroid gland
Neural crest		Parathyroid glands
Adrenal medulla		Glands of the GI tract
Ganglia		Submandibular gland
Sensory (unipolar)		Sublingual gland
Autonomic (postganglionic)		
Pigment cells (melanocytes)		
Schwann cells (PNS myelin)		
Meninges		
Pia and arachnoid mater		
Pharyngeal arch cartilage (First Arch Syndromes)		
Odontoblasts		
Parafollicular (C) cells		
Aorticopulmonary septum (Tetrology of Fallot)		
Endocardial cushions (Down Syndrome)		

Yolk sac derivatives:

  Primordial germ cells

  Early blood and blood vessels

Smooth msle
Cardiac
Glands

AUTONOMIC NERVOUS SYSTEM: GENERAL ORGANIZATION

The autonomic nervous system (ANS) is responsible for the motor innervation of smooth muscle, cardiac muscle, and glands of the body. The ANS is composed of 2 divisions: (*1*) sympathetic and (*2*) parasympathetic.

In both divisions there are 2 neurons in the peripheral distribution of the motor innervation.

1. Preganglionic neuron with cell body in CNS
2. Postganglionic neuron with cell body in a ganglion in the PNS

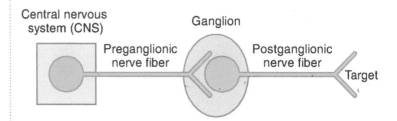

Figure III-1-3. **Autonomic Nervous System**

Peripheral Nervous System

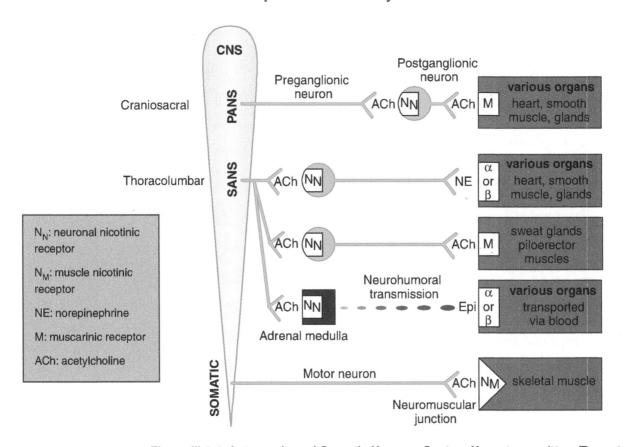

Figure III-1-4. **Autonomic and Somatic Nervous System Neurotransmitters/Receptors**

- **Somatic nervous system:** 1 neuron (from CNS → effector organ)
- **ANS:** 2 neurons (from CNS → effector organ)
  - **Preganglionic** neuron: cell body in CNS
  - **Postganglionic** neuron: cell body in ganglia in PNS
  - **Parasympathetic:** long preganglionic, short postganglionic
  - **Sympathetic:** short preganglionic, long postganglionic (except adrenal medulla)

Parasympathetic Nervous System

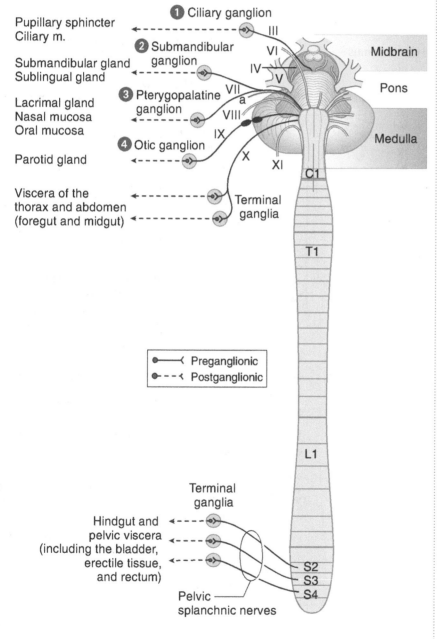

Figure III-1-5. Overview of Parasympathetic Outflow

Clinical Correlate

Hirschsprung's disease results from missing terminal ganglia in wall of rectum. Infant cannot pass meconium.

Table III-1-4. Parasympathetic = Craniosacral Outflow

Origin	Site of Synapse	Innervation
Cranial nerves III, VII, IX	Four cranial ganglia	Glands and smooth muscle of the head
Cranial nerve X	Terminal ganglia (in or near the walls of viscera)	Viscera of the neck, thorax, foregut, and midgut
Pelvic splanchnic nerves (S2, S3, S4)	Terminal ganglia (in or near the walls of viscera)	Hindgut and pelvic viscera (including bladder and erectile tissue)

Sympathetic Nervous System

Note

Horner's syndrome results in *ipsilateral* ptosis, miosis, anhydrosis

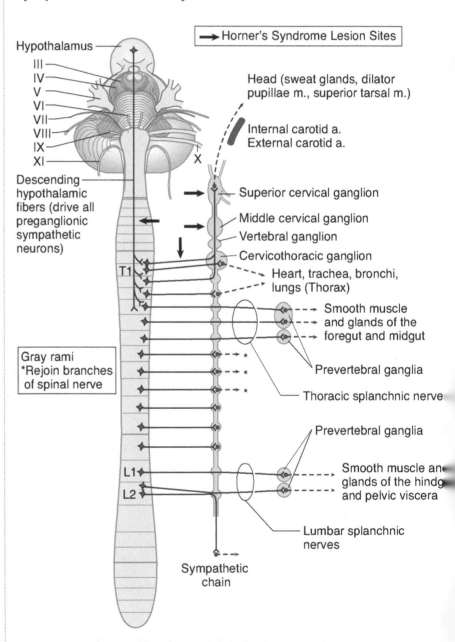

Figure III-1-6. **Overview of Sympathetic Outflow**

Table III-1-5. Sympathetic = Thoracolumbar Outflow

Origin	Site of Synapse	Innervation
Spinal cord levels T1–L2	Sympathetic chain ganglia (paravertebral ganglia)	Smooth muscle and glands of body wall and limbs; head and thoracic viscera
Thoracic splanchnic nerves T5–T12	Prevertebral ganglia (collateral; e.g., celiac, aorticorenal superior mesenteric ganglia)	Smooth muscle and glands of the foregut and midgut
Lumbar splanchnic nerves L1, L2	Prevertebral ganglia (collateral; e.g., inferior mesenteric and pelvic ganglia)	Smooth muscle and glands of the pelvic viscera and hindgut

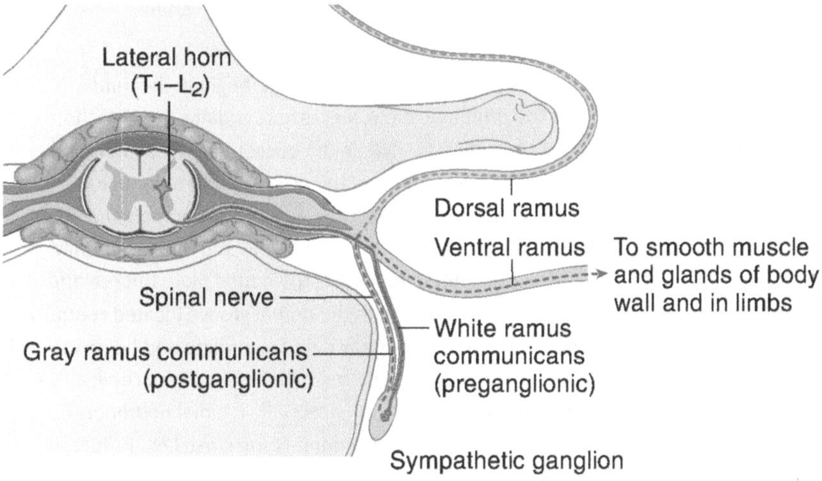

Note

Gray rami are postganglionics that rejoin spinal nerves to go to the body wall.

Figure III-1-7. Cross Section of Spinal Cord Showing Sympathetic Outflow

Chapter Summary

- The peripheral nervous system (PNS) consists of 12 pairs of cranial nerves, 31 pairs of spinal nerves with their related sensory and motor ganglia, and the peripheral part of the autonomic nervous system. The afferent and efferent neurons in the PNS convey somatic and visceral (autonomic) functions to and from the central nervous system (CNS).

Cells of Nervous System

- The basic functional cell for conducting motor and sensory functions within the nervous system is the neuron. Neurons in the CNS are myelinated by oligodendrocytes, and in the PNS neurons are myelinated by Schwann cells. Oligodendrocytes myelinate multiple axons but Schwann cells myelinate only a segment of one axon.

- The skeletal motor neurons and preganglionic motor neurons in the CNS develop from the neural tube, whereas the sensory neurons and postganglionic neurons located in sensory or autonomic ganglia, respectively, in the PNS derive from neural crest cells.

- Neurulation and the development of the nervous system begin in the third week of development. As the primitive streak regresses caudally, the notochord develops in the midaxis of the embryo between the buccopharyngeal membrane and the cloacal membrane. The appearance of the notochord then induces the ectoderm overlying the notochord to form the neural plate composed of neuroectoderm. The neural plate is wide at the cranial end and tapers caudally. By the end of the third week, the lateral margins of the neural plate thicken and become elevated to form the neural folds with the neural groove located centrally between the 2 folds. The neural folds then grow over the midline and begin to fuse to form the neural tube. Closure of the neural tube begins in the cervical region and continues cranially and caudally. The cephalic (cranial neuropore) and the caudal (caudal neuropore) ends of the neural tube close last. Failure of closure of the cranial and caudal neuropores results in anencephaly and spina bifida, respectively. Alpha-fetoprotein levels are increased with the neural tube defects. During closure of the neural tube, neural crest cells are formed from neuroectoderm at the margins of the neural folds. The neural crest cells migrate throughout the embryo and form a number of cell types.

- The neural tube forms 3 primary vesicles at its cranial end:
  - Forebrain (prosencephalon)
  - Midbrain
  - Hindbrain (rhombencephalon)

- These primary vesicles then develop into 5 secondary vesicles that form the adult derivatives of the CNS.
  - The telencephalon forms the cerebral hemispheres
  - The diencephalon forms 4 thalamic derivatives
  - The mesencephalon forms the midbrain
  - The metencephalon forms the pons and cerebellum
  - The myelencephalon forms the medulla

- The remainder of the neural tube forms the spinal cord. The lumen of the neural tube will develop into the ventricular system.

Histology of the Nervous System 2

Learning Objectives

❏ Explain information related to neurons

❏ Solve problems concerning disorders of myelination

NEURONS

Neurons are cells that are morphologically and functionally polarized so that information may pass from one end of the cell to the other.

Neurons may be classified by the form and number of their processes as bipolar, unipolar, or multipolar. The cell body of the neuron contains the nucleus and membrane-bound cytoplasmic organelles typical of a eukaryotic cell, including endoplasmic reticulum (ER), Golgi apparatus, mitochondria, and lysosomes. The nucleus and nucleolus are prominent in neurons.

The cytoplasm contains Nissl substance, clumps of rough ER with bound polysomes. The cytoplasm also contains free polysomes; free and bound polysomes in the Nissl substance are sites of protein synthesis.

Multipolar Neuron

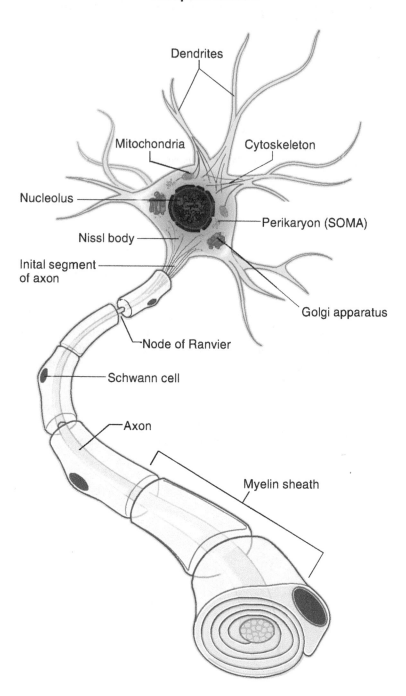

Figure III-2-1. Neuron Structure

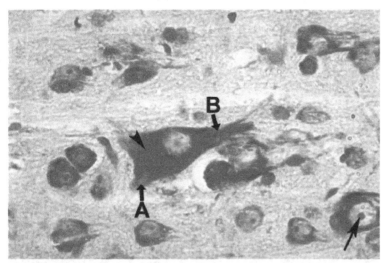

Copyright McGraw-Hill Companies. Used with permission.

Figure III-2-2. Neural Tissue with Nissl stain that stains rough ER in cell body (arrowhead) and proximal parts of dendrites (B)

The axon (A) lacks Nissl substance. The nucleus of an adjacent neuron has a prominent nucleolus (arrow).

Clinical Correlate

CNS Disease and Cytoplasmic Inclusions in Neurons

Lewy bodies are cytoplasmic inclusions of degenerating neurons of the substantia nigra, pars compacta, evident in patients with Parkinson's disease and in cortical and brain-stem neurons in patients with certain forms of dementia.

Negri bodies are eosinophilic cytoplasmic inclusions seen in degenerating neurons in the hippocampus and cerebellar cortex in patients with rabies.

Cytoskeleton

The **cytoskeleton of the neuron** consists of microfilaments, neurofilaments, and microtubules.

Neurofilaments provide structural support for the neuron and are most numerous in the axon and the proximal parts of dendrites.

Microfilaments form a matrix near the periphery of the neuron. A microfilament matrix is prominent in growth cones of neuronal processes and functions to aid in the motility of growth cones during development. A microfilament matrix is prominent in dendrites and forms structural specializations at synaptic membranes. **Microtubules** are found in all parts of the neuron, and are the cytoplasmic organelles used in axonal transport.

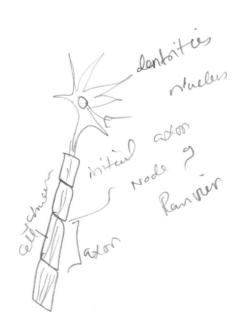

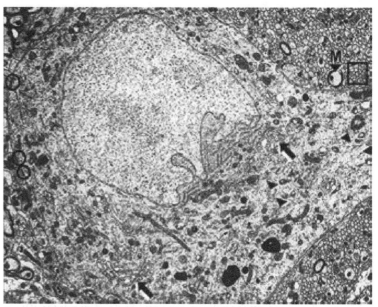

Figure III-2-3. EM of Neuropil including the Cell Body of a Neuron with Rough ER (arrowheads) and Golgi (arrows)

Surrounding neuropil has myelinated axons(M) and unmyelinated bare axons (box).

Clinical Correlate

Microtubules and Neuronal Degenerative Diseases

In degenerative neuronal diseases of the CNS, a **tau protein** becomes excessively phosphorylated, which prevents crosslinking of microtubules. The affected microtubules form helical filaments and neurofibrillary tangles and senile plaques in the cell body and dendrites of neurons. **Neurofibrillary tangles** are prominent features of degenerating neurons in Alzheimer's disease, amyotrophic lateral sclerosis, and Down syndrome patients.

Dendrites taper from the cell body and provide the major surface for synaptic contacts with axons of other neurons. **Dendrites may contain spines**, which are small cytoplasmic extensions that dramatically increase the surface area of dendrites. Dendrites may be highly branched; the branching pattern of dendrites may be used to define a particular neuronal cell type.

The **axon has a uniform diameter and may branch at right angles into collaterals** along the length of the axon, in particular near its distal end. The proximal part of the axon is usually marked by an **axon hillock**, a tapered extension of the cell body that lacks Nissl substance.

The initial segment is adjacent to the axon hillock. The membrane of the initial segment contains numerous voltage-sensitive sodium ion channels. The initial segment is the "trigger zone" of an axon where conduction of electrical activity as an action potential is initiated.

If the axon is myelinated, the myelin sheath begins at the initial segment. The cytoplasm of the entire axon lacks free polysomes, Nissl substance, and Golgi apparatus but contains mitochondria and smooth ER.

Anterograde axonal transport moves proteins and membranes that are synthesized in the cell body through the axon to the synaptic terminal. In **fast anterograde transport**, there is a rapid (100–400 mm/day) movement of materials from the cell body to the axon terminal.

Fast anterograde transport is dependent on **kinesin**, which acts as the motor molecule.

Fast anterograde transport delivers precursors of peptide neurotransmitters to synaptic terminals. In **slow anterograde transport**, there is a slow (1–2 mm/day) anterograde movement of soluble cytoplasmic components. Cytoskeletal proteins, enzymes, and precursors of small molecule neurotransmitters are transported to synaptic terminals by slow anterograde transport. Slow transport is not dependent on microtubules or ATPase motor molecules.

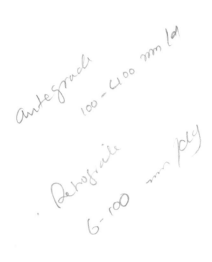

Clinical Correlate

Neuropathies and Axonal Transport

- Disruption of fast anterograde transport may result in an axonal polyneuropathy and may be caused by anoxia, which affects mitochondrial oxidative phosphorylation; or by anticancer agents, such as colchicine and vinblastine, which depolymerize microtubules.

- In patients with diabetes, hyperglycemia results in an alteration of proteins that form microtubules, which may disrupt axonal transport. Patients may develop axonal polyneuropathies in long axons in nerves that produces a "glove-and-stocking" pattern of altered sensation and pain in the feet and then in the hands.

Retrograde axonal transport returns intracellular material from the synaptic terminal to the cell body to be recycled or digested by lysosomes.

Retrograde transport uses microtubules and is slower than anterograde transport (60–100 mm/day). It is dependent on dynein, an ATPase, which acts as the retrograde motor molecule. Retrograde transport also permits communication between the synaptic terminal and the cell body by transporting trophic factors emanating from the postsynaptic target or in the extracellular space.

Glial and Supporting Cells in the CNS and PNS

The supporting, or glial, cells of the CNS are small cells, which differ from neurons. Supporting cells have only one kind of process and do not form chemical synapses. Unlike neurons, supporting cells readily divide and proliferate; gliomas are the most common type of primary tumor of the CNS.

Astrocytes are the most numerous glial cells in the CNS and have large numbers of radiating processes. They provide the structural support or scaffolding for the CNS and contain large bundles of intermediate filaments that consist of **glial fibrillary acidic protein** (GFAP). Astrocytes have uptake systems that

Clinical Correlate

Retrograde Axonal Transport and Neurological Disorders

The polio, herpes, and rabies viruses and tetanus toxins are taken up and retrogradely transported by axons that innervate skeletal muscle.

Herpes is taken up and retrogradely transported in sensory fibers and remains dormant in sensory ganglia.

remove the neurotransmitter glutamate and K^+ ions from the extracellular space. Astrocytes have foot processes that contribute to the blood–brain barrier by forming a glial-limiting membrane. Astrocytes hypertrophy and proliferate after an injury to the CNS; they fill up the extracellular space left by degenerating neurons by forming an astroglial scar. **Radial glia** are precursors of astrocytes that guide neuroblast migration during CNS development.

Microglia cells are the smallest glial cells in the CNS. Unlike the rest of the CNS neurons and glia, which are derived from neuroectoderm, microglia are derived from bone marrow monocytes and enter the CNS after birth. Microglia provide a link between cells of the CNS and the immune system. Microglia proliferate and migrate to the site of a CNS injury and phagocytose neuronal debris after injury. Pericytes are microglia that contribute to the blood–brain barrier.

Microglia determine the chances of survival of a CNS tissue graft and are the cells in the CNS that are targeted by the HIV-1 virus in patients with AIDS. The affected microglia may produce cytokines that are toxic to neurons.

CNS microglia that become phagocytic in response to neuronal tissue damage may secrete toxic free radicals. Accumulation of free radicals, such as superoxide, may lead to disruption of the calcium homeostasis of neurons.

Oligodendrocytes form myelin for axons in the CNS. Each of the processes of the oligodendrocyte can myelinate individual segments of many axons. Unmyelinated axons in the CNS are not ensheathed by oligodendrocyte cytoplasm.

Schwann cells are the supporting cells of the peripheral nervous system (PNS), and are derived from neural crest cells. Schwann cells form the myelin for axons and processes in the PNS. Each Schwann cell forms myelin for only a single internodal segment of a single axon. Unmyelinated axons in the PNS are enveloped by the cytoplasmic processes of a Schwann cell. Schwann cells act as phagocytes and remove neuronal debris in the PNS after injury. A **node of Ranvier** is the region between adjacent myelinated segments of axons in the CNS and the PNS.

In all myelinated axons, nodes of Ranvier are sites that permit action potentials to jump from node to node (saltatory conduction). Saltatory conduction dramatically increases the conduction velocity of impulses in myelinated axons.

DISORDERS OF MYELINATION

Demyelinating diseases are acquired conditions involving selective damage to myelin. Other diseases (e.g., infectious, metabolic, inherited) can also affect myelin and are generally called leukodystrophies.

Table III-2-1. Conditions of Impaired Myelination

Disease	Symptoms	Notes
Multiple sclerosis (MS)	Symptoms separated in space and time	Occurs twice as often in women
	Vision loss (optic neuritis)	Onset often in third or fourth decade
	Internuclear ophthalmoplegia (MLF)	Higher prevalence in temperate zones
	Motor and sensory deficits	Relapsing–remitting course is most common
	Vertigo	Well-circumscribed demyelinated plaques often in periventricular areas
	Neuropsychiatric	Chronic inflammation; axons initially preserved
		Increased IgG (oligoclonal bands) in CSF
		Treatment: high-dose steroids, interferon-beta, glatiramer (Copaxone®)
Metachromatic leukodystrophy (MLD)	Four types; motor and cognitive issues with seizures	Arylsulfatase A deficiency in lysosomes affects both CNS and PNS myelin
Progressive multifocal leukoencephalopathy (PML)	Cortical myelin commonly affected; causes limb weakness, speech problems	Caused by JC virus
		Affects immunocompromised, especially AIDS
		Demyelination, astrogliosis, lymphohistiocytosis
Central pontine myelin-olysis (CPM)	Pseudobulbar palsy	Focal demyelination of central area of basis pontis (affects corticospinal, corticobulbar tracts)
	Spastic quadriparesis	Seen in severely malnourished, alcoholics, liver disease
	Mental changes	
	May produce the "locked-in" syndrome	Probably caused by overly aggressive correction of hyponatremia
	Often fatal	
Guillain-Barré syndrome	Acute symmetric ascending inflammatory neuropathy of PNS myelin	Two-thirds of patients have history of respiratory or GI illness 1–3 weeks prior to onset
	Weakness begins in lower limbs and ascends; respiratory failure can occur in severe cases	Elevated CSF protein with normal cell count (albuminocytologic dissociation)
	Autonomic dysfunction may be prominent	
	Cranial nerve involvement is common	
	Sensory loss, pain, and paresthesias rarely occur	
	Reflexes invariably decreased or absent	

Abbreviations: CJD, Jacob-Creutzfeldt; MLF, medial longitudinal fasciculus

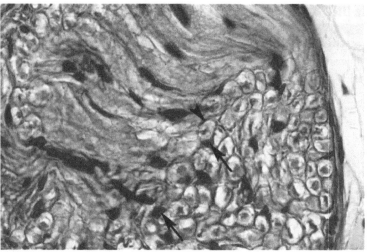

Figure III-2-4. Section of a Peripheral Nerve

Endoneurial border of an individual axon (arrowhead)
and two Schwann cell nuclei (arrows) are shown.

Myelin

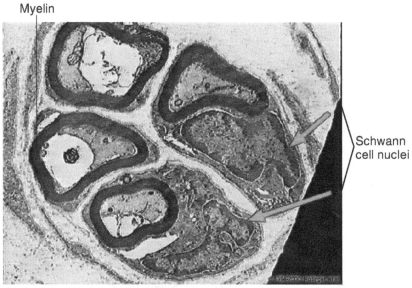

Schwann
cell nuclei

Figure III-2-5. Axons Cut in Cross-Section

Ependymal cells line the ventricles in the adult brain. Some ependymal cells differentiate into choroid epithelial cells, forming part of the choroid plexus, which produces cerebrospinal fluid (CSF). Ependymal cells are ciliated; ciliary action helps circulate CSF.

Tanycytes are specialized ependymal cells that have basal cytoplasmic processes in contact with blood vessels; these processes may transport substances between a blood vessel and a ventricle.

Blood–Brain Barrier

- The blood–brain barrier restricts access of micro-organisms, proteins, cells, and drugs to the nervous system.
- The blood–brain barrier consists of capillary endothelial cells, an underlying basal lamina, astrocytes, and pericytes.
- Cerebral capillary endothelial cells and their intercellular tight junctions are the most important elements of the blood–brain barrier.
- Astrocytes and pericytes are found at the blood–brain barrier outside the basal lamina. Astrocytes have processes with "end feet" that cover more than 95% of the basal lamina adjacent to the capillary endothelial cells.

Substances cross the blood–brain barrier into the CNS by diffusion, by selective transport, and via ion channels. Oxygen and carbon dioxide are lipid-soluble gases that readily diffuse across the blood–brain barrier. Glucose, amino acids, and vitamins K and D are selectively transported across the blood–brain barrier. Sodium and potassium ions move across the blood–brain barrier through ion channels.

Clinical Correlate

Drugs of Addiction and the Blood–Brain Barrier

Heroin, ethanol, and nicotine are lipid-soluble compounds that readily diffuse across the blood–brain barrier.

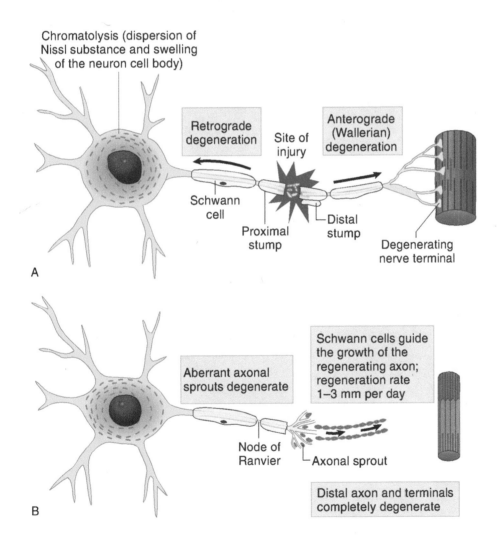

Figure III-2-6. Neuron Undergoing Axotomy, Chromatolysis, and Regeneration in the PNS

Response of Axons to Destructive Lesions (Severing an Axon or Axotomy) or Irritative Lesions (Compression of an Axon)

Anterograde or Wallerian degeneration distal to the cut occurs when an axon is severed in either the CNS or PNS. The closer the destructive lesion is to the neuronal cell body, the more likely the neuron is to die. In the PNS, anterograde degeneration of axons is rapid and complete after several weeks. In the PNS, the endoneurial Schwann cell sheath that envelops a degenerating axon does not degenerate and provides a scaffold for regeneration and remyelination of the axon.

Neurons with severed axons in the PNS are capable of complete axonal regeneration. Successful sprouts from the cut axon grow into and through endoneurial sheaths and are guided by Schwann cells back to their targets. Regeneration proceeds at the rate of 1–2 mm/day, which corresponds to the rate of slow anterograde transport.

Half of brain and spinal cord tumors are metastatic.

Clinical Correlate

Schwannomas typically affect VIII nerve fibers seen in neurofibromatosis type 2.

pseudo palisading necrosis

Table III-2-2. Primary Tumors

Tumor	Features	Pathology
Glioblastoma multiforme (grade IV astrocytoma)	• **Most common primary brain tumor** • **Highly malignant** • Usually lethal in 8–12 months	• Can cross the midline via the corpus callosum ("**butterfly glioma**") • Areas of necrosis surrounded by rows of neoplastic cells (**pseudopalisading necrosis**)
Astrocytoma (pilocytic)	• Benign tumor of children and young adults • Usually in **posterior fossa in children**	• **Rosenthal fibers** • Immunostaining with **GFAP**
Oligodendroglioma	• Slow growing • Long survival (average 5–10 years)	• **"Fried-egg" appearance**—perinuclear halo
Ependymoma	• Ependymal origin • Can arise in IV ventricle and lead to **hydrocephalus**	Rosettes and pseudorosettes
Medulloblastoma	• Highly malignant cerebellar tumor • A type of primitive neuroectodermal tumor (PNET)	Blue, small, round cells with pseudorosettes
Meningioma	• Second most common primary brain tumor • Dural convexities; parasagittal region	• Attaches to the dura, compresses underlying brain without invasion • Microscopic—**psammoma bodies**
Schwannoma	• Third most common primary brain tumor • Most frequent location: **CN VIII at cerebellopontine angle** • **Hearing loss, tinnitus, CN V + VII signs** • Good prognosis after surgical resection	• Antoni A (hypercellular) and B (hypocellular) areas • **Bilateral acoustic schwannomas—pathognomonic for neurofibromatosis type 2**
Retinoblastoma	• Sporadic—unilateral • **Familial—bilateral; associated with osteosarcoma**	Small, round, blue cells; may have rosettes
Craniopharyngioma	• Derived from oral epithelium (remnants of **Rathke pouch**) • Usually children and young adults • Often calcified • Symptoms due to encroachment on pituitary stalk or **Oral cavity** • Benign but may recur	Histology resembles **adamantinoma** (most common tumor of tooth)

Abbreviation: GFAP, glial fibrillary acidic protein

Chapter Summary

- **Neurons** are composed of a cell body, dendrites, and an axon. They contain pigments such as melanin and lipofuscin.

- The **cell body** (soma or perikaryon) contains a nucleus, other cellular components, and rough endoplasmic reticulum (ER). Microtubules and neurofilaments form the cytoskeleton. They are important for axonal transport.

- **Dendrites** receive and transmit information to the cell body.

- **Axons** arise from the perikaryon or proximal dendrite. They contain microtubules and neurofilaments. Rapid axonal transport utilizes microtubules. Kinesins promote anterograde transport, whereas dynein promotes retrograde transport.

- **Myelin** is the covering of axons and is composed of phospholipids and cholesterol. Axons may be myelinated or nonmyelinated. Schwann cells myelinate a single peripheral nervous system (PNS) axon.

- **Neurons** may also associate with several axons (unmyelinated) without forming myelin. Oligodendrocytes form myelin in the central nervous system (CNS). One oligodendrocyte myelinates many axons.

- The **node of Ranvier** is a collar of naked axon between a proximal and distal bundle of myelin that has myelinated the axon. Its purpose is to allow rapid signal transport by rapidly moving from one node to the next. This process is called saltatory conduction.

Ventricular System 3

Learning Objectives

❏ Demonstrate understanding of ventricular system and venous drainage

❏ Explain information related to CSF distribution, secretion, and circulation

The brain and spinal cord float within a protective bath of cerebrospinal fluid (CSF), which is produced continuously by the choroid plexus within the ventricles of the brain.

Each part of the CNS contains a component of the ventricular system. There are 4 interconnected ventricles in the brain: 2 lateral ventricles, a third ventricle, and a fourth ventricle. A lateral ventricle is located deep within each cerebral hemisphere. Each lateral ventricle communicates with the third ventricle via an interventricular foramen (foramen of Monro). The third ventricle is found in the midline within the diencephalon and communicates with the fourth ventricle via the cerebral aqueduct (of Sylvius), which passes through the midbrain. The fourth ventricle is located between the dorsal surfaces of the pons and upper medulla and the ventral surface of the cerebellum. The fourth ventricle is continuous with the central canal of the lower medulla and spinal cord (Figure III-3-1).

VENTRICULAR SYSTEM AND VENOUS DRAINAGE

The brain and spinal cord float within a protective bath of cerebrospinal fluid (CSF), which is produced by the lining of the ventricles, the choroid plexus. CSF circulation begins in the ventricles and then enters the subarachnoid space to surround the brain and spinal cord.

In A Nutshell

Choroid plexus secretes CSF into all ventricles. Arachnoid granulations are sites of CSF resorption.

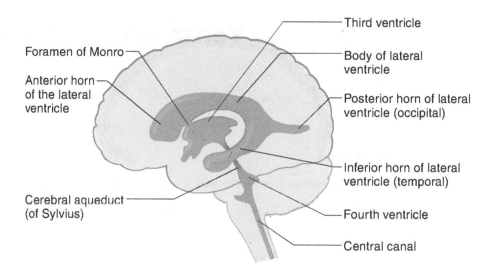

Foramen of Monro

Anterior horn
of the lateral
ventricle

Cerebral aqueduct
(of Sylvius)

Third ventricle

Body of lateral
ventricle

Posterior horn of lateral
ventricle (occipital)

Inferior horn of lateral
ventricle (temporal)

Fourth ventricle

Central canal

Figure III-3-1. Ventricles and CSF Circulation

Note

A total of 400–500 cc of CSF is
produced per day; ventricles and
subarachnoid space contain 90–150 cc,
so all of CSF is turned over 2–3 times
per day.

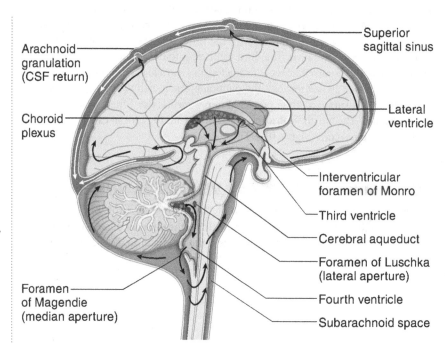

Arachnoid
granulation
(CSF return)

Choroid
plexus

Foramen
of Magendie
(median aperture)

Superior
sagittal sinus

Lateral
ventricle

Interventricular
foramen of Monro

Third ventricle

Cerebral aqueduct

Foramen of Luschka
(lateral aperture)

Fourth ventricle

Subarachnoid space

Figure III-3-2. Sagittal Section of the Brain

interventricular foramen of Monro   cerebral aqueduct
Lateral ventricles $\overset{\lor}{\to}$ third ventricle $\overset{\lor}{\to}$ fourth ventricle → subarachnoid space
(via foramina of Luschka and foramen of Magendie)

CSF Production and Barriers

Choroid plexus—contains **choroid epithelial cells** and is in the lateral, third, and fourth ventricles. **Secretes CSF.** Tight junctions form **blood-CSF barrier.**

Blood-brain barrier—formed by capillary endothelium with tight junctions; astrocyte foot processes contribute.

Once CSF is in the subarachnoid space, it goes up over convexity of the brain and enters the venous circulation by passing through **arachnoid granulations** into **dural venous sinuses.**

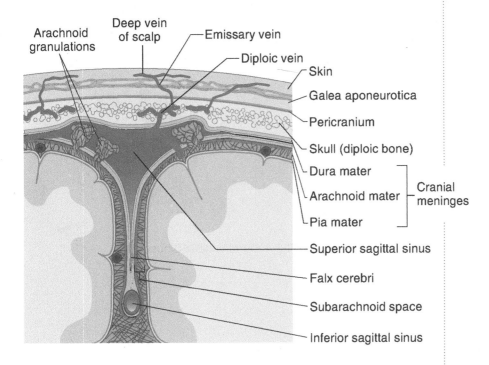

Figure III-3-3. Coronal Section of the Dural Sinuses

Sinuses

Superior sagittal sinus (in superior margin of falx cerebri)—drains into 2 **transverse sinuses.** Each of these drains blood from the **confluence of sinuses** into **sigmoid sinuses.** Each sigmoid sinus exits the skull (via **jugular foramen**) as the **internal jugular veins.**

Inferior sagittal sinus (in inferior margin of falx cerebri)— terminates by joining with the great cerebral vein of Galen to form the **straight sinus** at the falx cerebri and tentorium cerebelli junction. This drains into the confluence of sinuses.

Cavernous sinus—a plexus of veins on either side of the **sella turcica.** Surrounds internal carotid artery and cranial nerves III, IV, V, and VI. It drains into the transverse sinus (via the **superior petrosal sinus**) and the internal jugular vein (via the **inferior petrosal sinus**).

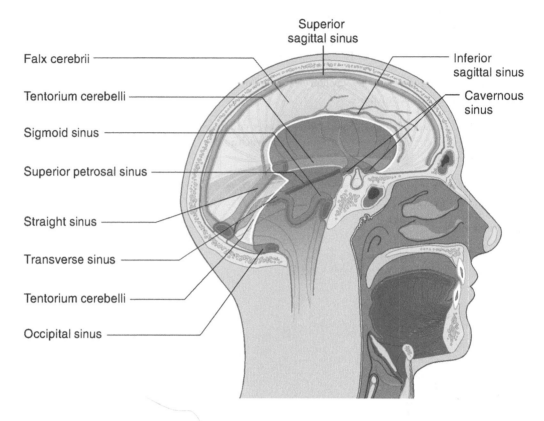

Figure III-3-4. Dural Venous Sinuses

Hydrocephalus

Excess volume or pressure of CSF, leading to dilated ventricles

Table III-3-1. Types and Features of Hydrocephalus

Type of Hydrocephalus	Description
Noncommunicating	**Obstruction of flow within ventricles**; most commonly occurs at narrow points, e.g., foramen of Monro, cerebral aqueduct and/or openings of fourth ventricle
Communicating	**Impaired CSF reabsorption** in arachnoid granulations or obstruction of flow in subarachnoid space
Normal pressure (chronic)	CSF is not absorbed by arachnoid villi (a form of communicating hydrocephalus). CSF pressure is usually normal. Ventricles chronically dilated. Produces **triad** of **dementia, apraxic (magnetic) gait,** and **urinary incontinence.** Peritoneal shunt.
Ex vacuo	Descriptive term referring to excess CSF in regions where brain tissue is lost due to atrophy, stroke, surgery, trauma, etc. Results in dilated ventricles but normal CSF pressure.

CSF DISTRIBUTION, SECRETION, AND CIRCULATION

CSF fills the subarachnoid space and the ventricles of the brain. The average adult has 90 to 150 mL of total CSF, although 400 to 500 mL is produced daily. Only 25 mL of CSF is found in the ventricles themselves.

Approximately 70% of the CSF is secreted by the choroid plexus, which consists of glomerular tufts of capillaries covered by ependymal cells that project into the ventricles (the remaining 30% represents metabolic water production). The choroid plexus is located in parts of each lateral ventricle, the third ventricle, and the fourth ventricle.

CSF from the lateral ventricles passes through the interventricular foramina of Monro into the third ventricle. From there, CSF flows through the aqueduct of Sylvius into the fourth ventricle. The only sites where CSF can leave the ventricles and enter the subarachnoid space outside the CNS are through 3 openings in the fourth ventricle, 2 lateral foramina of Luschka and the median foramen of Magendie.

Within the subarachnoid space, CSF also flows up over the convexity of the brain and around the spinal cord. Almost all CSF returns to the venous system by draining through arachnoid granulations into the superior sagittal dural venous sinus.

Normal CSF is a **clear** fluid, isotonic with serum (290–295 mOsm/L).

The pH of CSF is 7.33 (arterial blood pH, 7.40; venous blood pH, 7.36).

Sodium ion (Na^+) concentration is equal in serum and CSF ($\approx$138 mEq/L).

CSF has a higher concentration of chloride (Cl^-) and magnesium (Mg^{2+}) ions than does serum.

CSF has a lower concentration of potassium (K^+), calcium (Ca^{2+}), and bicarbonate (HCO_3^-) ions, as well as glucose, than does serum.

The Blood–CSF Barrier

The blood–CSF barrier is a mechanism that protects the chemical integrity of the brain. Tight junctions located along the epithelial cells of the choroid plexus form the blood–CSF barrier. Transport systems are similar but not identical to the those of blood–brain barrier. The ability of a substance (drug) to enter the CSF does not guarantee it will gain access to the brain.

Chapter Summary

- The ventricular system is continuous throughout each part of the central nervous system (CNS) and contains cerebrospinal fluid (CSF), which provides a protective bath for the brain and spinal cord. The system consists of 2 lateral ventricles in the cerebral hemispheres, a third ventricle in the midbrain, and a fourth ventricle in the pons and medulla. CSF is produced in the choroid plexuses of the lateral, third, and fourth ventricles. CSF leaves the fourth ventricle through the foramen of Magendie and the foramina of Luschka to enter the subarachnoid space. From the subarachnoid space, CSF returns to the venous system by passing through arachnoid granulations into the superior sagittal dural venous sinus.

- Hydrocephalus results from excess volume and pressure of CSF, producing ventricular dilatation. Noncommunicating hydrocephalus is caused by obstruction to CSF flow inside the ventricular system, and communicating hydrocephalus is caused by oversecretion or reduced absorption of CSF.

The Spinal Cord 4

Learning Objectives

❑ Solve problems concerning general features

❑ Interpret scenarios on neural systems

GENERAL FEATURES

The spinal cord is housed in the vertebral canal. It is continuous with the medulla below the pyramidal decussation and terminates as the conus medullaris at the second lumbar vertebra of the adult. The roots of 31 pairs of spinal nerves arise segmentally from the spinal cord.

There are **8 cervical pairs** of spinal nerves (C1 through C8). The cervical enlargement (C5 through T1) gives rise to the rootlets that form the brachial plexus, which innervates the upper limbs.

There are **12 thoracic pairs** of spinal nerves (T1 through T12). Spinal nerves emanating from thoracic levels innervate most of the trunk.

There are **5 lumbar pairs** of spinal nerves (L1 through L5). The lumbar enlargement (L1 through S2) gives rise to rootlets that form the lumbar and sacral plexuses, which innervate the lower limbs.

There are **5 sacral pairs** of spinal nerves (S1 through S5). Spinal nerves at the sacral level innervate part of the lower limbs and the pelvis.

There is **one coccygeal pair** of spinal nerves. The cauda equina consists of the dorsal and ventral roots of the lumbar, sacral, and coccygeal spinal nerves.

Inside the spinal cord, gray matter is centrally located and shaped like a butterfly. It contains neuronal cell bodies, their dendrites, and the proximal parts of axons. White matter surrounds the gray matter on all sides. White matter contains bundles of functionally similar axons called tracts or fasciculi, which ascend or descend in the spinal cord (Figures III-4-1 and III-4-2).

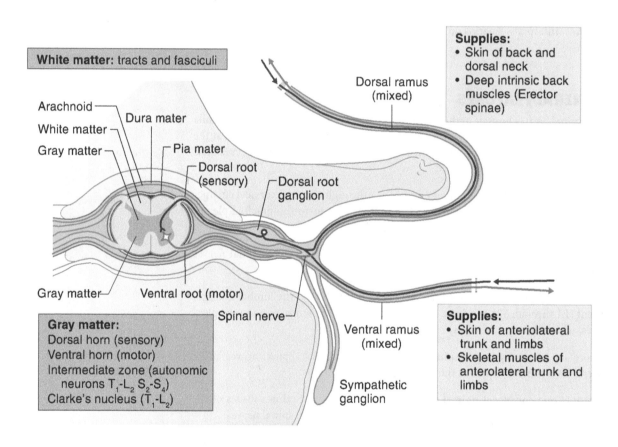

Figure III-4-1. Cross Section of Spinal Cord and Parts of Spinal Nerve

Table III-4-1. General Spinal Cord Features

Conus medullaris	Caudal end of the spinal cord (S3–S5). In adult, ends at the L2 vertebra
Cauda equina	Nerve roots of the lumbar, sacral, and coccygeal spinal nerves
Filum terminale	Slender pial extension that tethers the spinal cord to the bottom of the vertebral column
Doral root ganglia	Cell bodies of primary sensory neurons
Dorsal and ventral roots	Each segment has a pair
Dorsal horn	**Sensory neurons**
Ventral horn	**Motor neurons**
Spinal nerve	Formed from dorsal and ventral roots (mixed nerve)
Cervical enlargement	(C5–T1) → branchial plexus → upper limbs
Lumbar enlargement	(L2–S3) → lumbar and sacral plexuses → lower limbs

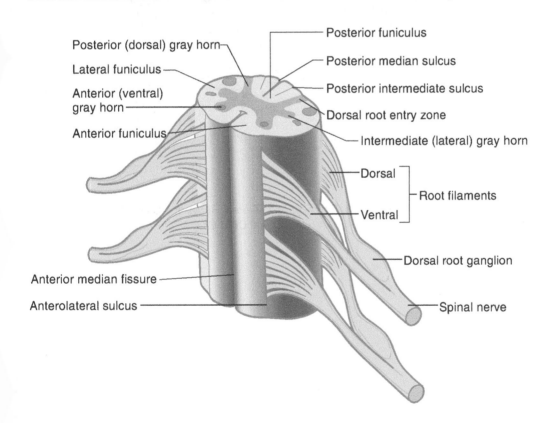

Figure III-4-2. General Spinal Cord Features

Dorsal Horn

The dorsal horn is dominated by neurons that respond to sensory stimulation. All incoming sensory fibers in spinal nerves enter the dorsolateral part of the cord adjacent to the dorsal horn in a dorsal root. Neurons in the dorsal horn project to higher levels of the CNS to carry sensations to the brain stem, cerebral cortex, or cerebellum. Other dorsal horn neurons participate in reflexes.

Dorsal horn: rexed laminae I–VI

Ventral horn: rexed laminae VIII–IX

Intermediate zone: lamina VII

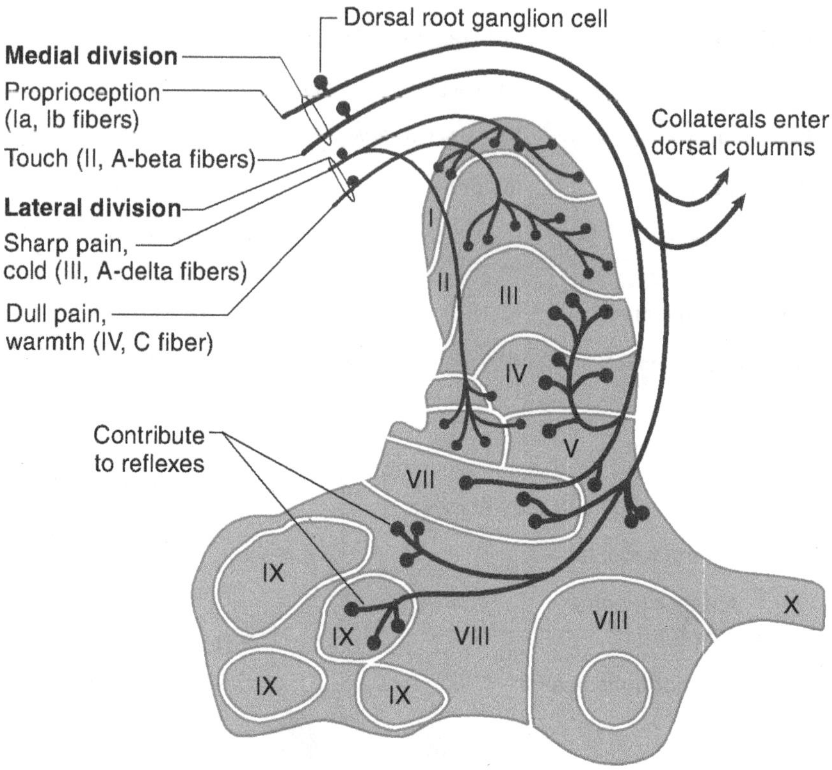

Figure III-4-3. Fiber Types in Dorsal Roots and Sites of Termination in the Spinal Cord Gray Matter

Ventral Horn

The ventral horn contains **alpha and gamma motoneurons**. The alpha motoneurons innervate skeletal muscle (extrafusal fibers) by way of a specialized synapse at a neuromuscular junction, and the gamma motoneurons innervate the contractile intrafusal muscle fibers of the muscle spindle. Within the ventral horn, alpha and gamma motoneurons that innervate flexors are dorsal to those that innervate extensors. Alpha and gamma motoneurons that innervate the proximal musculature are medial to those that innervate the distal musculature. Axons of alpha and gamma motoneurons and axons of preganglionic autonomic neurons leave the cord by way of a ventral root.

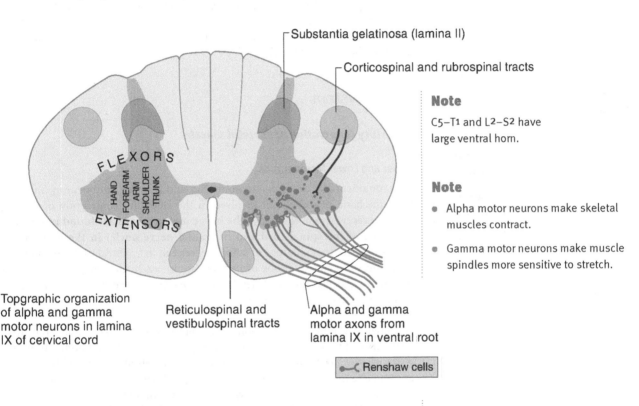

Note

C5–T1 and L2–S2 have large ventral horn.

Note

- Alpha motor neurons make skeletal muscles contract.

- Gamma motor neurons make muscle spindles more sensitive to stretch.

Substantia gelatinosa (lamina II)

Corticospinal and rubrospinal tracts

FLEXORS

HAND FOREARM ARM SHOULDER TRUNK

EXTENSORS

Topgraphic organization of alpha and gamma motor neurons in lamina IX of cervical cord

Reticulospinal and vestibulospinal tracts

Alpha and gamma motor axons from lamina IX in ventral root

Renshaw cells

Figure III-4-4. Topographic Organization of Alpha and Gamma Motoneurons (LMNs) in Lamina IX

Intermediate Zone

The intermediate zone of the spinal cord from T1 to L2 contains preganglionic sympathetic neuron cell bodies and Clarke nucleus, which sends unconscious proprioception to the cerebellum.

NEURAL SYSTEMS

There are 3 major neural systems in the spinal cord that use neurons in the gray matter and tracts or fasciculi of axons in the white matter. These neural systems have components that can be found at all levels of the CNS from the cerebral cortex to the tip of the spinal cord. An understanding of these 3 neural systems is essential to understanding the effects of lesions in the spinal cord and brain stem, and at higher levels of the CNS.

Motor System

Voluntary innervation of skeletal muscle

Upper and Lower Motoneurons

Two motoneurons, an upper motoneuron and a lower motoneuron, together form the basic neural circuit involved in the voluntary contraction of skeletal muscle everywhere in the body. **The lower motoneurons are found in the ventral horn of the spinal cord** and in **cranial nerve nuclei in the brain stem**. Axons of lower motoneurons of spinal nerves exit in a ventral root, then join the spinal nerve to course in one of its branches to reach and synapse directly at a neuromuscular junction in skeletal muscle. Axons of lower motoneurons in the brain stem exit in a cranial nerve.

To initiate a voluntary contraction of skeletal muscle, a lower motoneuron must be innervated by an upper motoneuron (Figure III-4-5). The **cell bodies of upper motoneurons are found in the brain stem and cerebral cortex**, and their axons descend into the spinal cord in a tract to reach and synapse on lower motoneurons, or on interneurons, which then synapse on lower motoneurons. At a minimum, therefore, to initiate a voluntary contraction of skeletal muscle, 2 motoneurons, an upper and a lower, must be involved. The upper motoneuron innervates the lower motoneuron, and the lower motoneuron innervates the skeletal muscle.

The cell bodies of upper motoneurons are found in the red nucleus, reticular formation, and lateral vestibular nuclei of the brain stem, but the **most important location of upper motoneurons is in the cerebral cortex**. Axons of these cortical neurons course in the *corticospinal tract*.

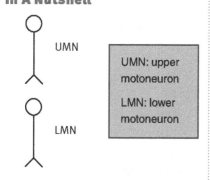

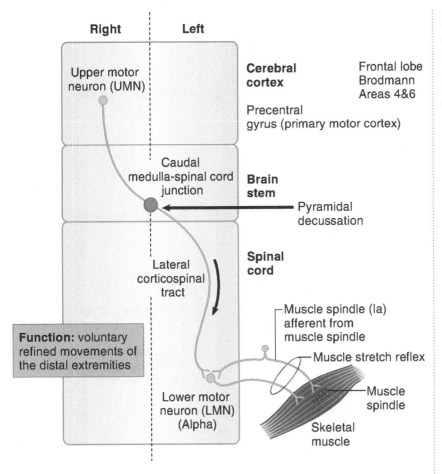

Figure III-4-5. Voluntary Contraction of Skeletal Muscle: UMN and LMNs

Corticospinal Tract

The primary motor cortex, located in the precentral gyrus of the frontal lobe, and the premotor area, located immediately anterior to the primary motor cortex, give rise to about 60% of the fibers of the corticospinal tract (Figure III-4-4). Primary and secondary somatosensory cortical areas located in the parietal lobe give rise to about 40% of the fibers of the corticospinal tract.

Fibers in the corticospinal tract leave the cerebral cortex in the internal capsule, which carries all axons in and out of the cortex. Corticospinal fibers then descend through the length of the brain stem in the ventral portion of the midbrain, pons, and medulla.

In the lower medulla, 80 to 90% of corticospinal fibers cross at the decussation of the pyramids and continue in the contralateral spinal cord as the lateral cortico-spinal tract. The lateral corticospinal tract descends the full length of the cord in the lateral part of the white matter. As it descends, axons leave the tract and enter the gray matter of the ventral horn to synapse on lower motoneurons.

Clinical Correlate

Lesions of the Corticospinal Tract

The crossing or decussation of axons of the corticospinal tract at the medulla/spinal cord junction has significant clinical implications. If lesions of the corticospinal tract occur above the pyramidal decussation, a weakness is seen in muscles on the contralateral side of the body; lesions below this level produce an ipsilateral muscle weakness. In contrast to upper motoneurons, the cell bodies of lower motoneurons are ipsilateral to the skeletal muscles that their axons innervate. A lesion to any part of a lower motoneuron will result in an ipsilateral muscle weakness at the level of the lesion.

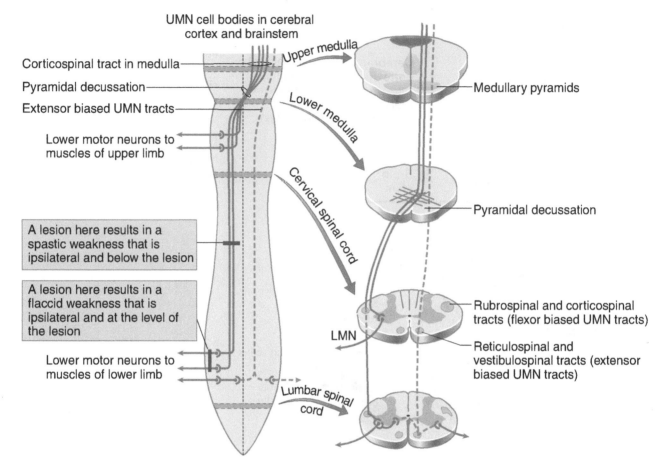

UMN cell bodies in cerebral cortex and brainstem

Corticospinal tract in medulla

Pyramidal decussation

Extensor biased UMN tracts

Lower motor neurons to muscles of upper limb

Upper medulla

Lower medulla

Cervical spinal cord

Medullary pyramids

Pyramidal decussation

A lesion here results in a spastic weakness that is ipsilateral and below the lesion

A lesion here results in a flaccid weakness that is ipsilateral and at the level of the lesion

LMN

Lower motor neurons to muscles of lower limb

Lumbar spinal cord

Rubrospinal and corticospinal tracts (flexor biased UMN tracts)

Reticulospinal and vestibulospinal tracts (extensor biased UMN tracts)

Figure III-4-6. Course of Axons of Upper Motor Neurons in the Medulla and Spinal Cord with Representative Cross-Sections

Reflex innervation of skeletal muscle

A reflex is initiated by a stimulus of a sensory neuron, which in turn innervates a motoneuron and produces a motor response. In reflexes involving skeletal muscles, the sensory stimulus arises from receptors in the muscle, and the motor response is a contraction or relaxation of one or more skeletal muscles. In the spinal cord, lower motoneurons form the specific motor component of skeletal muscle reflexes. **Upper motoneurons provide descending control over the reflexes.**

Both alpha and gamma motoneurons are lower motoneurons that participate in reflexes.

- Alpha motoneurons are large cells in the ventral horn that innervate extrafusal muscle fibers. A single alpha motoneuron innervates a group of muscle fibers, which constitutes a motor unit, the basic unit for voluntary, postural, and reflex activity.

- Gamma motoneurons supply intrafusal muscle fibers, which are modified skeletal muscle fibers. The intrafusal muscle fibers form the muscle spindle, which acts as a sensory receptor in skeletal muscle stretch reflexes.

Both ends of the muscle spindle are connected in parallel with the extrafusal fibers, so these receptors monitor the length and rate of change in length of extrafusal fibers. Muscles involved with fine movements contain a greater density of spindles than those used in coarse movements.

Commonly tested muscle stretch reflexes

The **deep tendon (stretch, myotatic) reflex** is monosynaptic and ipsilateral. The **afferent limb** consists of a **muscle spindle, Ia sensory neuron,** and **efferent limb (lower motor neuron)**. These reflexes are useful in the clinical exam.

Reflex	Cord Segment Involved	Muscle Tested
Knee (patellar)	L2–L4 (femoral n.)	Quadriceps
Ankle	S1 (tibial n.)	Gastrocnemius
Elbow	C5–C6 (musculocutaneous n.)	Biceps
Elbow	C7–C8 (radial n.)	Triceps
Forearm	C5–C6 (radial n.)	Brachioradialis

Muscle stretch (myotatic) reflex

The muscle stretch (myotatic) reflex is the stereotyped contraction of a muscle in response to stretch of that muscle. **The stretch reflex is a basic reflex that occurs in all muscles and is the primary mechanism for regulating muscle tone.** Muscle tone is the tension present in all resting muscles. Tension is controlled by the stretch reflexes.

The best example of a muscle stretch or deep tendon reflex is the knee-jerk reflex. Tapping the patellar ligament stretches the quadriceps muscle and its muscle spindles. Stretch of the spindles activates sensory endings (Ia afferents), and afferent impulses are transmitted to the cord. Some impulses from stretch receptors carried by Ia fibers monosynaptically stimulate the alpha motoneurons that supply the quadriceps. This causes contraction of the muscle and a sudden extension of the leg at the knee. Afferent impulses simultaneously inhibit antagonist muscles through interneurons (in this case, hamstrings).

Inverse muscle stretch reflex

The inverse muscle stretch reflex monitors muscle tension. This reflex uses Golgi tendon organs (GTOs). These are encapsulated groups of nerve endings that terminate between collagenous tendon fibers at the junction of muscle and tendon. GTOs are oriented in series with the extrafusal fibers and respond to increases in force or tension generated in that muscle. Increases in force in a muscle increase the firing rate of Ib afferent neurons that innervate the GTOs, which, in turn, polysynaptically facilitate antagonists and inhibit agonist muscles.

Muscle tone and reflex activity can be influenced by **gamma motoneurons** and by upper motoneurons. Gamma motoneurons directly innervate the muscle spindles and regulate their sensitivity to stretch. Upper motoneurons innervate gamma motoneurons and also influence the sensitivity of muscle spindles to stretch. Stimulation of gamma motoneurons causes intrafusal muscle fibers located at the pole of each muscle spindle to contract, which activates alpha motoneurons, causing an increase in muscle tone.

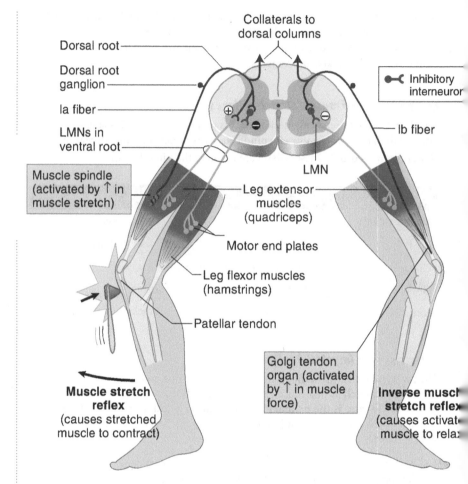

Figure III-4-7. Muscle Stretch and Golgi Tendon Reflex Components

Note:

UMN lesions result in:

- Hyperactive muscle stretch reflexes

- Clasp knife reflex due to oversensitive Golgi tendon organs

Flexor withdrawal reflex

The flexion withdrawal reflex is a protective reflex in which a stimulus (usually painful) causes withdrawal of the stimulated limb. This reflex may be accompanied by a crossed extension reflex in which the contralateral limb is extended to help support the body.

Clinical Correlate

Upper Motoneuron Versus Lower Motoneuron Muscle Lesions

A fundamental requirement of interpreting the cause of motor weakness in neuroscience cases is the ability to distinguish between a lesion of an upper versus a lower motoneuron. Because a lesion to either an upper or a lower motoneuron produces a weakness in the ability to voluntarily contract skeletal muscles, the key to distinguishing an upper from a lower motoneuron lesion will be the condition of reflexes of the affected muscles (Figure III-4-5).

A lesion of any part of a lower motoneuron will result in hypoactive muscle stretch reflexes and a reduction in muscle tone (hypotonicity) because lower motoneurons form the motor component of the reflex. Therefore, lower motoneuron lesions result in a paresis combined with suppressed or absent muscle stretch reflexes. An early sign of a lower motoneuron lesion is muscle fasciculations, which are twitches or contractions of groups of muscle fibers, that may produce a twitch visible on the skin. Later, lower motoneuron lesions produce fibrillations, which are invisible 1- to 5-ms potentials, detected with electromyography. Muscles denervated by a lower motoneuron lesion undergo pronounced wasting or atrophy. The constellation of lower motoneuron lesion signs combining paresis with suppressed or absent reflexes, fasciculations, and atrophy is known as a **flaccid paralysis**. With few exceptions, lower motoneuron lesions produce a flaccid paralysis ipsilateral and at the level of the lesion.

Neurologically, upper motoneurons including the corticospinal tract have a net overall inhibitory effect on muscle stretch reflexes. As a result, upper motoneuron lesions combine paresis of skeletal muscles with muscle stretch or deep tendon reflexes that are hyperactive or hypertonic. The hypertonia may be seen as decorticate rigidity (i.e., postural flexion of the arm and extension of the leg) or decerebrate rigidity (i.e., postural extension of the arm and leg) depending on the location of the lesion. Lesions above the midbrain produce decorticate rigidity; lesions below the midbrain produce decerebrate rigidity. Upper motoneuron lesions result in atrophy of weakened muscles only as a result of disuse, because these muscles can still be contracted by stimulating muscle stretch reflexes.

Upper motoneuron lesions are also accompanied by reversal of cutaneous reflexes, which normally yield a flexor motor response. The best known of the altered flexor reflexes is the **Babinski sign**. The test for the Babinski reflex is performed by stroking the lateral surface of the sole of the foot with a slightly painful stimulus. Normally, there is plantar flexion of the big toe. With a lesion of the corticospinal tract, the Babinski reflex is present, which is characterized by extension of the great toe and fanning of the other toes. Two other flexor reflexes, the abdominal and cremasteric, are also lost in upper motoneuron lesions. The constellation of upper motoneuron lesion signs combining paresis with increases or hyperactive reflexes, disuse atrophy of skeletal muscles, and altered cutaneous reflexes is known as a spastic paresis.

In contrast to lower motoneuron lesions, lesions of upper motoneurons result in a **spastic paresis** that is ipsilateral or contralateral and below the site of the lesion. Upper motoneuron lesions anywhere in the spinal cord will result in an ipsilateral spastic paresis below the level of the lesion. Upper motoneuron lesions between the cerebral cortex and the medulla above the decussation of the pyramids will result in a contralateral spastic paresis below the level of the lesion.

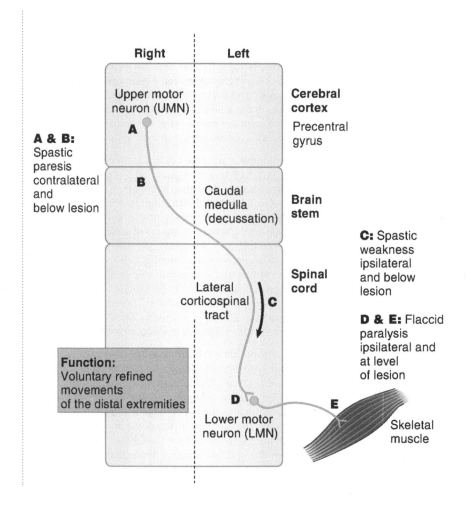

A & B: Spastic paresis contralateral and below lesion

C: Spastic weakness ipsilateral and below lesion

D & E: Flaccid paralysis ipsilateral and at level of lesion

Figure III-4-8. Upper Versus Lower Motor Neuron Lesions

Table III-4-2. Upper Versus Lower Motoneuron Lesions

Upper Motor Neuron Lesion[*]	Lower Motor Neuron Lesion[†]
Spastic paresis	Flaccid paralysis
Hyperreflexia	Areflexia
Babinski sign present	No Babinski
Increased muscle tone	Fasciculations
Clasp knife reflex	Decreased muscle tone or atonia
Disuse atrophy of muscles	Atrophy of muscle(s)
Decreased speed of voluntary movements	Loss of voluntary movements
Large area of the body involved	Small area of the body affected

*Deficits contralateral or ipsilateral and below the lesion
†Deficits ipsilateral and at the level of lesion

Sensory Systems

Two sensory systems, the dorsal column–medial lemniscal system and the antero-lateral (spinothalamic) system, use 3 neurons to convey sensory information from peripheral sensory receptors to conscious levels of cerebral cortex. In both systems, the first sensory neuron that innervates a sensory receptor has a cell body in the dorsal root ganglion and carries the information into the spinal cord in the dorsal root of a spinal nerve. The first neuron synapses with a second neuron in the brain stem or the spinal cord, and the axon of the second neuron crosses the midline and is carried in a tract in the CNS. The axon of the second neuron then synapses on a third neuron that is in the thalamus. The axon of the third neuron projects to primary somatosensory cortex (Figure III-4-9).

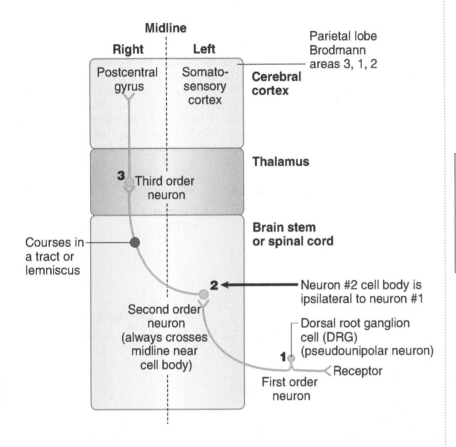

1: first-order neuron in sensory ganglion

2: second-order neuron in CNS (axon always crosses midline)

3: third-order neuron in thalamus

Figure III-4-9. General Sensory Pathways

Ascending Pathways

The 2 most important ascending pathways use a 3-neuron system to convey sensory information to the cortex. Key general features are listed below.

Pathway	Function	Overview
Dorsal column–medial lemniscal system	Discriminative touch, conscious proprioception, vibration, pressure	**3-neuron system:** 1° neuron: cell body in **DRG** 2° neuron: **decussates** 3° neuron: **thalamus** **(VPL)** → **cortex**
Anterolateral system (spinothalamic)	Pain and temperature	

Abbreviations: DRG, dorsal root ganglia; VPL, ventral posterolateral nucleus.

Dorsal column–medial lemniscal system

The dorsal column–medial lemniscal system carries sensory information for discriminative touch, joint position (kinesthetic or conscious proprioceptive) sense, vibratory, and pressure sensations from the trunk and limbs (Figures III-4-10 and III-4-11). The primary afferent neurons in this system have their cell bodies in the dorsal root ganglia, enter the cord via class II or A-beta dorsal root fibers, and then coalesce in the fasciculus gracilis or fasciculus cuneatus in the dorsal funiculus of the spinal cord. The fasciculus gracilis, found at all spinal cord levels, is situated closest to the midline and carries input from the lower extremities and lower trunk. The fasciculus cuneatus, found only at upper thoracic and cervical spinal cord levels, is lateral to the fasciculus gracilis and carries input from the upper extremities and upper trunk. These 2 fasciculi form the dorsal columns of the spinal cord that carry the central processes of dorsal root ganglion cells and ascend the length of the spinal cord to reach their second neurons in the lower part of the medulla.

In the lower part of the medulla, fibers in the fasciculus gracilis and fasciculus cuneatus synapse with the second neurons found in the nucleus gracilis and nucleus cuneatus, respectively. Cells in these medullary nuclei give rise to fibers that cross the midline as internal arcuate fibers and ascend through the brain stem in the medial lemniscus. Fibers of the medial lemniscus terminate on cells of the ventral posterolateral (VPL) nucleus of the thalamus. From the VPL nucleus, thalamocortical fibers project to the primary somesthetic (somatosensory) area of the postcentral gyrus, located in the most anterior portion of the parietal lobe.

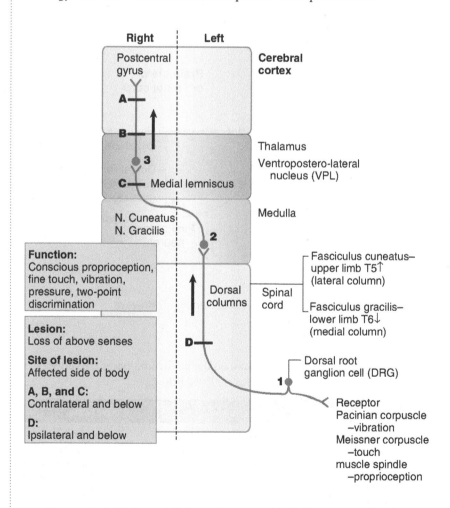

Figure III-4-10. Dorsal Column Pathway–Medial Lemniscal System

Clinical Correlate

Lesions of the dorsal columns result in a loss of joint position sensation, vibratory and pressure sensations, and 2-point discrimination. There is loss of the ability to identify the characteristics of an object, called astereognosis (e.g., size, consistency, form, shape), using only the sense of touch. Typically, dorsal column–medial lemniscal lesions are evaluated by testing vibratory sense using a 128-Hz tuning fork. Romberg sign is also used to distinguish between lesions of the dorsal columns and the midline (vermal area) of the cerebellum.

Romberg sign is tested by asking the patients to place their feet together. If there is a marked deterioration of posture (if the patient sways) with the eyes closed, this is a positive Romberg sign, suggesting that the lesion is in the dorsal columns (or dorsal roots of spinal nerves). With the eyes open, interruption of proprioceptive input carried by the dorsal columns can be compensated for by visual input to the cerebellum. Therefore, if the patient has balance problems and tends to sway with the eyes open, this is indicative of cerebellar damage.

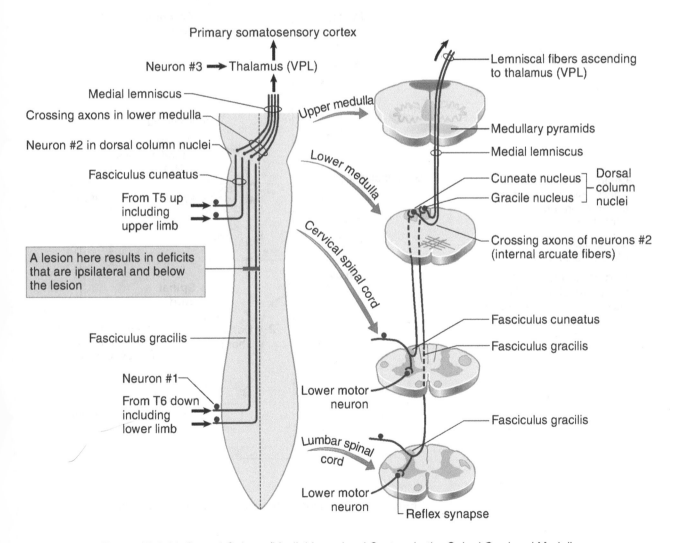

Figure III-4-11. Dorsal Column/Medial Lemniscal System in the Spinal Cord and Medulla

Clinical Correlate

Because the pain and temperature information crosses almost as soon as it enters the spinal cord, any unilateral **lesion of the spinothalamic tract** in the spinal cord or brain stem will result in a contralateral loss of pain and temperature. This is an extremely useful clinical sign because it means that if a patient presents with analgesia on one side of the trunk or limbs, the location of the lesion must be on the contralateral side of the spinal cord or brain stem. The analgesia begins 1 to 2 segments below the lesion and includes everything below that level.

Anterolateral (spinothalamic tract) system

The anterolateral system carries pain, temperature, and crude touch sensations from the extremities and trunk.

Pain and temperature fibers have cell bodies in the dorsal root ganglia and enter the spinal cord via A-delta and C or class III and class IV dorsal root fibers (Figure III-4-12). Their fibers ascend or descend a couple of segments in the dorsolateral tract of Lissauer before entering and synapsing in the dorsal horn. The second neuron cell bodies are located in the dorsal horn gray matter. Axons from these cells cross in the ventral white commissure just below the central canal of the spinal cord and coalesce to form the spinothalamic tract in the ventral part of the lateral funiculus. The spinothalamic tract courses through the entire length of the spinal cord and the brain stem to terminate in the VPL nucleus of the thalamus. Cells in the VPL nucleus send pain and temperature information to the primary somatosensory cortex in the postcentral gyrus.

Lesion:
Anesthesia (loss of pain and temperature sensations)

Site of lesion:
Affected side of body

A, B, C, and D:
Contralateral below the lesion; tract intact rostral to the lesion

---

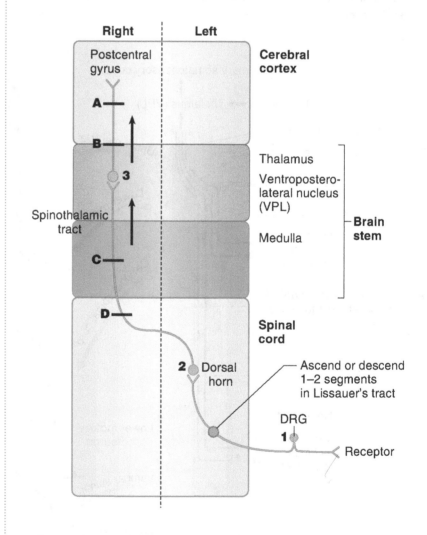

Figure III-4-12. Spinothalamic Tract (Anterolateral System)

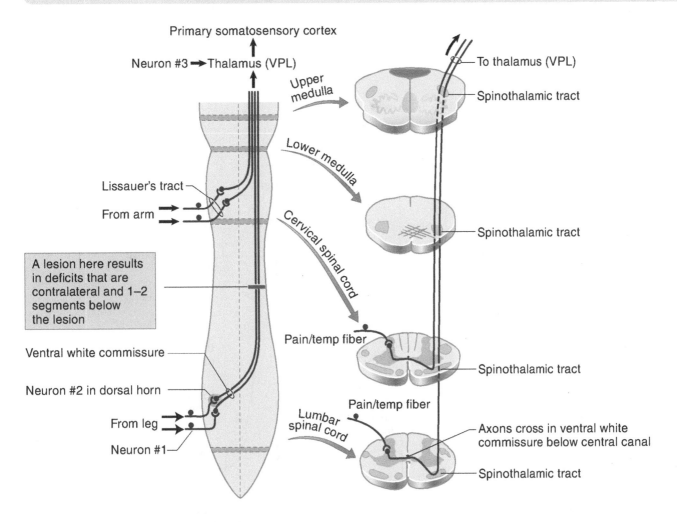

Figure III-4-13. Anterolateral System in the Spinal Cord and Medulla

Spinocerebellar pathways

The spinocerebellar tracts mainly carry unconscious proprioceptive input from muscle spindles and GTOs to the cerebellum, where this information is used to help monitor and modulate movements. There are 2 major spinocerebellar pathways:

- Dorsal spinocerebellar tract—carries input from the lower extremities and lower trunk.
- Cuneocerebellar tract—carries proprioceptive input to the cerebellum from the upper extremities and upper trunk.

The cell bodies of the dorsal spinocerebellar tract are found in Clarke's nucleus, which is situated in the spinal cord from T1 to L2. The cell bodies of the cuneocerebellar tract are found in the medulla in the external cuneate nucleus.

Clinical Correlate

Lesions that affect only the spinocerebellar tracts are uncommon, but there are a group of hereditary diseases in which degeneration of spinocerebellar pathways is a prominent feature. The most common of these is Friedreich ataxia, which is usually inherited as an autosomal recessive trait. The spinocerebellar tracts, dorsal columns, corticospinal tracts, and cerebellum may be involved. Ataxia of gait is the most common initial symptom of this disease.

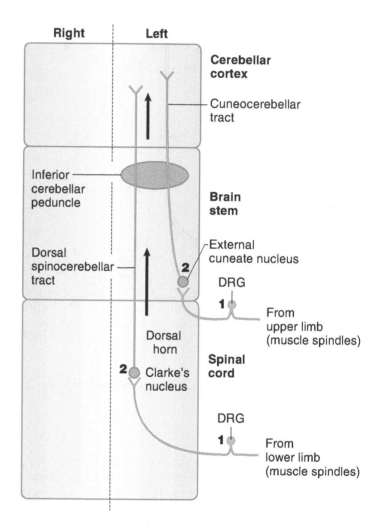

Figure III-4-14. Spinocerebellar Tracts

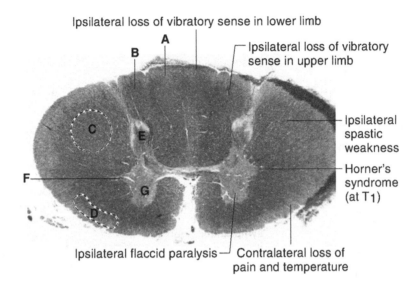

Ipsilateral loss of vibratory sense in lower limb

Ipsilateral loss of vibratory sense in upper limb

Ipsilateral spastic weakness

Horner's syndrome (at T1)

Contralateral loss of pain and temperature

Ipsilateral flaccid paralysis

Figure III-4-15. Major spinal cord neural components and clinical anatomy depicted in myelin-stained section of upper thoracic cord.

A Fasciculus Gracilis, B Fasciculus Cuneatus, C Corticospinal tract, D Anterolateral system, E Dorsal Horn, F Lateral horn (preganglionic sympathetic neurons), G Ventral horn (lower motor neurons)

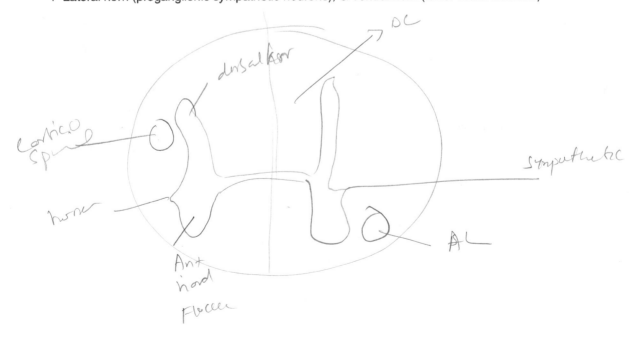

Features to look for to identify a cord section:

- Is there a large ventral horn?

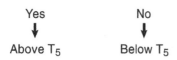

C$_5$–T$_1$, or L$_2$–S$_2$ T$_2$–L$_1$, C$_1$–C$_4$

- Are both dorsal columns present?

Yes   No

Above T$_5$ Below T$_5$

- Is there a lateral horn present?

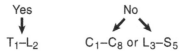

T$_1$–L$_2$ C$_1$–C$_8$ or L$_3$–S$_5$

Note

In Argyll Robertson pupil, the pupil reacts to accommodation but not to light.

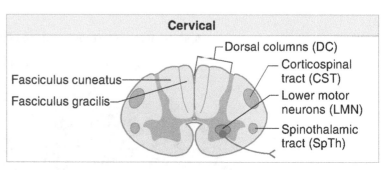

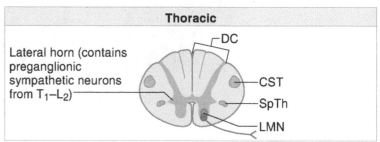

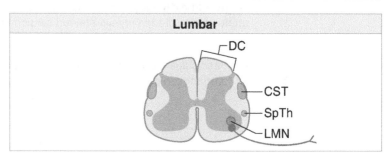

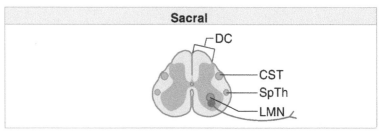

Figure III-4-16. Spinal Cord: Levels

Spinal Cord Lesions

Figure III-4-17 provides an overview of the spinal cord tracts, and Figures III-4-18 and III-4-19 show lesions at different sites, which are discussed below.

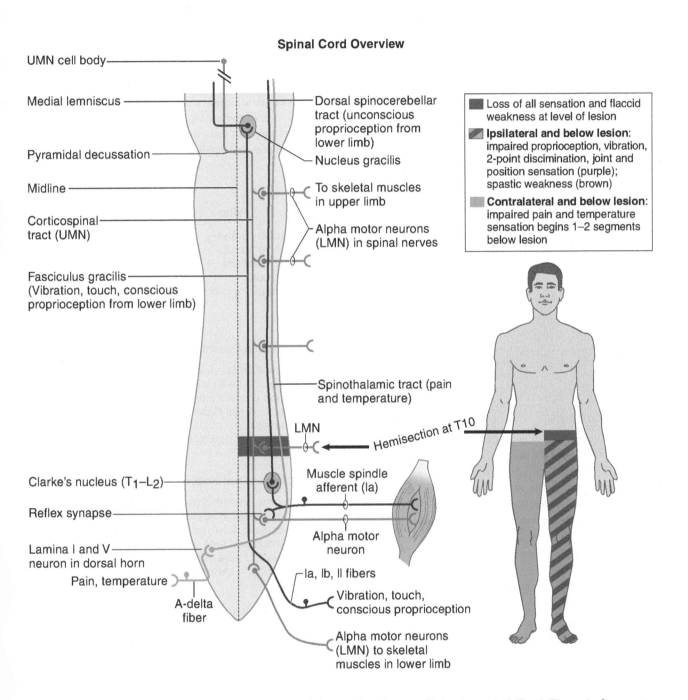

Spinal Cord Overview

UMN cell body

Medial lemniscus

Pyramidal decussation

Midline

Corticospinal tract (UMN)

Fasciculus gracilis (Vibration, touch, conscious proprioception from lower limb)

Clarke's nucleus (T₁–L₂)

Reflex synapse

Lamina I and V neuron in dorsal horn

Pain, temperature

A-delta fiber

Dorsal spinocerebellar tract (unconscious proprioception from lower limb)

Nucleus gracilis

To skeletal muscles in upper limb

Alpha motor neurons (LMN) in spinal nerves

Spinothalamic tract (pain and temperature)

LMN

Muscle spindle afferent (Ia)

Alpha motor neuron

Ia, Ib, II fibers

Vibration, touch, conscious proprioception

Alpha motor neurons (LMN) to skeletal muscles in lower limb

Hemisection at T10

Loss of all sensation and flaccid weakness at level of lesion

Ipsilateral and below lesion: impaired proprioception, vibration, 2-point discrimination, joint and position sensation (purple); spastic weakness (brown)

Contralateral and below lesion: impaired pain and temperature sensation begins 1–2 segments below lesion

Figure III-4-17. Spinal Cord Overview and Brown-Séquard Syndrome with Lesion at Left Tenth Thoracic Segment

Brown-Séquard syndrome

Hemisection of the cord results in a lesion of each of the 3 main neural systems: the principal upper motoneuron pathway of the corticospinal tract, one or both dorsal columns, and the spinothalamic tract. The hallmark of a lesion to these 3 long tracts is that the patient presents with 2 ipsilateral signs and one contralateral sign. Lesion of the corticospinal tract results in an ipsilateral spastic paresis below the level of the injury. Lesion to the fasciculus gracilis or cuneatus results in an ipsilateral loss of joint position sense, tactile discrimination, and vibratory sensations below the lesion. Lesion of the spinothalamic tract results in a contralateral loss of pain and temperature sensation starting one or 2 segments below the level of the lesion. At the level of the lesion, there will be an ipsilateral loss of all sensation, including touch modalities as well as pain and temperature, and an ipsilateral flaccid paralysis in muscles supplied by the injured spinal cord segments (Figure III-4-15).

Clinical Correlate

Tabes patients present with paresthesias (pins-and-needles sensations), pain, polyuria, Romberg sign.

Clinical Correlate

Spastic bladder results from lesions of the spinal cord **above the sacral spinal cord levels**. There is a loss of inhibition of the parasympathetic nerve fibers that innervate the detrusor muscle during the filling stage. Thus, the detrusor muscle responds to a minimum amount of stretch, causing urge incontinence.

Clinical Correlate

Atonic bladder results from lesions **to the sacral spinal cord segments** or the sacral spinal nerve roots. Loss of pelvic splanchnic motor innervation with loss of contraction of the detrusor muscle results in a full bladder with a continuous dribble of urine from the bladder.

Polio

a. Flaccid paralysis
b. Muscle atrophy
c. Fasciculations
d. Areflexia
e. Common at lumbar levels

Tabes Dorsalis

a. "Paresthesias, pain, polyuria"
b. Associated with late-stage syphilis, sensory ataxia, positive Romberg sign: sways with eyes closed, Argyll Robertson pupils, suppressed reflexes
c. Common at lumbar cord levels

Amyotrophic Lateral Sclerosis (ALS)

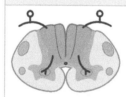
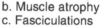

a. Progressive spinal muscular atrophy (ventral horn)
b. Primary lateral sclerosis (corticospinal tract)
 • Spastic paralysis in lower limbs
 • Increased tone and reflexes
 • Flaccid paralysis in upper limbs
c. Common in cervical enlargement

Anterior Spinal Artery (ASA) Occlusion

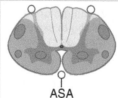

a. DC spared
b. All else bilateral signs
c. Common at mid thoracic levels
d. Spastic bladder

ASA

Figure III-4-18. Lesions of the Spinal Cord I

Subacute Combined Degeneration

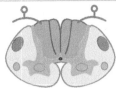

a. Vitamin B12, pernicious anemia
b. Demyelination of the:
- Dorsal columns (central and peripheral myelin)
- Spinocerebellar tracts
- Corticospinal tracts (CST)
c. Upper thoracic or lower cervical cord

Clinical Correlate

Subacute combined degeneration patients present paresthesias, bilateral spastic weakness, Babinski signs, and antibodies to intrinsic factor.

Syringomyelia

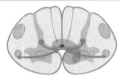

a. Cavitation of the cord (usually cervical)
b. Bilateral loss of pain and temperature at the level of the lesion
c. As the disease progresses, there is muscle weakness; eventually flaccid paralysis and atrophy of the upper limb muscles due to destruction of ventral horn cells

Clinical Correlate

Syringomyelia may present with hydrocephalus and Arnold-Chiari I malformation.

Hemisection: Brown-Séquard Syndrome (cervical)

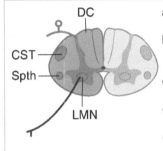

a. DC: Ipsilateral loss of position and vibratory senses at and below level of the lesion
b. Spinothalamic tract: Contralateral loss of pain and temp 1–2 segments below lesion and ipsilateral loss at the level of the lesion
c. CST: Ipsilateral paresis below the level of the lesion
d. LMN: Flaccid paralysis at the level of the lesion
e. Descending hypothalamics: Ipsilateral Horner syndrome (if cord lesion is above T1)
- Facial hemianhydrosis
- Ptosis (slight)
- Miosis

Note

Syringomyelia results in a "belt-like" or "cape-like" loss of pain and temperature.

Figure III-4-19. Lesions of the Spinal Cord II

Poliomyelitis

Poliomyelitis results from a relatively selective destruction of lower motoneurons in the ventral horn by the poliovirus. The disease causes a flaccid paralysis of muscles with the accompanying hyporeflexia and hypotonicity. Some patients may recover most function, whereas others progress to muscle atrophy and permanent disability (Figure III-4-18).

Amyotrophic lateral sclerosis

Amyotrophic lateral sclerosis (ALS, Lou Gehrig disease) is a relatively pure motor system disease that affects both upper and lower motoneurons. The disease typically begins at cervical levels of the cord and progresses either up or down the cord. Patients present with bilateral flaccid weakness of the upper limbs and bilateral spastic weakness of the lower limbs. Lower motoneurons in the brainstem nuclei may be involved later (Figure III-4-18).

Occlusion of the anterior spinal artery

This artery lies in the anterior median sulcus of the spinal cord. Occlusion of the anterior spinal artery interrupts blood supply to the ventrolateral parts of the cord, including the corticospinal tracts and spinothalamic tracts. Below the level of the lesion, the patient exhibits a bilateral spastic paresis and a bilateral loss of pain and temperature (Figure III-4-18).

Syringomyelia

Syringomyelia is a disease characterized by progressive cavitation of the central canal, usually in the cervical spinal cord but may involve other cord regions or the medulla. Early in the disease, there is a bilateral loss of pain and temperature sensation in the hands and forearms as a result of the destruction of spinothalamic fibers crossing in the anterior white commissure. When the cavitation expands, lower motoneurons in the ventral horns are compressed, resulting in bilateral flaccid paralysis of upper limb muscles. A late manifestation of cavitation is **Horner syndrome**, which occurs as a result of involvement of descending hypothalamic fibers innervating preganglionic sympathetic neurons in the T1 through T4 cord segments. Horner syndrome consists of miosis (pupillary constriction), ptosis (drooping eyelids), and anhidrosis (lack of sweating) in the face (Figure III-4-19).

Tabes dorsalis

Tabes dorsalis is one possible manifestation of neurosyphilis. It is caused by bilateral degeneration of the dorsal roots and secondary degeneration of the dorsal columns. There may be impaired vibration and position sense, astereognosis, paroxysmal pains, and ataxia, as well as diminished stretch reflexes or incontinence. Owing to the loss of proprioceptive pathways, individuals with tabes dorsalis are unsure of where the ground is and walk with a characteristic and almost diagnostic "high-step stride" (Figure III-4-18). Tabetic patients may also present with abnormal pupillary responses (Argyll Robertson pupils).

Subacute combined degeneration

Subacute combined degeneration is seen most commonly in cases of vitamin B12 deficiency, sometimes related to pernicious anemia. The disease is characterized by patchy losses of myelin in the dorsal columns and lateral corticospinal tracts, resulting in a bilateral spastic paresis and a bilateral alteration of touch, vibration, and pressure sensations below the lesion sites (Figure III-4-19). Myelin in both CNS and PNS is affected.

Chapter Summary

- The spinal cord is internally divided into 31 segments that give rise to 31 pairs of spinal nerves: 8 cervical, 12 thoracic, 5 lumbar, 5 sacral, and 1 coccygeal. Each segment is divided into an inner gray matter containing neuron cell bodies. The ventral horn of gray contains alpha and gamma motoneurons, the intermediate horn contains preganglionic neurons and Clarke nucleus, and the dorsal horn contains sensory neurons. The outer part of the spinal cord is the white matter containing ascending and descending axons that form tracts located within funiculi.

Motor Pathways

- The corticospinal tract is involved in the voluntary contraction of skeletal muscle, especially in the distal extremities. This pathway consists of 2 neurons, an upper motor neuron, and a lower motor neuron. Most of the upper motor neurons have their cell bodies in the primary motor cortex and premotor cortex of the frontal lobe. These axons leave the cerebral hemispheres through the posterior limb of the internal capsule and descend medially through the midbrain, pons, and medulla. In the medulla, 80–90% of these fibers decussate at the pyramids and then descend in the spinal cord as the lateral corticospinal tract in the lateral funiculus of the white matter. These enter the ventral horn of gray at each cord segment and synapse upon the lower motor neurons. Axons of the lower neurons (final common pathway) leave via the ventral root of the spinal nerves and innervate the skeletal muscles. Lesions above the decussation (in the brain stem or cortex) produce contralateral deficits, and lesions below the decussation (in the spinal cord) produce ipsilateral findings. Patients with upper motor neuron lesions present with spastic paralysis, hyperreflexia, a clasp-knife reflex, and a positive Babinski. Lower motor neuron lesions present with flaccid paralysis, areflexia, atonia, muscle atrophy, and fasciculations.

Sensory Pathways

- Most sensory systems use 3 neurons to project sensory modalities to the cerebral cortex. The first neuron (primary afferent neuron) has its cell body in the dorsal root ganglion of the spinal nerve. This axon enters the spinal cord and either synapses in the spinal cord or the brain stem. The second neuron will decussate and project to the thalamus. The third neuron then projects from the thalamus to the somatosensory cortex of the parietal lobe.

(Continued)

Chapter Summary (*Cont'd*)

Dorsal Column–Medial Lemniscal System

- This pathway conducts sensory information for touch, proprioception, vibration, and pressure. The primary afferent neurons of this pathway have their cell bodies in the dorsal root ganglia. Their axons enter the spinal cord and ascend in the dorsal columns of the white matter as the fasciculus gracilis (from lower limb) or the fasciculus cuneatus (from upper limb). They synapse with the second neuron in the same named nuclei in the lower medulla. Axons of the second neuron decussate (internal arcuate fibers) and ascend the midline of the brain stem in the medial lemniscus to reach the ventral posterolateral (VPL) nucleus of the thalamus. The third neuron then projects through the posterior limb of the internal capsule to the somatosensory cortex. Lesions above the decussation (in the brain stem or cortex) produce contralateral loss of joint position, vibration, and touch, whereas lesions below decussations (in the spinal cord) produce ipsilateral deficits below the level of the lesion. A positive Romberg test indicates lesions of the sensory input to the cerebellum.

Anterolateral System

- The anterolateral pathway carries pain and temperature sensations. The first neuron fibers enter the spinal cord and synapse in the dorsal horn with the second neurons. The first neuron often ascends or descends one or 2 segments before they synapse. The second neuron axons then decussate (ventral white commissure) and ascend the spinal cord and form the spinothalamic tract in the lateral funiculus of the white matter. The spinothalamic tract ascends the lateral aspect of the brain stem and synapses in the VPL nucleus of the thalamus where the third neuron projects to the cortex. All lesions of the spinothalamic tract in the spinal cord, brain stem, or cortex produce contralateral loss of pain and temperature below the lesion. Note that a central cord lesion at the spinal canal (syringomyelia) produces bilateral loss of pain and temperature at the level of the lesion.

- Lesions of the spinal cord that involve the above-mentioned tracts include poliomyelitis, tabes dorsalis, amyotrophic lateral sclerosis, anterior spinal artery occlusion, subacute combined degeneration, syringomyelia, and Brown-Sequard syndrome.

The Brain Stem 5

Learning Objectives

❏ Answer questions about cranial nerves

❏ Answer questions about sensory and motor neural systems

❏ Solve problems concerning medulla

❏ Demonstrate understanding of pons

❏ Interpret scenarios on midbrain

❏ Interpret scenarios on components of the ear, auditory, and vestibular systems

❏ Demonstrate understanding of horizontal conjugate gaze

❏ Solve problems concerning blood supply to the brain stem

❏ Interpret scenarios on brain-stem lesions

❏ Interpret scenarios on reticular formation

The brain stem is divisible into 3 continuous parts: the midbrain, the pons, and the medulla. The midbrain is most rostral and begins just below the diencephalon. The pons is in the middle and is overlain by the cerebellum.

The medulla is caudal to the pons and is continuous with the spinal cord.

The brain stem is the home of the origins or sites of termination of fibers in 9 of the 12 cranial nerves (CNs).

CRANIAL NERVES

Two cranial nerves, the oculomotor and trochlear (CN III and IV), arise from the midbrain (Figure III-5-3).

Four cranial nerves—the trigeminal, abducens, facial, and vestibulocochlear nerves (CN V, VI, VII, and VIII)—enter or exit from the pons.

Three cranial nerves—the glossopharyngeal, vagus, and hypoglossal nerves (CN IX, X, and XII)— enter or exit from the medulla. Fibers of the accessory nerve arise from the cervical spinal cord.

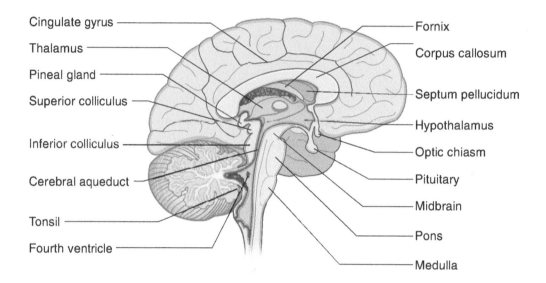

Cingulate gyrus

Thalamus

Pineal gland

Superior colliculus

Inferior colliculus

Cerebral aqueduct

Tonsil

Fourth ventricle

Fornix

Corpus callosum

Septum pellucidum

Hypothalamus

Optic chiasm

Pituitary

Midbrain

Pons

Medulla

Figure III-5-1. Brain: Mid-Sagittal Section

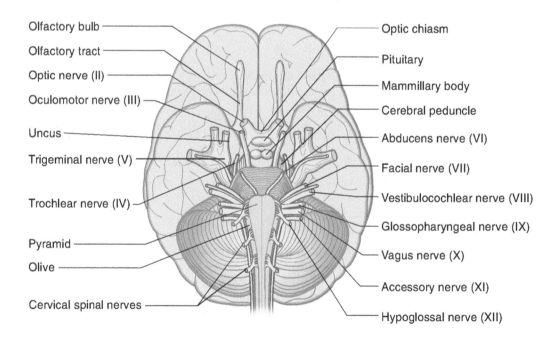

Olfactory bulb

Olfactory tract

Optic nerve (II)

Oculomotor nerve (III)

Uncus

Trigeminal nerve (V)

Trochlear nerve (IV)

Pyramid

Olive

Cervical spinal nerves

Optic chiasm

Pituitary

Mammillary body

Cerebral peduncle

Abducens nerve (VI)

Facial nerve (VII)

Vestibulocochlear nerve (VIII)

Glossopharyngeal nerve (IX)

Vagus nerve (X)

Accessory nerve (XI)

Hypoglossal nerve (XII)

Figure III-5-2. Brain: Inferior View

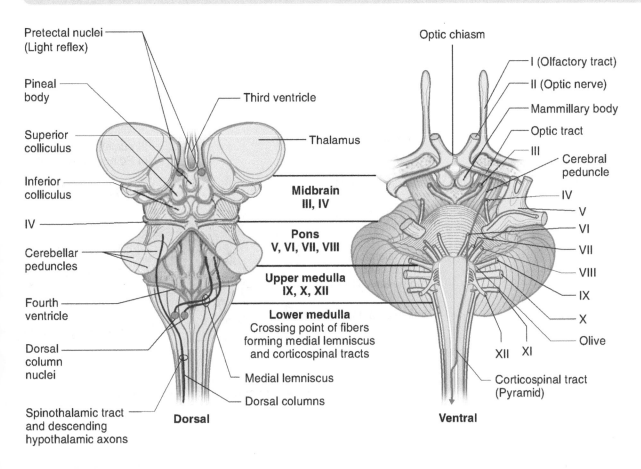

Pretectal nuclei
(Light reflex)

Pineal
body

Superior
colliculus

Inferior
colliculus

IV

Cerebellar
peduncles

Fourth
ventricle

Dorsal
column
nuclei

Spinothalamic tract
and descending
hypothalamic axons

Third ventricle

Thalamus

**Midbrain
III, IV**

**Pons
V, VI, VII, VIII**

**Upper medulla
IX, X, XII**

Lower medulla
Crossing point of fibers
forming medial lemniscus
and corticospinal tracts

Medial lemniscus

Dorsal columns

Dorsal

Optic chiasm

I (Olfactory tract)

II (Optic nerve)

Mammillary body

Optic tract

III

Cerebral
peduncle

IV

V

VI

VII

VIII

IX

X

Olive

XII   XI

Corticospinal tract
(Pyramid)

Ventral

Figure III-5-3. Brain Stem and Cranial Nerve: Surface Anatomy

Afferent fibers of cranial nerves enter the central nervous system (CNS) and terminate in relation to aggregates of neurons in sensory nuclei. Motor or efferent components of cranial nerves arise from motor nuclei. All motor and sensory nuclei that contribute fibers to cranial nerves are organized in a series of discontinuous columns according to the functional component that they contain. Motor nuclei are situated medially, closest to the midline, and sensory nuclei are situated lateral to the motor nuclei. A cranial nerve nucleus or nerve will be found at virtually every transverse sectional level of the brain stem (Figure III-5-4).

Note

The descending hypothalamic fibers course with the spinothalamic tract.

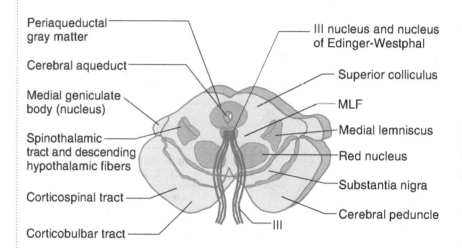

Periaqueductal gray matter

Cerebral aqueduct

Medial geniculate body (nucleus)

Spinothalamic tract and descending hypothalamic fibers

Corticospinal tract

Corticobulbar tract

III nucleus and nucleus of Edinger-Westphal

Superior colliculus

MLF

Medial lemniscus

Red nucleus

Substantia nigra

Cerebral peduncle

III

Figure III-5-4A. Upper Midbrain; Level of Nerve III

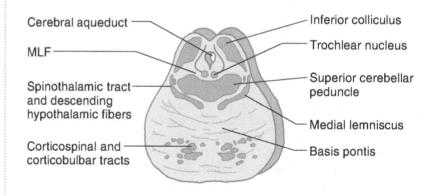

Cerebral aqueduct

MLF

Spinothalamic tract and descending hypothalamic fibers

Corticospinal and corticobulbar tracts

Inferior colliculus

Trochlear nucleus

Superior cerebellar peduncle

Medial lemniscus

Basis pontis

Figure III-5-4B. Lower Midbrain; Level of Nucleus CN IV

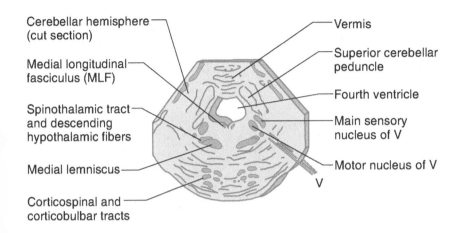

Cerebellar hemisphere (cut section)

Medial longitudinal fasciculus (MLF)

Spinothalamic tract and descending hypothalamic fibers

Medial lemniscus

Corticospinal and corticobulbar tracts

Vermis

Superior cerebellar peduncle

Fourth ventricle

Main sensory nucleus of V

Motor nucleus of V

V

Figure III-5-4C. Middle Pons; Level of Nerve V

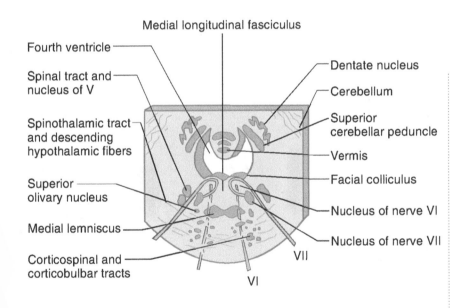

Medial longitudinal fasciculus

Fourth ventricle

Spinal tract and nucleus of V

Spinothalamic tract and descending hypothalamic fibers

Superior olivary nucleus

Medial lemniscus

Corticospinal and corticobulbar tracts

Dentate nucleus

Cerebellum

Superior cerebellar peduncle

Vermis

Facial colliculus

Nucleus of nerve VI

Nucleus of nerve VII

VII

VI

Figure III-5-4D. Lower Pons; Level of Nerves VI and VII

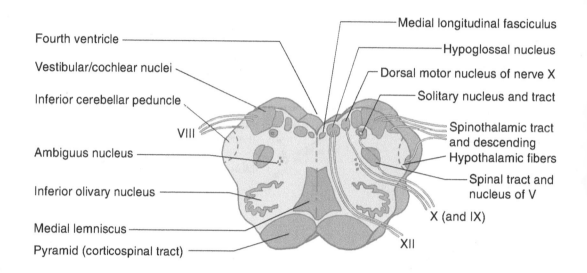

Fourth ventricle

Vestibular/cochlear nuclei

Inferior cerebellar peduncle

VIII

Ambiguus nucleus

Inferior olivary nucleus

Medial lemniscus

Pyramid (corticospinal tract)

Medial longitudinal fasciculus

Hypoglossal nucleus

Dorsal motor nucleus of nerve X

Solitary nucleus and tract

Spinothalamic tract and descending

Hypothalamic fibers

Spinal tract and nucleus of V

X (and IX)

XII

Figure III-5-4E. Open Medulla

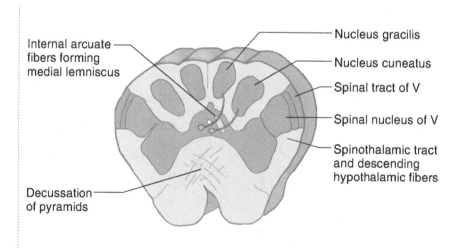

Internal arcuate fibers forming medial lemniscus

Decussation of pyramids

Nucleus gracilis

Nucleus cuneatus

Spinal tract of V

Spinal nucleus of V

Spinothalamic tract and descending hypothalamic fibers

Figure III-5-4F. Closed Medulla

Table III-5-1. Cranial Nerves: Functional Features

CN	Name	Type	Function	Results of Lesions
I	Olfactory	Sensory	Smells	Anosmia
II	Optic	Sensory	Sees	Visual field deficits (anopsia)
				Loss of light reflex with III
				Only nerve to be affected by MS
III	Oculomotor	Motor	Innervates SR, IR, MR, IO extraocular muscles: adduction (MR) most important action	Diplopia, external strabismus
				Loss of parallel gaze
			Raises eyelid (levator palpebrae superioris)	Ptosis
			Constricts pupil (sphincter pupillae)	Dilated pupil, loss of light reflex with II
			Accommodates (ciliary muscle)	Loss of near response
IV	Trochlear	Motor	Superior oblique—depresses and abducts eyeball (makes eyeball look down and out)	Weakness looking down with adducted eye
				Trouble going down stairs
			Intorts	Head tilts away from lesioned side
V	Trigeminal	Mixed	General sensation (touch, pain, temperature) of forehead/scalp/cornea	V1—loss of general sensation in skin of forehead/scalp
	Ophthalmic (V1)			Loss of blink reflex with VII
	Maxillary (V2)		General sensation of palate, nasal cavity, maxillary face, maxillary teeth	V2—loss of general sensation in skin over maxilla, maxillary teeth
	Mandibular (V3)		General sensation of anterior two-thirds of tongue, mandibular face, mandibular teeth	V3—loss of general sensation in skin over mandible, mandibular teeth, tongue, weakness in chewing
			Motor to muscles of mastication (temporalis, masseter, medial and lateral pterygoids) and anterior belly of digastric, mylohyoid, tensor tympani, tensor palati	Jaw deviation toward weak side
				Trigeminal neuralgia—intractable pain in V2 or V3 territory

Abbreviations: CN, cranial nerve; IO, inferior oblique; IR, inferior rectus; MR, medial rectus; MS, multiple sclerosis; SR, superior rectus

(Continued)

Table III-5-1. Cranial Nerves: Functional Features (*Cont'd.*)

CN	Name	Type	Function	Results of Lesions
VI	Abducens	Motor	Lateral rectus—abducts eyeball	Diplopia, internal strabismus Loss of parallel gaze, "pseudoptosis"
VII	Facial	Mixed	To muscles of facial expression, posterior belly of digastric, stylohyoid, stapedius Salivation (submandibular, sublingual glands) Skin behind ear Taste in anterior ⅔ of tongue/palate Tears (lacrimal gland)	Corner of mouth droops, cannot close eye, cannot wrinkle forehead, loss of blink reflex, hyperacusis; Bell palsy—lesion of nerve in facial canal Pain behind ear Alteration or loss of taste (ageusia) Eye dry and red
VIII	Vestibulocochlear	Sensory	Hearing Angular acceleration (head turning) Linear acceleration (gravity)	Sensorineural hearing loss Loss of balance, nystagmus
IX	Glossopharyngeal	Mixed	Oropharynx sensation, carotid sinus/body Salivation (parotid gland) All sensation of posterior one-third of tongue Motor to one muscle—stylopharyngeus	Loss of gag reflex with X
X	Vagus	Mixed	To muscles of palate and pharynx for swallowing except tensor palati (V) and stylopharyngeus (IX) To all muscles of larynx (phonates) Sensory of larynx and laryngopharynx Sensory of GI tract To GI tract smooth muscle and glands in foregut and midgut	Nasal speech, nasal regurgitation Dysphagia, palate droop Uvula pointing away from affected side Hoarseness/fixed vocal cord Loss of gag reflex with IX Loss of cough reflex
XI	Accessory	Motor	Head rotation to opposite side (sternocleidomastoid) Elevates and rotates scapula (trapezius)	Weakness turning chin to opposite side Shoulder droop
XII	Hypoglossal	Motor	Tongue movement (styloglossus, hyoglossus, genioglossus, and intrinsic tongue muscles—palatoglossus is by X)	Tongue pointing toward same (affected) side on protrusion

SENSORY AND MOTOR NEURAL SYSTEMS

Each of the following 5 ascending or descending neural tracts, fibers, or fasciculi courses through the brain stem and will be found at every transverse sectional level.

Medial Lemniscus

The medial lemniscus (ML) contains the axons from cell bodies found in the dorsal column nuclei (gracilis and cuneatus) in the caudal medulla and represents the second neuron in the pathway to the thalamus and cortex for discriminative touch, vibration, pressure, and conscious proprioception. The axons in the ML cross the midline of the medulla immediately after emerging from the dorsal column nuclei. Lesions in the ML, in any part of the brain stem, result in a loss of discriminative touch, vibration, pressure, and conscious proprioception from the **contralateral** side of the body.

Spinothalamic Tract (Part of Anterolateral System)

The spinothalamic tract has its cells of origin in the spinal cord and represents the crossed axons of the second neuron in the pathway conveying pain and temperature to the thalamus and cortex. Lesions of the spinothalamic tract, in any part of the brain stem, results in a loss of pain and temperature sensations from the **contralateral** side of the body.

Corticospinal Tract

The corticospinal tract controls the activity of lower motoneurons, and interneuron pools for lower motoneurons course through the brain stem on their way to the spinal cord. Lesions of this tract produce a spastic paresis in skeletal muscles of the body **contralateral** to the lesion site in the brain stem.

Descending Hypothalamic Fibers

The descending hypothalamic fibers arise in the hypothalamus and course without crossing through the brain stem to terminate on preganglionic sympathetic neurons in the spinal cord. Lesions of this pathway produce an ipsilateral **Horner syndrome.** Horner syndrome consists of miosis (pupillary constriction), ptosis (drooping eyelid), and anhidrosis (lack of sweating) in the face ipsilateral to the side of the lesion.

Descending hypothalamic fibers course with the spinothalamic fibers in the lateral part of the brain stem. Therefore, brain stem lesions producing Horner syndrome may also result in a contralateral loss of pain and temperature sensations from the limbs and body.

Medial Longitudinal Fasciculus

The medial longitudinal fasciculus is a fiber bundle interconnecting centers for horizontal gaze, the vestibular nuclei, and the nerve nuclei of CN III, IV, and VI, which innervate skeletal muscles that move the eyeball. This fiber bundle courses close to the dorsal midline of the brain stem and also contains vestibulospinal fibers, which course through the medulla to the spinal cord. Lesions of the fasciculus produce **internuclear ophthalmoplegia** and disrupt the vestibulo-ocular reflex.

MEDULLA

In the caudal medulla, 2 of the neural systems—the corticospinal and dorsal column–medial lemniscal pathways—send axons across the midline. The nucleus gracilis and nucleus cuneatus give rise to axons that decussate in the caudal medulla (the crossing axons are the internal arcuate fibers), which then form and ascend in the medial lemniscus.

The corticospinal (pyramidal) tracts, which are contained in the pyramids, course ventromedially through the medulla. Most of these fibers decussate in the caudal medulla just below the crossing of axons from the dorsal column nuclei, and then travel down the spinal cord as the (lateral) corticospinal tract.

The olives are located lateral to the pyramids in the rostral two-thirds of the medulla. The olives contain the convoluted inferior olivary nuclei. The olivary nuclei send climbing (olivocerebellar) fibers into the cerebellum through the inferior cerebellar peduncle. The olives are a key distinguishing feature of the medulla.

The spinothalamic tract and the descending hypothalamic fibers course together in the lateral part of the medulla below the inferior cerebellar peduncle and near the spinal nucleus and tract of CN V.

Cranial Nerve Nuclei

Spinal nucleus of V

The spinal nucleus of the trigeminal nerve (CN V) is located in a position analogous to the dorsal horn of the spinal cord. The spinal tract of the trigeminal nerve lies just lateral to this nucleus and extends from the upper cervical cord (C2) to the point of entry of the fifth cranial nerve in the pons. Central processes from cells in the trigeminal ganglion conveying pain and temperature sensations from the face enter the brain stem in the rostral pons but descend in the spinal tract of CN V and synapse on cells in the spinal nucleus (Figure IV-5-3).

Solitary nucleus

The solitary nucleus receives the axons of all general and special visceral afferent fibers carried into the CNS by CN VII, IX, and X. These include taste, cardiorespiratory, and gastrointestinal sensations carried by these cranial nerves. Taste and visceral sensory neurons all have their cell bodies in ganglia associated with CN VII, IX, and X outside the CNS.

Nucleus ambiguus

The nucleus ambiguus is a column of large motoneurons situated dorsal to the inferior olive. Axons arising from cells in this nucleus course in the ninth and tenth cranial nerves. The component to the ninth nerve is insignificant. In the tenth nerve, these fibers supply muscles of the soft palate, larynx, pharynx, and upper esophagus. A unilateral lesion will produce ipsilateral paralysis of the soft palate causing the uvula to deviate away from the lesioned nerve and nasal regurgitation of liquids, weakness of laryngeal muscles causing hoarseness, and pharyngeal weakness resulting in difficulty in swallowing.

Dorsal motor nucleus of CN X

These visceral motoneurons of CN X are located lateral to the hypoglossal nucleus in the floor of the fourth ventricle. This is a major parasympathetic nucleus of the brain stem, and it supplies preganglionic fibers innervating terminal ganglia in the thorax and the foregut and midgut parts of the gastrointestinal tract.

Hypoglossal nucleus

The hypoglossal nucleus is situated near the midline just beneath the central canal and fourth ventricle. This nucleus sends axons into the hypoglossal nerve to innervate all of the tongue muscles except the palatoglossus.

The accessory nucleus

The accessory nucleus is found in the cervical spinal cord. The axons of the spinal accessory nerve arise from the accessory nucleus, pass through the foramen magnum to enter the cranial cavity, and join the fibers of the vagus to exit the cranial cavity through the jugular foramen. As a result, intramedullary lesions do not affect fibers of the spinal accessory nerve. The spinal accessory nerve supplies the sternocleidomastoid and trapezius muscles.

The rootlets of the glossopharyngeal (CN IX) and vagus (CN X) nerves exit between the olive and the fibers of the inferior cerebellar peduncle. The hypoglossal nerve (CN XII) exits more medially between the olive and the medullary pyramid.

PONS

The pons is located between the medulla (caudally) and the midbrain (rostrally). The cerebellum overlies the pons. It is connected to the brain stem by 3 pairs of cerebellar peduncles. The fourth ventricle is found between the dorsal surface of the pons and the cerebellum. The ventral surface of the pons is dominated by fibers, which form a large ventral enlargement that carries fibers from pontine nuclei to the cerebellum in the middle cerebellar peduncle. This ventral enlargement is the key distinguishing feature of the pons.

The corticospinal tracts are more diffuse in the pons than in the medulla and are embedded in the transversely coursing fibers that enter the cerebellum in the middle cerebellar peduncle.

The medial lemniscus is still situated near the midline but is now separated from the corticospinal tracts by the fibers forming the middle cerebellar peduncle. The medial lemniscus has changed from a dorsoventral orientation in the medulla to a more horizontal orientation in the pons.

The spinothalamic tract and the descending hypothalamic fibers continue to course together in the lateral pons.

The lateral lemniscus, an ascending auditory pathway, is lateral and just dorsal to the medial lemniscus. The lateral lemniscus carries the bulk of ascending auditory fibers from both cochlear nuclei to the inferior colliculus of the midbrain.

The medial longitudinal fasciculus (MLF) is located near the midline just beneath the fourth ventricle.

Cranial Nerve Nuclei

Abducens nucleus

The abducens nucleus is found near the midline in the floor of the fourth ventricle just lateral to the MLF.

Facial motor nucleus

The facial motor nucleus is located ventrolateral to the abducens nucleus. Fibers from the facial nucleus curve around the posterior side of the abducens nucleus (the curve forms the internal genu of the facial nerve), then pass ventrolaterally to exit the brain stem at the pontomedullary junction.

Superior olivary nucleus

The superior olivary nucleus lies immediately ventral to the nucleus of CN VII and receives auditory impulses from both ears by way of the cochlear nuclei. The cochlear nuclei are found at the pontomedullary junction just lateral to the inferior cerebellar peduncle.

Vestibular nuclei

The vestibular nuclei are located near the posterior surface of the pons lateral to the abducens nucleus, and extend into the medulla.

Cochlear nuclei

The dorsal and ventral cochlear nuclei are found at the pontomedullary junction. All of the fibers of the cochlear part of CN VIII terminate here.

Trigeminal nuclei

Motor Nucleus—Pons

The motor nucleus of CN V is located in the pons just medial to the main sensory nucleus of the trigeminal and adjacent to the point of exit or entry of the trigeminal nerve fibers. These motor fibers supply the muscles of mastication (masseter, temporalis, and medial and lateral pterygoid (Figure IV-5-3).

Main Sensory Nucleus—Pons

The main sensory nucleus is located just lateral to the motor nucleus.

The main sensory nucleus receives tactile and pressure sensations from the face, scalp, oral cavity, nasal cavity, and dura.

Spinal Trigeminal Nucleus—Spinal cord to pons

The spinal trigeminal nucleus is a caudal continuation of the main sensory nucleus, extending from the mid pons through the medulla to the cervical cord. Central processes from cells in the trigeminal ganglion conveying pain and temperature sensations from the face descend in the spinal tract of V and synapse on cells in the spinal nucleus.

Mesencephalic Nucleus—Midbrain

The mesencephalic nucleus of CN V is located at the point of entry of the fifth nerve and extends into the midbrain. It receives proprioceptive input from joints, muscles of mastication, extraocular muscles, teeth, and the periodontium. Some of these fibers synapse monosynaptically on the motoneurons, forming the sensory limb of the jaw jerk reflex.

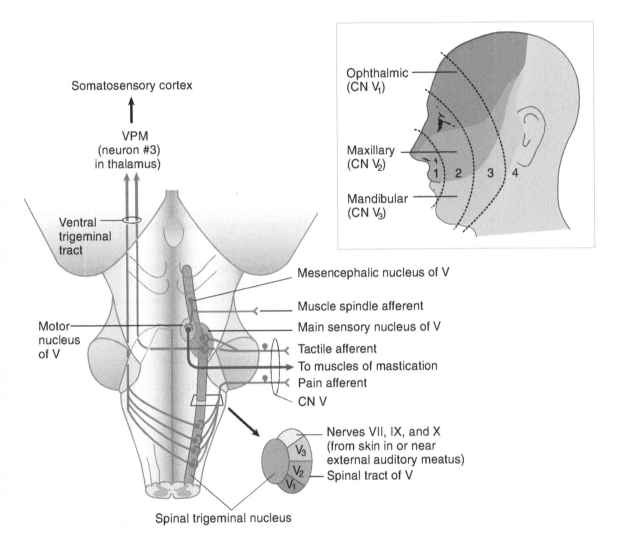

Figure III-5-5. Shaded areas indicate regions of face and scalp innervated by branches of the 3 divisions of CN V. Dotted lines indicate concentric numbered "onion-skin" regions emanating posteriorly from nose and mouth that have a rostral to caudal representation in the spinal nucleus of V in the brain stem.

Note

VPM relays touch, pain, temperature (CN V) and taste (CN VII, IX) sensations to cortex.

Cranial Nerves V, VI, VII, and VIII

Four cranial nerves emerge from the pons. Cranial nerves VI, VII, and VIII emerge from the pontomedullary junction. The facial nerve is located medial to the vestibulocochlear nerve. The abducens nerve (CN VI) emerges near the midline lateral to the corticospinal tract. The trigeminal nerve (CN V) emerges from the middle of the pons.

MIDBRAIN

The midbrain (mesencephalon) is located between the pons and diencephalon. The cerebral aqueduct, a narrow channel that connects the third and fourth ventricles, passes through the midbrain. The inferior colliculi and superior colliculi are found on the dorsal aspect of the midbrain above the cerebral aqueduct. The inferior colliculus processes auditory information received bilaterally from the cochlear nuclei by axon fibers of the lateral lemniscus. The superior colliculi help direct movements of both eyes in gaze. The pretectal region is located just beneath the superior colliculi and in front of the oculomotor complex. This area contains interneurons involved in the pupillary light reflex. The massive cerebral peduncles extend ventrally from the midbrain. The cerebral peduncles contain corticospinal and corticobulbar fibers. The interpeduncular fossa is the space between the cerebral peduncles.

The substantia nigra is the largest nucleus of the midbrain. It appears black to dark brown in the freshly cut brain because nigral cells contain melanin pigments. Neurons in the substantia nigra utilize Dopamine and GABA as neurotransmitters.

The medial lemniscus and spinothalamic tract and descending hypothalamic fibers course together ventrolateral to the periaqueductal gray.

The MLF continues to be located near the midline, just beneath the cerebral aqueduct.

The mesencephalic nuclei of the trigeminal nerve are located on either side of the central gray.

Cranial Nerve Nuclei

The trochlear nucleus is located just beneath the periaqueductal gray near the midline between the superior and inferior colliculi. The oculomotor nucleus and the nucleus of Edinger-Westphal are found just beneath the periaqueductal gray near the midline at the level of the superior colliculus.

Two cranial nerves emerge from the midbrain: the oculomotor (CN III) and the trochlear (CN IV) nerves.

The **oculomotor nerve** arises from the oculomotor nucleus and exits ventrally from the midbrain in the interpeduncular fossa. CN III also contains preganglionic parasympathetic axons that arise from the nucleus of Edinger-Westphal, which lies adjacent to the oculomotor nucleus.

Axons of the **trochlear nerve** decussate in the superior medullary velum and exit the brain stem near the posterior midline just inferior to the inferior colliculi.

Corticobulbar (Corticonuclear) Innervation of Cranial Nerve Nuclei

Corticobulbar fibers serve as the source of upper motoneuron innervation of lower motoneurons in cranial nerve nuclei (Figure III-5-6). Corticobulbar fibers arise in the motor cortex and influence lower motoneurons in all brain stem nuclei that innervate skeletal muscles. This includes:

- Muscles of mastication (CN V)
- Muscles of facial expression (CN VII) – (partially bilateral)
- Palate, pharynx, and larynx (CN X)
- Tongue (CN XII)
- Sternocleidomastoid and trapezius muscles (CN XI)

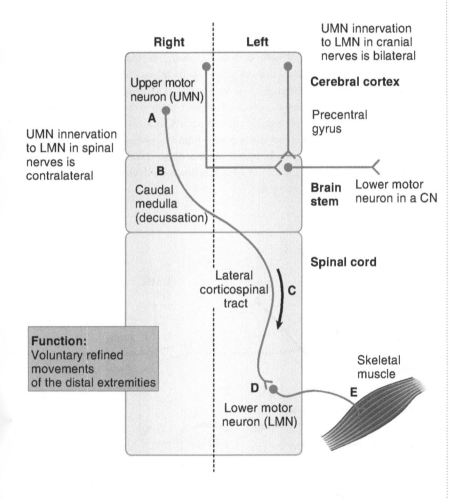

Figure III-5-6. Upper Motor Neuron Innervation of Spinal Nerves and Cranial Nerves

The corticobulbar innervation of cranial nerve lower motoneurons is predominantly bilateral, in that each lower motoneuron in a cranial nerve nucleus receives input from corticobulbar axons arising from both the right and the left cerebral cortex. The major exception is that only some of the LMNs of the facial nerve (CN VII) receive a contralateral innervation.

Clinical Correlate

Facial Paralysis

The upper motoneuron innervation of lower motoneurons in the facial motor nucleus is different and clinically significant. Like most cranial nerve lower motoneurons, the corticobulbar innervation of facial motoneurons to muscles of the upper face (which wrinkle the forehead and shut the eyes) is bilateral. The corticobulbar innervation of facial motoneurons to muscles of the mouth, however, is contralateral only. Clinically, this means that one can differentiate between a lesion of the seventh nerve and a lesion of the corticobulbar fibers to the facial motor nucleus.

A facial nerve lesion (as in **Bell Palsy**) will result in a complete ipsilateral paralysis of muscles of facial expression, including an inability to wrinkle the forehead or shut the eyes and a drooping of the corner of the mouth. A corticobulbar lesion will result in only a drooping of the corner of the mouth on the contralateral side of the face and no other facial motor deficits. Generally, no other cranial deficits will be seen with corticobulbar lesions because virtually every other cranial nerve nucleus is bilaterally innervated. In some individuals, the hypoglossal nucleus may receive mainly contralateral corticobulbar innervation. If these corticobulbar fibers are lesioned, the tongue muscles undergo transient weakness without atrophy or fasciculations and may deviate away from the injured corticobulbar fibers. If, for example, the lesion is in corticobulbar fibers on the left, there is transient weakness of the right tongue muscles, causing a deviation of the tongue toward the right side upon protrusion.

Clinical Correlate

Lesion A: left lower face weakness

Lesion B: complete left face weakness

Abbreviations

UMN = upper motoneuron

LMN = lower motoneuron

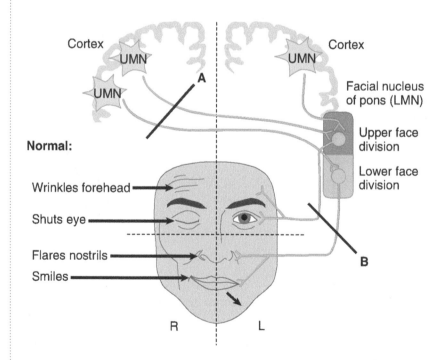

Figure III-5-7. Corticobulbar Innervation of the Facial Motor Nucleus

COMPONENTS OF THE EAR, AUDITORY, AND VESTIBULAR SYSTEMS

Each ear consists of 3 components: 2 air-filled spaces, the external ear and the middle ear; and the fluid-filled spaces of the inner ear (Figures III-5-8 and III-5-9).

The external ear includes the pinna and the external auditory meatus, which extends to the tympanic membrane. Sound waves travel through the external auditory canal and cause the tympanic membrane (eardrum) to vibrate. Movement of the eardrum causes vibrations of the ossicles in the middle ear (i.e., the malleus, incus, and stapes). Vibrations of the ossicles are transferred through the oval window and into the inner ear.

The middle ear lies in the temporal bone, where the chain of 3 ossicles connect the tympanic membrane to the oval window. These auditory ossicles amplify the vibrations received by the tympanic membrane and transmit them to the fluid of the inner ear with minimal energy loss. The malleus is inserted in the tympanic membrane, and the stapes is inserted into the membrane of the oval window. Two small skeletal muscles, the tensor tympani and the stapedius, contract to prevent damage to the inner ear when the ear is exposed to loud sounds. The middle-ear cavity communicates with the nasopharynx via the eustachian tube, which allows air pressure to be equalized on both sides of the tympanic membrane.

The inner ear consists of a labyrinth (osseous and membranous) of interconnected sacs (utricle and saccule) and channels (semicircular ducts and the cochlear duct) that contain patches of receptor or hair cells that respond to airborne vibrations or movements of the head. Both the cochlear duct and the sacs and channels of the vestibular labyrinth are filled with endolymph, which bathes the hairs of the hair cells. Endolymph is unique because it has the inorganic ionic composition of an intracellular fluid but it lies in an extracellular space. The intracellular ionic composition of endolymph is important for the function of hair cells. Perilymph, ionically like a typical extracellular fluid, lies outside the endolymph-filled labyrinth (Figure III-5-8).

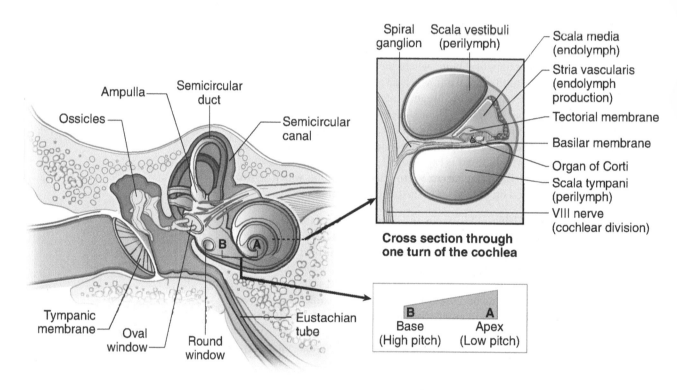

Figure III-5-8. Structures of the Inner Ear

Clinical Correlate

Middle-ear diseases (otitis media, otosclerosis) result in a conductive hearing loss because of a reduction in amplification provided by the ossicles.

Lesions of the facial nerve in the brain stem or temporal bone (Bell palsy) may result in hyperacusis, an increased sensitivity to loud sounds.

Clinical Correlate

Presbycusis results from a loss of hair cells at the base of the cochlea.

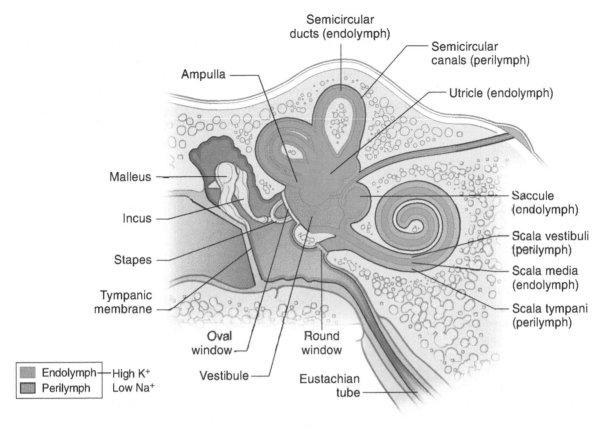

Figure III-5-9. Distribution of Endolymph and Perilymph in Inner Ear

Auditory System

Cochlear duct

The cochlear duct is the auditory receptor of the inner ear. It contains hair cells, which respond to airborne vibrations transmitted by the ossicles to the oval window. The cochlear duct coils 2 and a quarter turns within the bony cochlea and contains hair cells situated on an elongated, highly flexible, basilar membrane. High-frequency sound waves cause maximum displacement of the basilar membrane and stimulation of hair cells at the base of the cochlea, whereas low-frequency sounds maximally stimulate hair cells at the apex of the cochlea.

Spiral ganglion

The spiral ganglion contains cell bodies whose peripheral axons innervate auditory hair cells of the organ of Corti. The central axons from these bipolar cells form the cochlear part of the eighth cranial nerve. All of the axons in the cochlear part of the eighth nerve enter the pontomedullary junction and synapse in the ventral and dorsal cochlear nuclei. Axons of cells in the ventral cochlear nuclei bilaterally innervate the superior olivary nuclei in the pons. The superior olivary nuclei are the first auditory nuclei to receive binaural input and use the binaural input to localize sound sources. The lateral lemniscus carries auditory input from the cochlear nuclei and the superior olivary nuclei to the inferior colliculus in the midbrain. Each lateral lemniscus carries information derived from both ears; however, input from the contralateral ear predominates (Figure III-5-9).

Clinical Correlate

Sensorineural hearing loss:
air conduction > bone conduction

Conductive hearing loss:
bone conduction > air conduction

Inferior colliculus

The inferior colliculus sends auditory information to the medial geniculate body (MGB) of the thalamus. From the MGB, the auditory radiation projects to the primary auditory cortex located on the posterior portion of the transverse temporal gyrus (Heschl's gyrus; Brodmann areas 41 and 42). The adjacent auditory association area makes connections with other parts of the cortex, including Wernicke's area, the cortical area for the comprehension of language.

Clinical Correlate

Lesions Causing Hearing Loss

Lesions of the cochlear part of the eighth nerve or cochlear nuclei inside the brain stem at the pontomedullary junction result in a profound unilateral sensorineural hearing loss (A). All other lesions to auditory structures in the brain stem, thalamus, or cortex result in a bilateral suppression of hearing and a decreased ability to localize a sound source (B). If a patient presents with a significant hearing loss in one ear, the lesion is most likely in the middle ear, inner ear, eighth nerve, or cochlear nuclei, and not at higher levels of the auditory system.

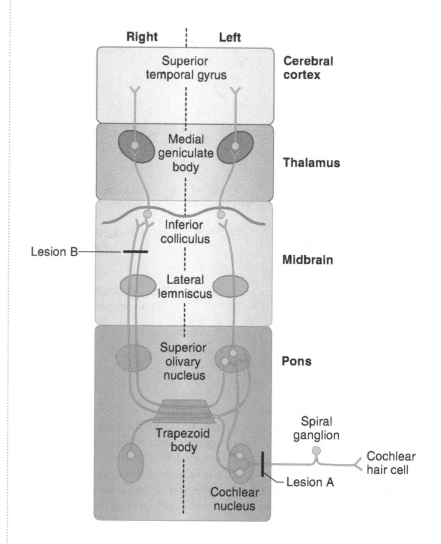

Figure III-5-10. Auditory System

Hearing Loss

Conductive: passage of sound waves through external or middle ear is interrupted. Causes: obstruction, otosclerosis, otitis media

Sensorineural: damage to cochlea, CN VIII, or central auditory connections

Auditory Tests

Weber test: place tuning fork on vertex of skull. If **unilateral conductive loss** → vibration is louder in affected ear; if **unilateral sensorineural loss** → vibration is louder in normal ear.

Rinne test: place tuning fork on mastoid process (bone conduction) until vibration is not heard, then place fork in front of ear (air conduction). If **unilateral conductive loss** → no air conduction after bone conduction is gone; if **unilateral sensorineural loss** → air conduction present after bone conduction is gone.

Vestibular System

Sensory receptors

The vestibular system contains 2 kinds of sensory receptors, one kind in the utricle and the saccule and the other in the semicircular ducts.

The utricle and the saccule are 2 large sacs, each containing a patch of hair cells in a macula. Each macula responds to linear acceleration and detects positional changes in the head relative to gravity. There are 3 semicircular ducts in the inner ear, each lying in a bony semicircular canal. Each semicircular duct contains an ampullary crest of hair cells that detect changes in angular acceleration resulting from circular movements of the head. The 3 semicircular ducts—anterior, posterior, and horizontal—are oriented such that they lie in the 3 planes of space. Circular movements of the head in any plane will depolarize hair cells in a semicircular duct in one labyrinth and hyperpolarize hair cells in the corresponding duct in the opposite labyrinth.

Vestibular nuclei

There are 4 vestibular nuclei located in the rostral medulla and caudal pons. The vestibular nuclei receive afferents from the vestibular nerve, which innervates receptors located in the semicircular ducts, utricle, and saccule. Primary vestibular fibers terminate in the vestibular nuclei and the flocculonodular lobe of the cerebellum.

Vestibular fibers

Secondary vestibular fibers, originating in the vestibular nuclei, join the MLF and supply the motor nuclei of CN III, IV, and VI. These fibers are involved in the production of conjugate eye movements. These compensatory eye movements represent the efferent limb of the vestibulo-ocular reflex, which enables the eye to remain focused on a stationary target during movement of the head or neck. Most of our understanding of the vestibulo-ocular reflex is based on horizontal head turning and a corresponding horizontal movement of the eyes in the direction opposite to that of head turning. For example, when the head turns horizontally to the right, both eyes will move to the left using the following vestibulo-ocular structures. Head turning to the right stimulates hairs cells in the right semicircular ducts. The right eighth nerve increases its firing rate to the right vestibular nuclei. These nuclei then send axons by way of the MLF to the right oculomotor nucleus and to the left abducens nucleus. The right oculomotor nerve to the right medial rectus adducts the right eye, and the left abducens nerve to the left lateral rectus abducts the left eye. The net effect of stimulating these nuclei is that both eyes will look to the left.

In A Nutshell

Vestibular Functions:
    Equilibrium
    Posture
    VOR

Clinical Correlate

A lesion of the vestibular nuclei or nerve (in this example, on the left) produces a vestibular nystagmus with a slow deviation of the eyes toward the lesion and a fast correction back to the right.

Vestibular System (VIII)

Three semicircular ducts respond to **angular acceleration and deceleration** of the head. The **utricle** and **saccule** respond to **linear acceleration** and the pull of **gravity**. There are 4 **vestibular nuclei** in the medulla and pons, which receive information from CN VIII. Fibers from the vestibular nuclei join the MLF and supply the motor nuclei of CNs III, IV, and VI, thereby regulating conjugate eye movements. Vestibular nuclei also receive and send information to the **flocculonodular lobe** of the cerebellum.

Vestibulo-Ocular Reflex

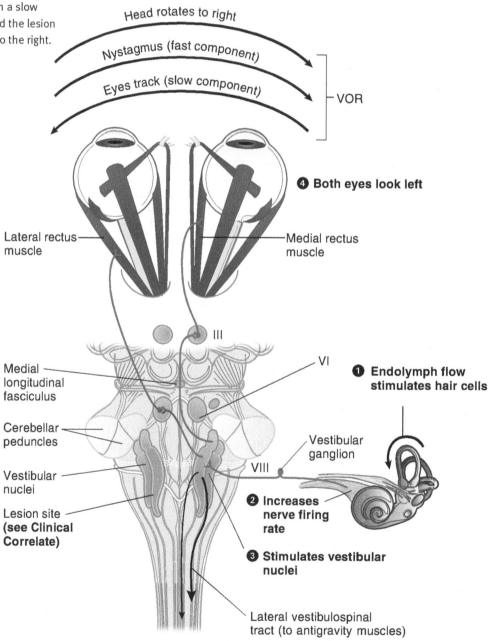

Figure III-5-11. Vestibulo-Ocular Reflex (VOR)

Caloric Test

This stimulates the horizontal semicircular ducts; can be used as a test of brain-stem function in unconscious patients.

Normal results:

- **Cold water** irrigation of ear → nystagmus to opposite side
- **Warm water** irrigation of ear → nystagmus to same side
- COWS: cold opposite, warm same

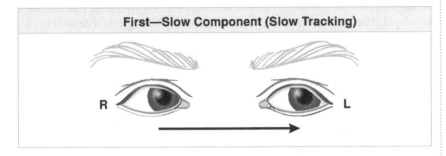

First—Slow Component (Slow Tracking)

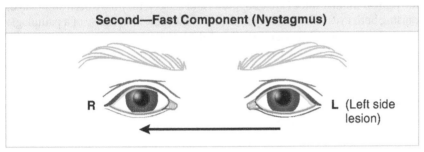

Second—Fast Component (Nystagmus)

Figure III-5-12. Vestibular System

Clinical Correlate

Vertigo: the perception of rotation. Usually severe in peripheral disease and mild in brain-stem disease. Chronic vertigo suggests a central lesion.

Ménière disease: characterized by abrupt, recurrent attacks of vertigo lasting minutes to hours; accompanied by deafness or tinnitus and is usually in one ear. Nausea and vomiting may occur. Due to distention of fluid spaces in the cochlear and vestibular parts of the labyrinth.

Eye Movement Control Systems

For the eyes to move together (**conjugate gaze**), the oculomotor nuclei and abducens nuclei are interconnected by the **medial longitudinal fasciculus (MLF)**.

Horizontal gaze is controlled by 2 gaze centers:

1. **Frontal eye field** (contralateral gaze)
2. **PPRF** (paramedian pontine reticular formation, ipsilateral gaze)

Nystagmus

Nystagmus refers to rhythmic oscillations of the eyes slowly to one side followed by a rapid reflex movement in the opposite direction. Nystagmus is defined by the direction of the rapid reflex movement or the fast phase. It is usually horizontal, although rotatory or vertical nystagmus may also occur.

Unilateral vestibular nerve or vestibular nucleus lesions may result in a vestibular nystagmus. In a pathologic vestibular nystagmus, the initial slow phase is the response to the pathology, and the fast phase is the correction attempt made by the cortex in response to the pathology. Consider this example: if the left vestibular nerve or nuclei are lesioned, because of the loss of balance between the 2 sides, the right vestibular nuclei are unopposed and act as if they have been stimulated, causing both eyes to look slowly to the left. This is the slow phase of a pathologic vestibular nystagmus. Because the head did not move, the cortex responds by moving both eyes quickly back to the right, the direction of the fast phase of the nystagmus.

Tests for Nystagmus

The integrity of the vestibulo-ocular reflex can be an indicator of brain-stem integrity in comatose patients. To test this reflex, a vestibular nystagmus is induced by performing a **caloric test** in which an examiner introduces warm or cool water into an external auditory meatus. Warm water introduced into the external ear stimulates the horizontal semicircular duct and causes the eyes to move slowly in the opposite direction. Because the head did not turn, the eyes are moved quickly back by the cortex (if intact) toward the same ear where the warm water was introduced, producing a fast phase of nystagmus to the same side. Introduction of cool water into the external ear mimics a lesion; the horizontal duct activity is inhibited on the cool water side, and the opposite vestibular complex moves the eyes slowly toward the cool-water ear. The corrective or fast phase of the nystagmus moves the eyes quickly away from the ear where the cool water was introduced. A mnemonic which summarizes the direction of the fast phase of vestibular nystagmus in a caloric test toward the warm-water side and away from the cool-water side is COWS; cool, opposite; warm, same.

HORIZONTAL CONJUGATE GAZE

The eyeballs move together in conjugate gaze. The ocular muscles function to move and position both eyes as a unit so that an image falls on a corresponding spot on the retina of each eye. The slightest weakness in the movements of one eye causes diplopia, the presence of a double image, indicating that the image has been shifted to a different position on the retina of the affected side. Although gaze in all planes is possible, the muscles and cranial nerves involved in horizontal conjugate gaze, or abduction and adduction of both eyes together, are the most important eye movements (Figure III-5-13).

Abduction of each eyeball is performed largely by the lateral rectus muscle, which is innervated by the abducens nerve (CN VI). Adduction of the eyeball is performed by the medial rectus muscle, which is innervated by the oculomotor nerve (CN III). Therefore, for both eyes to look to the right in horizontal gaze, the right abducens nerve and the right lateral rectus muscle must be active to abduct the right eye, and the left oculomotor nerve and the left medial rectus muscle must be active to adduct the left eye. The net effect is that both eyes will look to the right.

In the brain stem, the abducens nucleus (CN VI) and the oculomotor nucleus (CN III) are situated close to the midline just beneath the fourth ventricle or the cerebral aqueduct, in the pons and midbrain. These nuclei are interconnected by the fibers in the MLF. It is the fibers in the MLF that permit conjugate gaze, either when the target moves or when the head moves, through their interconnections to gaze centers and the vestibular system.

Control of Horizontal Gaze

Horizontal gaze is controlled by 2 interconnected gaze centers. One control center is in the frontal lobe, the frontal eye field (Brodmann area 8). This area acts as a center for **contralateral** horizontal gaze. In the pons is a second gaze center, known as the pontine gaze center or the PPRF, the paramedian pontine reticular formation. This is a center for **ipsilateral** horizontal gaze. When activated by neurons in the frontal eye field, the pontine gaze center neurons send axons to synapse with cell bodies in the abducens nucleus, which is actually contained within the pontine gaze center. The pontine gaze center also sends axons that cross immediately and course in the contralateral MLF to reach the contralateral oculomotor nucleus. The net effect of stimulation of the left frontal eye field, therefore, is activation of the pontine gaze center on the right and a saccadic horizontal eye movement of both eyes to the right. Horizontal gaze to the right results from activation of the right abducens nucleus and the left oculomotor nucleus by fibers in the MLF.

Lesions in the MLF result in an internuclear ophthalmoplegia in which there is an inability to adduct one eye on attempted gaze to the opposite side. For example, a lesion in the right MLF results in an inability to adduct the right eye on an attempted gaze to the left. The left eye abducts normally but exhibits a nystagmus. If the MLF is lesioned bilaterally (as might be the case in multiple sclerosis), neither eye adducts on attempted gaze (Figures III-5-13 and III-5-14), and the abducting eye exhibits a nystagmus.

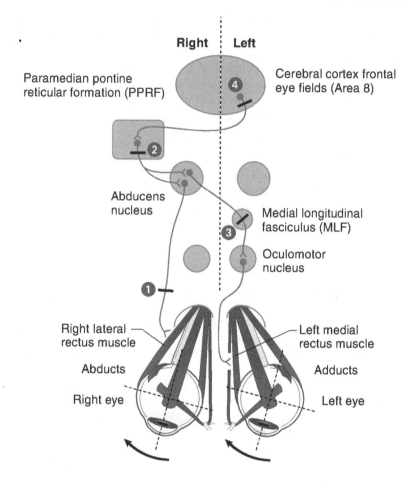

Lesion sites are indicated by 1–4.

Figure III-5-13. Voluntary Horizontal Conjugate Gaze

Table III-5-2. Clinical Correlate

Lesion Examples	Symptoms
1. Right CN VI	Right eye cannot look right
2. Right PPRF	Neither eye can look right
3. Left MLF	**Internuclear ophthalmoplegia (INO)**
	Left eye cannot look right; convergence is intact (this is how to distinguish an INO from an oculomotor lesion); right eye has nystagmus; seen in multiple sclerosis
4. Left frontal eye field	Neither eye can look right; but slow drift to left

Abbreviations: MLF, medial longitudinal fasciculus; PPRF, paramedian pontine reticular formation

Ask patient to look to the right—response shown below

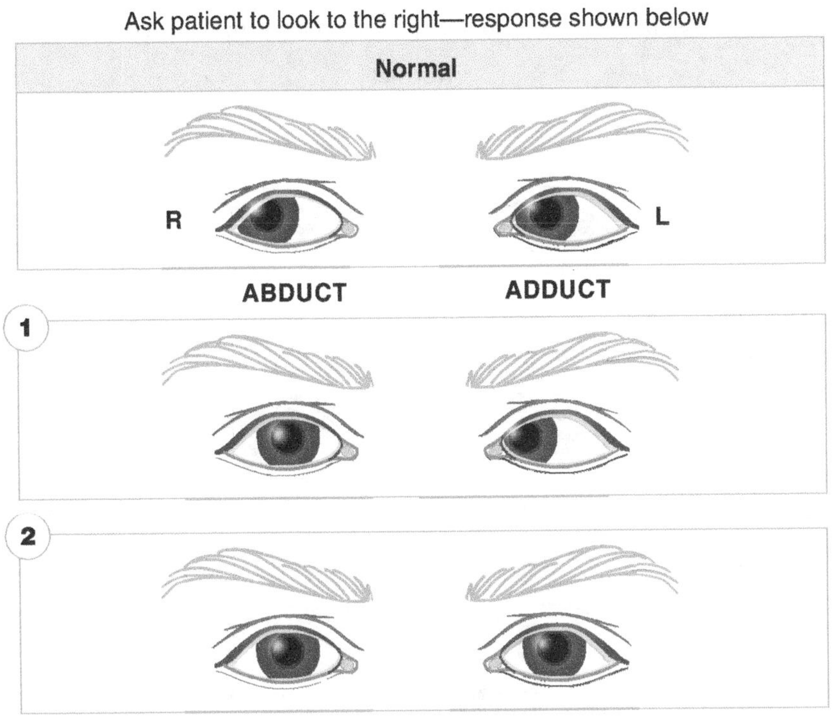

Figure III-5-14. Normal and Abnormal Horizontal Gaze

Clinical Correlate

The abducens nucleus is coexistent with the PPRF, the center for ipsilateral horizontal gaze. Lesions result in an inability to look to the lesion side, and may include a complete ipsilateral facial paralysis because the VIIth nerve fibers loop over the CN VI nucleus.

Table III-5-3. Normal/Abnormal Responses to Horizontal Conjugate Gaze: Part 1

Lesion Location	Symptoms (Results)
Right Abducens nerve, #1	Right eye cannot look right (abduct)
Right Abducens nucleus, #2	Neither eye can look right (lateral gaze paralysis)—may be slow drift left and complete **right facial paralysis**

Ask patient to look to the right—response shown below

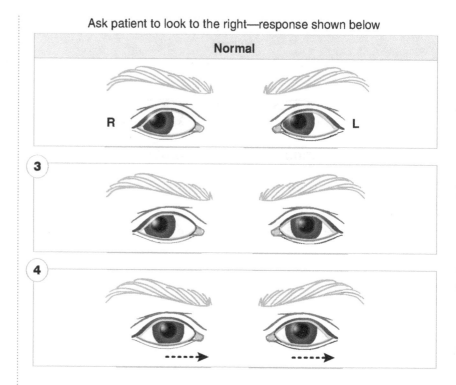

Figure III-5-15. Normal and Abnormal Horizontal Gaze

Table III-5-4. Normal/Abnormal Responses to Horizontal Gaze: Part 2

Lesion Location	Symptoms (Results)
Left MLF, #3 Internuclear ophthalmoplegia	Left eye cannot look right; convergence intact; right eye exhibits nystagmus
Left cerebral cortex, #4	Neither eye can look right: but slow drift to left; may be seen with right lower face weakness and right upper limb weakness

Abbreviation: MLF, medial longitudinal fasciculus

BLOOD SUPPLY TO THE BRAIN STEM

Vertebral Artery

This artery is a branch of the subclavian that ascends through the foramina of the transverse processes of the upper 6 cervical vertebrae. It enters the posterior fossa by passing through the foramen magnum. The vertebral arteries continue up the ventral surface of the medulla and, at the caudal border of the pons, join to form the basilar artery (Figure III-5-16).

> AICA: anterior inferior cerebellar artery
>
> PICA: posterior inferior cerebellar artery

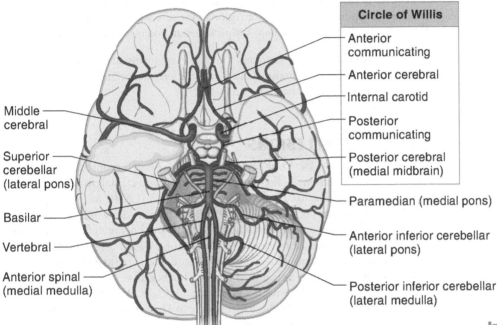

Circle of Willis
Anterior communicating
Anterior cerebral
Internal carotid
Posterior communicating
Posterior cerebral (medial midbrain)

Middle cerebral

Superior cerebellar (lateral pons)

Basilar

Vertebral

Anterior spinal (medial medulla)

Paramedian (medial pons)

Anterior inferior cerebellar (lateral pons)

Posterior inferior cerebellar (lateral medulla)

Figure III-5-16. Arterial Supply of the Brain

Branches of the vertebral artery include: the anterior spinal artery, which supplies the ventrolateral two-thirds of the cervical spinal cord and the ventromedial part of the medulla; and the posterior inferior cerebellar artery (PICA), which supplies the cerebellum and the dorsolateral part of the medulla.

In A Nutshell

Brain stem:

Vertebral Artery:
1. ASA
2. PICA

Basilar:
1. AICA
2. Paramedian
3. Superior cerebellar
4. Posterior cerebral

Basilar Artery

The basilar artery is formed by the joining of the 2 vertebral arteries at the ponto-medullary junction. It ascends along the ventral midline of the pons and terminates near the rostral border of the pons by dividing into the 2 posterior cerebral arteries. Branches include the anterior inferior cerebellar arteries (AICA) and the paramedian arteries.

Branches of the basilar artery include: the labyrinthine artery, which follows the course of the eighth cranial nerve and supplies the inner ear; the anterior inferior cerebellar artery, which supplies part of the pons and the anterior and inferior regions of the cerebellum; the superior cerebellar artery, which supplies part of the rostral pons and the superior region of the cerebellum; and pontine branches, which supply much of the pons via paramedian and circumferential vessels.

At the rostral end of the midbrain, the basilar artery divides into a pair of posterior cerebral arteries. Paramedian and circumferential branches of the posterior cerebral artery supply the midbrain.

BRAIN-STEM LESIONS

There are 2 keys to localizing brain-stem lesions. First, it is uncommon to injure parts of the brain stem without involving one or more cranial nerves. The cranial nerve signs will localize the lesion to the midbrain (CN III or IV), upper pons (CN V), lower pons (CN VI, VII, or VIII), or upper medulla (CN IX, X, or XII). Second, if the lesion is in the brain stem, the cranial nerve deficits will be seen with a lesion to one or more of the descending or ascending long tracts (corticospinal, medial lemniscus, spinothalamic, descending hypothalamic fibers). Lesions in the brain stem to any of the long tracts except for the descending hypothalamic fibers will result in a contralateral deficit. A unilateral lesion to the descending hypothalamic fibers that results in Horner syndrome is always seen ipsilateral to the side of the lesion.

Medial Medullary Syndrome

Medial medullary syndrome is most frequently the result of occlusion of the vertebral artery or the anterior spinal artery (Figure III-5-17). Medial medullary syndrome presents with a lesion of the hypoglossal nerve as the cranial nerve sign and lesions to both the medial lemniscus and the corticospinal tract. Corticospinal tract lesions produce contralateral spastic hemiparesis of both limbs.

Medial lemniscus lesions produce a contralateral deficit of proprioception and touch, pressure, and vibratory sensations in the limbs and body.

Lesions of the hypoglossal nerve in the medulla produce an ipsilateral paralysis of half the tongue with atrophy. Upon protrusion, the tongue deviates toward the side of the lesion.

Medulla

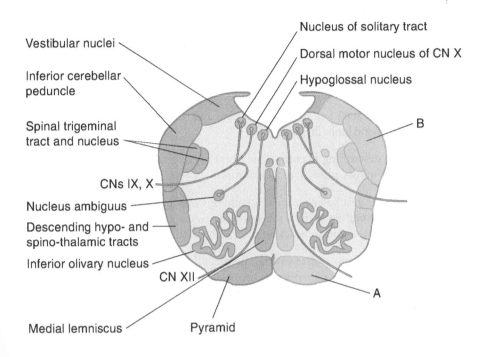

Vestibular nuclei

Inferior cerebellar peduncle

Spinal trigeminal tract and nucleus

CNs IX, X

Nucleus ambiguus

Descending hypo- and spino-thalamic tracts

Inferior olivary nucleus

CN XII

Medial lemniscus

Pyramid

Nucleus of solitary tract

Dorsal motor nucleus of CN X

Hypoglossal nucleus

B

A

Figure III-5-17. Medulla Lesions

Medial Medullary Syndrome A

Anterior Spinal Artery

- **Pyramid:** contralateral spastic paresis
- **Medial lemniscus:** contralateral loss of tactile, vibration, conscious proprioception
- **XII nucleus/fibers:** ipsilateral flaccid paralysis of tongue with tongue deviation on protrusion to lesion side.

Lateral Medullary Syndrome B

PICA, Wallenberg Syndrome

- **Inferior cerebellar peduncle:** ipsilateral limb ataxia
- **Vestibular nuclei:** vertigo, nausea/vomiting, nystagmus (away from lesion)
- **Nucleus ambiguus (CN IX, X):** ipsilateral paralysis of larynx, pharynx, palate → dysarthria, dysphagia, loss of gag reflex
- **Spinal V:** ipsilateral pain/temperature loss (face)
- **Spinothalamic tract:** Contralateral pain/temperature loss (body)
- **Descending hypothalamics:** ipsilateral Horner syndrome

Lateral Medullary (Wallenberg) Syndrome

Lateral medullary syndrome results from occlusion of the PICA (Figure IV-5-15).

The cranial nerves or nuclei involved in the lesion are the vestibular or the cochlear parts of CN VIII, the glossopharyngeal and the vagus nerves, and the spinal nucleus or tract of V. The long tracts involved are the spinothalamic tract and the descending hypothalamic fibers.

Spinothalamic tract lesions produce a pain and temperature sensation deficit in the contralateral limbs and body.

Lesions of descending hypothalamic fibers produce an ipsilateral Horner syndrome (i.e., miosis, ptosis, and anhidrosis).

Lesions of the vestibular nuclei and pathways may produce nystagmus, vertigo, nausea, and vomiting. If there is a vestibular nystagmus, the fast component will be away from the side of the lesion.

Lesions of the vagus nerves exiting the medulla may produce dysphagia (difficulty in swallowing) or hoarseness. The palate will droop on the affected side, and the uvula will deviate away from the side of the lesion.

Lesions of the glossopharyngeal nerve result in a diminished or absent gag reflex.

Lesions of the spinal tract and nucleus of the trigeminal nerve produce a loss of just pain and temperature sensations on the ipsilateral side of half the face. Touch sensations from the face and the corneal blink reflex will be intact. In lateral medullary syndrome, the pain and temperature losses are alternating; these sensations are lost from the face and scalp ipsilateral to the lesion but are lost from the contralateral limbs and trunk.

Taste sensations may be altered if the solitary nucleus is involved.

Medial Pontine Syndrome

Medial pontine syndrome results from occlusion of paramedian branches of the basilar artery (Figure III-5-18).

At a minimum, this lesion affects the exiting fibers of the abducens nerve and the corticospinal tract. The medial lemniscus may be affected if the lesion is deeper into the pons, and the facial nerve may be affected if the lesion extends laterally.

The long tract signs will be the same as in medial medullary syndrome, involving the corticospinal and medial lemniscus, but the abducens nerve and the facial nerve lesions localize the lesion to the caudal pons.

Corticospinal tract lesions produce contralateral spastic hemiparesis of both limbs.

Medial lemniscus lesions produce a contralateral deficit of proprioception and touch, pressure, and vibratory sensations in the limbs and body.

Lesions of the abducens nerve exiting the caudal pons produce an internal strabismus of the ipsilateral eye (from paralysis of the lateral rectus). This results in diplopia on attempted lateral gaze to the affected side.

Lesions of the facial nerve exiting the caudal pons produce complete weakness of the muscles of facial expression on the side of the lesion.

Lesions of the facial nerve may also include an alteration of taste from the anterior two-thirds of the tongue, loss of lacrimation (eye dry and red), and loss of the motor limb of the corneal blink reflex.

If a lesion extends dorsally to include the abducens nucleus (which includes the horizontal gaze center in the PPRF), there may be a lateral gaze paralysis in which both eyes are forcefully directed to the side contralateral to the lesion.

Lateral Pontine Syndrome

Lesions of the dorsolateral pons usually result from occlusion of the anterior inferior cerebellar artery (caudal pons) or superior cerebellar artery (rostral pons). The long tracts involved will be the same as in lateral medullary syndrome, the spinothalamic tract and the descending hypothalamic fibers. The cranial nerves involved will be the facial and vestibulocochlear in the caudal pons, the trigeminal nerve in the rostral pons, and the spinal nucleus and tract of V in both lesions (Figure III-5-19).

Spinothalamic tract lesions produce a pain and temperature sensation deficit in the contralateral limbs and body.

Lesions of descending hypothalamic fibers produce an ipsilateral Horner syndrome (i.e., miosis, ptosis, and anhidrosis).

Lesions of the vestibular nuclei and pathways (caudal pons) produce nystagmus, vertigo, nausea, and vomiting. Again, the fast phase of the nystagmus will be away from the side of the lesion. Lesions of the cochlear nucleus or auditory nerve produce an ipsilateral sensorineural hearing loss.

Lesions of the spinal tract and nucleus of the trigeminal nerve result only in a loss of pain and temperature sensations on the ipsilateral side of half the face.

Lesions of the facial nerve and associated structures produce ipsilateral facial paralysis, loss of taste from the anterior two-thirds of the tongue, loss of lacrimation and salivation, and loss of the corneal reflex.

Lesions of the trigeminal nerve (rostral pons) result in complete anesthesia of the face on the side of the lesion, weakness of muscles of mastication, and deviation of the jaw toward the lesioned side.

Pons

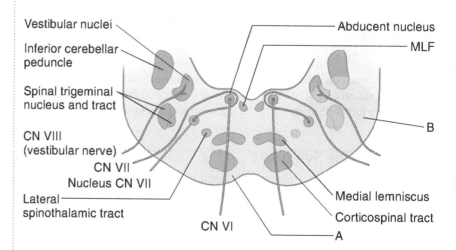

Figure III-5-18. Pons

Medial Pontine Syndrome (A)

Paramedian Branches of Basilar Artery

- **Corticospinal tract:** contralateral spastic hemiparesis
- **Medial lemniscus:** contralateral loss of tactile/position/vibration sensation
- **Fibers of VI:** medial strabismus

Lateral Pontine Syndrome (B)

AICA

- **Middle cerebellar peduncle:** ipsilateral ataxia
- **Vestibular nuclei:** vertigo, nausea and vomiting, nystagmus
- **Facial nucleus and fibers:** ipsilateral facial paralysis; ipsilateral loss of taste (anterior two-thirds of tongue), lacrimation, salivation, and corneal reflex; hyperacusis
- **Spinal trigeminal nucleus/tract:** ipsilateral pain/temperature loss (face)
- **Spinothalamic tract:** contralateral pain/temperature loss (body)
- **Cochlear nucleus/VIII fibers:** ipsilateral hearing loss
- **Descending hypothalamics:** ipsilateral Horner syndrome

Pontocerebellar Angle Syndrome

Pontocerebellar angle syndrome is usually caused by an acoustic neuroma (schwannoma) of CN VIII. This is a slow-growing tumor, which originates from Schwann cells in the vestibular nerve (or less commonly the auditory nerve). As the tumor grows, it exerts pressure on the lateral part of the caudal pons where CN VII emerges and may expand anteriorly to compress the fifth nerve. The cranial nerve deficits seen together localize the lesion to the brain stem, but the absence of long tract signs indicates that the lesion must be outside of the brain stem.

Medial Midbrain (Weber) Syndrome

Medial midbrain (Weber) syndrome results from occlusion of branches of the posterior cerebral artery (Figures III-5-19).

In medial midbrain syndrome, exiting fibers of CN III are affected, along with corticobulbar and corticospinal fibers in the medial aspect of the cerebral peduncle. Third-nerve lesions result in a ptosis, mydriasis (dilated pupil), and an external strabismus. As with any brain-stem lesion affecting the third cranial nerve, accommodation and convergence will also be affected. Corticospinal tract lesions produce contralateral spastic hemiparesis of both limbs. The involvement of the cortico-bulbar fibers results in a contralateral lower face weakness seen as a drooping of the corner of the mouth. The patient will be able to shut the eye (blink reflex is intact) and wrinkle the forehead.

Midbrain

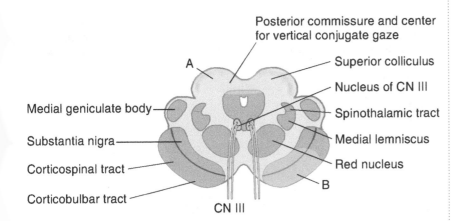

Figure III-5-19. Midbrain

Dorsal Midbrain (Parinaud) Syndrome (A)

Tumor in Pineal Region

- **Superior colliculus/pretectal area:** paralysis of upward gaze, various pupillary abnormalities
- **Cerebral aqueduct:** noncommunicating hydrocephalus

Medial Midbrain (Weber) Syndrome (B)

Branches of PCA

- **Fibers of III:** ipsilateral oculomotor palsy (lateral strabismus, dilated pupil, ptosis)
- **Corticospinal tract:** contralateral spastic hemiparesis
- **Corticobulbar tract:** contralateral hemiparesis of lower face

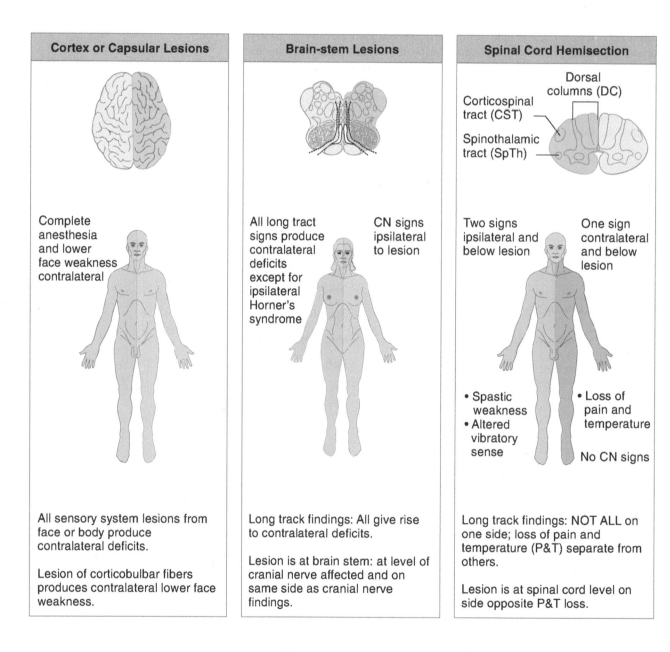

Cortex or Capsular Lesions	Brain-stem Lesions	Spinal Cord Hemisection

Dorsal columns (DC)

Corticospinal tract (CST)

Spinothalamic tract (SpTh)

Complete anesthesia and lower face weakness contralateral

All long tract signs produce contralateral deficits except for ipsilateral Horner's syndrome

CN signs ipsilateral to lesion

Two signs ipsilateral and below lesion

One sign contralateral and below lesion

• Spastic weakness
• Altered vibratory sense

• Loss of pain and temperature

No CN signs

All sensory system lesions from face or body produce contralateral deficits.

Lesion of corticobulbar fibers produces contralateral lower face weakness.

Long track findings: All give rise to contralateral deficits.

Lesion is at brain stem: at level of cranial nerve affected and on same side as cranial nerve findings.

Long track findings: NOT ALL on one side; loss of pain and temperature (P&T) separate from others.

Lesion is at spinal cord level on side opposite P&T loss.

Figure III-5-20. Strategy for the Study of Lesions

Parinaud Syndrome

Parinaud syndrome usually occurs as a result of a pineal tumor compressing the superior colliculi. The most common sign is paralysis of upward or vertical gaze, combined with bilateral pupillary abnormalities (e.g., slightly dilated pupils, which may show an impaired light or accommodation reaction) and signs of elevated intracranial pressure. Compression of the cerebral aqueduct can result in noncommunicating hydrocephalus.

RETICULAR FORMATION

The reticular formation is located in the brain stem and functions to coordinate and integrate the actions of different parts of the CNS. It plays an important role in the regulation of muscle and reflex activity and control of respiration, cardiovascular responses, behavioral arousal, and sleep.

Reticular Nuclei

Raphe nuclei

The raphe nuclei are a narrow column of cells in the midline of the brain stem, extending from the medulla to the midbrain. Cells in some of the raphe nuclei (e.g., the dorsal raphe nucleus) synthesize serotonin (5-hydroxytryptamine [5-HT]) from L-tryptophan and project to vast areas of the CNS. They play a role in mood, aggression, and the induction of non–rapid eye movement (non-REM) sleep.

Locus caeruleus

Cells in the locus caeruleus synthesize norepinephrine and send projections to most brain areas involved in the control of cortical activation (arousal). Decreased levels of norepinephrine are evident in REM (paradoxic) sleep.

Periaqueductal gray

The periaqueductal (central) gray is a collection of nuclei surrounding the cerebral aqueduct in the midbrain. Opioid receptors are present on many periaqueductal gray cells, the projections from which descend to modulate pain at the level of the dorsal horn of the spinal cord.

Clinical Correlate

Neurons in both the raphe and locus caeruleus degenerate in Alzheimer disease.

Chapter Summary

- The brain stem is divided into 3 major subdivisions—the medulla oblongata, pons, and midbrain. The brain stem contains many descending and ascending tracts, the reticular formation, and the sensory and motor cranial nuclei of CNs III–XII. Cranial nerve nuclei for CN III and IV are located in the midbrain; cranial nerve nuclei for CN V–VIII are located in the pons; and cranial nerve nuclei of IX–XII in the medulla. Most of the motor nuclei are located medially and the sensory nuclei are located more laterally in the brain stem. Normal functions of the cranial nerves and the clinical deficits resulting from lesions of the brain stem are listed in Table IV-5-1. Lesions affecting the 3 long tracts to and from the spinal cord will produce contralateral deficits, but lesions of the motor or sensory cranial nuclei result in ipsilateral findings.

- The motor nuclei of CNs III–VII and IX–XII are lower motor neurons that innervate most of the skeletal muscles of the head. These lower motor neurons are innervated by upper motor neurons (corticobulbar fibers). The cell bodies of the corticobulbar fibers are found primarily in the motor cortex of the frontal lobe. Corticobulbar innervation of lower motor neurons is primarily bilateral from both the right and left cerebral cortex, except for the innervation of the lower facial muscles around the mouth, which are derived only from the contralateral motor cortex. Generally, no cranial deficits will be seen with unilateral corticobulbar lesions, except for drooping of the corner of the mouth contralateral to the side of the lesion.

- CN VIII provides sensory pathways for auditory and vestibular systems. Auditory input depends on the stimulation of hair cells on the organ of Corti due to movement of endolymph within the membranous labyrinth of the inner ear. Axons from the organ of Corti enter the pons via CN VIII and synapse in the cochlear nuclei. From the cochlear nuclei, auditory projections bilaterally ascend the brain stem to the superior olivary nuclei, then via the lateral lemniscus to the inferior colliculus, and then to the medial geniculate body of the thalamus. Final auditory projections connect the thalamus with the primary auditory cortex of both temporal lobes. Thus, each auditory cortex receives input from both ears; however, input from the contralateral ear predominates. Lesions of the inner ear or of the cochlear nuclei in the pons will produce total deafness, whereas other lesions central to the cochlear nuclei will primarily affect the ability to localize sound direction.

(Continued)

Chapter Summary (*Continued*)

- Vestibular functions originate from endolymph movement that depolarizes hair cells in the macula of the utricle and saccule (linear acceleration and positional changes to gravity) and the ampulla of the semicircular ducts (angular acceleration). Input from these receptors project to the vestibular nuclei located in the rostral medulla and caudal pons. From these nuclei, neurons project (*1*) to the spinal cord via the lateral vestibulospinal tract to innervate the antigravity muscles, (*2*) to the flocculonodular lobe of the cerebellum, and (*3*) via the medial longitudinal fasciculus (MLF) to the ipsilateral oculomotor nucleus and the contralateral trochlear nucleus. This latter pathway to the ocular nuclei is the basis of the vestibuloocular reflex that allows horizontal movement of the head in one direction and the eyes moving in the direction opposite to that of head turning. Unilateral lesions of the vestibular nerve or vestibular nuclei may result in pathologic nystagmus. Nystagmus consists of 2 phases: first, a slow phase to the side of the lesion, and then a fast phase away from the side of the lesion. The direction of the fast phase is used to classify the direction of nystagmus. The caloric test is used to test the integrity of the vestibuloocular reflex.

- The eyes move together in horizontal conjugate gaze, which allows a focused image to fall on the same spot on the retina of each eye. Horizontal gaze requires the adduction (medial rectus muscle) and abduction (lateral rectus muscle) of both eyes together. There are 2 control centers for horizontal gaze. The frontal eye fields of the inferior frontal gyrus serves as a center for contralateral gaze, and the paramedian pontine reticular formation (PPRF) serves as a center for ipsilateral gaze. Neurons of the frontal eye fields cross the midline and synapse in the PPRF. This pontine center sends axons that synapse in the ipsilateral abducens nucleus. Other neurons cross the midline and course in the contralateral MLF to innervate the contralateral oculomotor nucleus. Thus, horizontal gaze to the right results from stimulation of the right abducens nucleus to abduct the right eye and the left oculomotor nucleus to adduct the left eye.

- Blood supply to the brain stem is provided by the anterior spinal and posterior inferior cerebellar (PICA) branches of the vertebral artery to the medulla, the paramedian and anterior inferior cerebellar branches of the basilar artery to the pons, and branches of the posterior cerebral artery to the midbrain.

- There are some key strategies for localizing brain-stem lesions. Lesions of cranial nerve nuclei produce ipsilateral findings; thus, looking at the cranial nerve deficits first will often identify the side and level of the brain-stem damage. Lesions of the long tracts from the spinal cord within the brain stem always produce contralateral findings. A unilateral lesion of the descending hypothalamic fibers results in ipsilateral Horner syndrome. Classic lesions of the brain stem include the medial medullary syndrome, lateral medullary (Wallenberg) syndrome, medial pontine syndrome, lateral pontine syndrome, and medial midbrain (Weber) syndrome.

The Cerebellum 6

Learning Objectives

❏ Use knowledge of general features

❏ Use knowledge of cerebellar cytoarchitecture

❏ Solve problems concerning circuitry

GENERAL FEATURES

The cerebellum is derived from the metencephalon and is located dorsal to the pons and the medulla. The fourth ventricle is found between the cerebellum and the dorsal aspect of the pons. The cerebellum functions in the planning and fine-tuning of skeletal muscle contractions. It performs these tasks by comparing an intended with an actual performance.

The cerebellum consists of a midline vermis and 2 lateral cerebellar hemispheres. The cerebellar cortex consists of multiple parallel folds that are referred to as folia. The cerebellar cortex contains several maps of the skeletal muscles in the body (Figure III-6-1).

The topographic arrangement of these maps indicates that the vermis controls the axial and proximal musculature of the limbs, the intermediate part of the hemisphere controls distal musculature, and the lateral part of the hemisphere is involved in motor planning.

The flocculonodular lobe is involved in control of balance and eye movements.

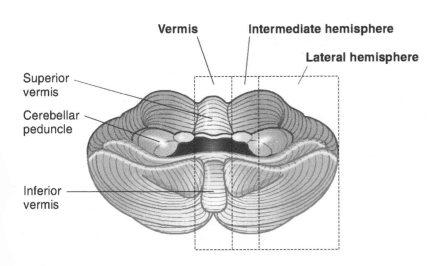

Figure III-6-1. Cerebellum

Anterior lobe
Flocculonodular lobe
Posterior lobe

Table III-6-1. Cerebellum

Region	Function	Principle Input
Vermis and intermediate zones	Ongoing motor execution	Spinal cord
Hemisphere (lateral)	Planning/coordination	Cerebral cortex and inferior olivary nucleus
Flocculonodular lobe	Balance and eye movements	Vestibular nuclei (VIII)

Major input to the cerebellum travels in the inferior cerebellar peduncle (ICP) (restiform body) and middle cerebellar peduncle (MCP). Major outflow from the cerebellum travels in the superior cerebellar peduncle (SCP).

Table III-6-2. Major Afferents to the Cerebellum

Name	Tract	Enter Cerebellum Via	Target and Function
Mossy fibers	Vestibulocerebellar	ICP	Excitatory terminals on granule cells (glutamate)
	Spinocerebellar	ICP and SCP	
	(Cortico) pontocerebellar	MCP (decussate)	
Climbing fibers	Olivocerebellar	ICP (decussate)	Excitatory terminals on Purkinje cells

Abbreviations: ICP, inferior cerebellar peduncle; MCP, middle cerebellar peduncle; SCP, superior cerebellar peduncle

CEREBELLAR CYTOARCHITECTURE

All afferent and efferent projections of the cerebellum traverse the ICP, MCP, or SCP. Most afferent input enters the cerebellum in the ICP and MCP; most efferent outflow leaves in the SCP (Figure III-6-2 and Table III-6-2).

Internally, the cerebellum consists of an outer cortex and an internal white matter (medullary substance).

The 3 cell layers of the cortex are the molecular layer, the Purkinje layer, and the granule cell layer.

The **molecular layer** is the outer layer and is made up of basket and stellate cells as well as parallel fibers, which are the axons of the granule cells. The extensive dendritic tree of the Purkinje cell extends into the molecular layer.

The **Purkinje layer** is the middle and most important layer of the cerebellar cortex. All of the inputs to the cerebellum are directed toward influencing the firing of Purkinje cells, and only axons of Purkinje cells leave the cerebellar cortex. A single axon exits from each Purkinje cell and projects to one of the deep cerebellar nuclei or to vestibular nuclei of the brain stem.

The **granule cell layer** is the innermost layer of cerebellar cortex and contains Golgi cells, granule cells, and glomeruli. Each glomerulus is surrounded by a glial capsule and contains a granule cell and axons of Golgi cells, which synapse with granule cells. The granule cell is the only excitatory neuron within the cerebellar cortex. All other neurons in the cerebellar cortex, including Purkinje, Golgi, basket, and stellate cells, are inhibitory.

Table III-6-3. Cerebellum: Cell Types

Name	Target (Axon Termination)	Transmitter	Function
Purkinje cell	Deep cerebellar nuclei	GABA	Inhibitory*
Granule cell	Purkinje cell	Glutamate	Excitatory
Stellate cell	Purkinje cell	GABA	Inhibitory
Basket cell	Purkinje cell	GABA	Inhibitory
Golgi cell	Granule cell	GABA	Inhibitory

*Purkinje cells are the only outflow from the cerebellar cortex.

The internal white matter contains the deep cerebellar nuclei.

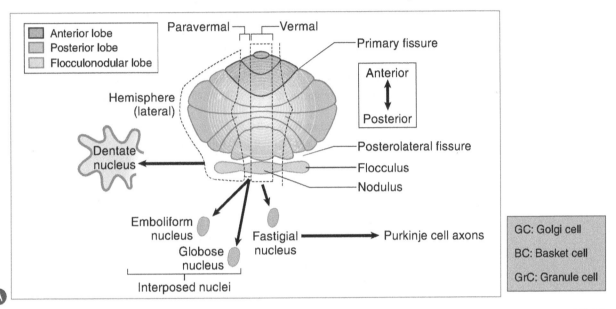

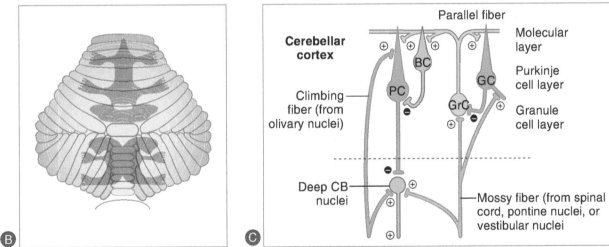

Figure III-6-2. Cerebellar Organization

(A) Parts of the cerebellar cortex and the deep cerebellar nuclei linked together by Purkinje cells

(B) Topographic arrangement of skeletal muscles controlled by parts of the cerebellum

(C) Cytology of the cerebellar cortex

From medial to lateral, the deep cerebellar nuclei in the internal white matter are the fastigial nucleus, interposed nuclei, and dentate nucleus.

Two kinds of excitatory input enter the cerebellum in the form of climbing fibers and mossy fibers. Both types influence the firing of deep cerebellar nuclei by axon collaterals.

Climbing fibers originate exclusively from the inferior olivary complex of nuclei on the contralateral side of the medulla. Climbing fibers provide a direct powerful monosynaptic excitatory input to Purkinje cells.

Mossy fibers represent the axons from all other sources of cerebellar input. Mossy fibers provide an indirect, more diffuse excitatory input to Purkinje cells.

All mossy fibers exert an excitatory effect on **granule cells**. Each granule cell sends its axon into the molecular layer, where it gives off collaterals at a 90-degree angle that run parallel to the cortical surface (i.e., parallel fibers). These granule cell axons stimulate the apical dendrites of the Purkinje cells. Golgi cells receive excitatory input from mossy fibers and from the parallel fibers of the granule cells. The Golgi cell in turn inhibits the granule cell, which activated it in the first place.

The **basket** and **stellate cells**, which also receive excitatory input from parallel fibers of granule cells, inhibit Purkinje cells.

CIRCUITRY

The basic cerebellar circuits begin with Purkinje cells that receive excitatory input directly from climbing fibers and from parallel fibers of granule cells.

Purkinje cell axons project to and inhibit the deep cerebellar nuclei or the vestibular nuclei in an orderly fashion (Figure III-6-3).

- Purkinje cells in the flocculonodular lobe project to the lateral vestibular nucleus.
- Purkinje cells in the vermis project to the fastigial nuclei.
- Purkinje cells in the intermediate hemisphere primarily project to the interposed (globose and emboliform) nuclei.
- Purkinje cells in the lateral cerebellar hemisphere project to the dentate nucleus.

Dysfunction

- **Hemisphere lesions** → ipsilateral symptoms: **intention** tremor, dysmetria, dysdiadochokinesia, scanning dysarthria, nystagmus, hypotonia
- **Vermal lesions** → truncal ataxia

Major Pathway

Purkinje cells → deep cerebellar nucleus; dentate nucleus → contralateral VL → first-degree motor cortex → pontine nuclei → contralateral cerebellar cortex

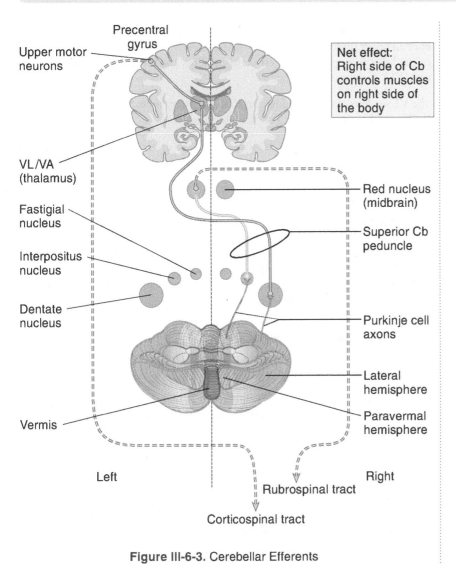

Net effect:
Right side of Cb controls muscles on right side of the body

Figure III-6-3. Cerebellar Efferents

Table III-6-4. Major Efferents From the Cerebellum

Cerebellar Areas	Deep Cerebellar Nucleus	Efferents to:	Function
Vestibulocerebellum (flocculonodular lobe)	Fastigial nucleus	Vestibular nucleus	Elicit positional changes of eyes and trunk in response to movement of the head
Spinocerebellum (intermediate hemisphere)	Interpositus nucleus	Red nucleus Reticular formation	Influence LMNs via the reticulospinal and rubrospinal tracts to adjust posture and effect movement
Pontocerebellum (lateral hemispheres)	Dentate nucleus	Thalamus (VA, VL) then cortex	Influence on LMNs via the corticospinal tract, which effect voluntary movements, especially sequence and precision

Efferents from the deep cerebellar nuclei leave mainly through the SCP and influence all upper motoneurons. In particular, axons from the dentate and interposed nuclei leave through the SCP, cross the midline, and terminate in the ventrolateral (VL) nucleus of the thalamus.

The VL nucleus of the thalamus projects to primary motor cortex and influences the firing of corticospinal and corticobulbar neurons.

Axons from other deep cerebellar nuclei influence upper motoneurons in the red nucleus and in the reticular formation and vestibular nuclei.

Cerebellar Lesions

The hallmark of cerebellar dysfunction is a tremor with intended movement without paralysis or paresis. Symptoms associated with cerebellar lesions are expressed ipsilaterally because the major outflow of the cerebellum projects to the contralateral motor cortex, and then the corticospinal fibers cross on their way to the spinal cord. Thus, unilateral lesions of the cerebellum will result in a patient falling toward the side of the lesion.

Lesions that include the hemisphere

Lesions that include the hemisphere produce a number of dysfunctions, mostly involving distal musculature.

An intention tremor is seen when voluntary movements are performed. For example, if a patient with a cerebellar lesion is asked to pick up a penny, a slight tremor of the fingers is evident and increases as the penny is approached. The tremor is barely noticeable or is absent at rest.

Dysmetria (past pointing) is the inability to stop a movement at the proper place. The patient has difficulty performing the finger-to-nose test.

Dysdiadochokinesia (adiadochokinesia) is the reduced ability to perform alternating movements, such as pronation and supination of the forearm, at a moderately quick pace.

Scanning dysarthria is caused by asynergy of the muscles responsible for speech. In scanning dysarthria, patients divide words into syllables, thereby disrupting the melody of speech.

Gaze dysfunction occurs when the eyes try to fix on a point: They may pass it or stop too soon and then oscillate a few times before they settle on the target. A nystagmus may be present, particularly with acute cerebellar damage. The nystagmus is often coarse, with the fast component usually directed toward the involved cerebellar hemisphere.

Hypotonia usually occurs with an acute cerebellar insult that includes the deep cerebellar nuclei. The muscles feel flabby on palpation, and deep tendon reflexes are usually diminished.

Lesions to the vermal region

Vermal lesions result in difficulty maintaining posture, gait, or balance (an ataxic gait). Patients with vermal damage may be differentiated from those with a lesion of the dorsal columns by the Romberg sign. In cerebellar lesions, patients will sway or lose their balance with their eyes open; in dorsal column lesions, patients sway with their eyes closed.

Chapter Summary

- The cerebellum controls posture, muscle tone, and learning of repeated motor functions, and coordinates voluntary motor activity. Diseases of the cerebellum result in disturbances of gait, balance, and coordinated motor actions, but there is no paralysis or inability to start or stop movement.

- The cerebellum is functionally divided into (1) the vermis and intermediate zone, (2) the hemisphere, and (3) the flocculonodular lobe. Each of these 3 areas receives afferent inputs mainly from the spinal cord, cortex and inferior olivary nucleus, and vestibular nuclei, respectively. These afferent fibers (mossy and climbing) reach the cerebellum via the inferior and middle cerebellar peduncles, which connect the cerebellum with the brain stem. The afferent fibers are excitatory and project directly or indirectly via granule cells to the Purkinje cells of the cerebellar cortex. The axons of the Purkinje cells are inhibitory and are the only outflow from the cerebellar cortex. They project to and inhibit the deep cerebellar nuclei (dentate, interposed, and fastigial nuclei) in the medulla. From the deep nuclei, efferents project mainly through the superior cerebellar peduncle and drive the upper motor neurons of the motor cortex. The efferents from the hemisphere project through the dentate nucleus, to the contralateral ventral lateral/ventral anterior nuclei of the thalamus, to reach the contralateral precentral gyrus. These influence contralateral lower motor neurons via the corticospinal tract.

- Symptoms associated with cerebellar lesions are expressed ipsilaterally. Unilateral lesions of the cerebellum will result in a patient falling toward the side of the lesion. Hallmarks of cerebellar dysfunction include ataxia, intention tremor, dysmetria, and dysdiadochokinesia.

Basal Ganglia   7

Learning Objectives

❏   Solve problems concerning general features

· ·

GENERAL FEATURES

The basal ganglia initiate and provide gross control over skeletal muscle movements. The major components of the basal ganglia include:

- Striatum, which consists of the caudate nucleus and the putamen (telencephalon)
- External and internal segments of the globus pallidus (telencephalon)
- Substantia nigra (in midbrain)
- Subthalamic nucleus (in diencephalon)

Together with the cerebral cortex and the ventrolateral (VL) nucleus of the thalamus, these structures are interconnected to form 2 parallel but antagonistic circuits known as the direct and indirect basal ganglia pathways (Figures III-7-1 and III-7-2). Both pathways are driven by extensive inputs from large areas of cerebral cortex, and both project back to the motor cortex after a relay in the VL nucleus of the thalamus. Both pathways use a process known as "disinhibition" to mediate their effects, whereby one population of inhibitory neurons inhibits a second population of inhibitory neurons.

Direct Basal Ganglia Pathway

In the direct pathway, excitatory input from the cerebral cortex projects to striatal neurons in the caudate nucleus and putamen. Through disinhibition, activated inhibitory neurons in the striatum, which use γ-aminobutyric acid (GABA) as their neurotransmitter, project to and inhibit additional GABA neurons in the internal segment of the globus pallidus.

The GABA axons of the internal segment of the globus pallidus project to the thalamus (VL). Because their input to the thalamus is disinhibited, the thalamic input excites the motor cortex. The net effect of the disinhibition in the direct pathway results in an **increased** level of cortical excitation and the promotion of movement.

Indirect Basal Ganglia Pathway

In the indirect pathway, excitatory input from the cerebral cortex also projects to striatal neurons in the caudate nucleus and putamen. These inhibitory neurons in the striatum, which also use GABA as their neurotransmitter, project to and inhibit additional GABA neurons in the external segment of the globus pallidus.

The GABA axons of the external segment of the globus pallidus project to the subthalamic nucleus. Through disinhibition, the subthalamic nucleus excites inhibitory GABA neurons in the internal segment of the globus pallidus, which inhibits the thalamus. This decreases the level of cortical excitation, inhibiting movement. The net effect of the disinhibition in the indirect pathway results in a **decreased** level of cortical excitation, and a suppression of unwanted movement.

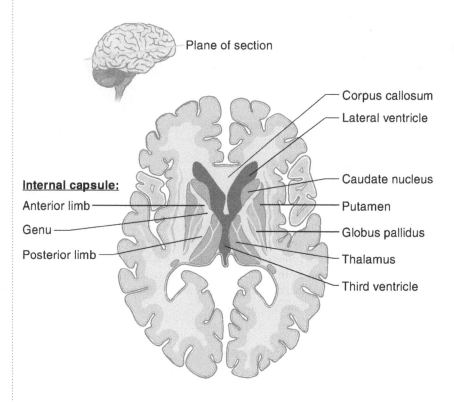

Plane of section

Corpus callosum

Lateral ventricle

Caudate nucleus

Putamen

Globus pallidus

Thalamus

Third ventricle

Internal capsule:

Anterior limb

Genu

Posterior limb

Figure III-7-1.

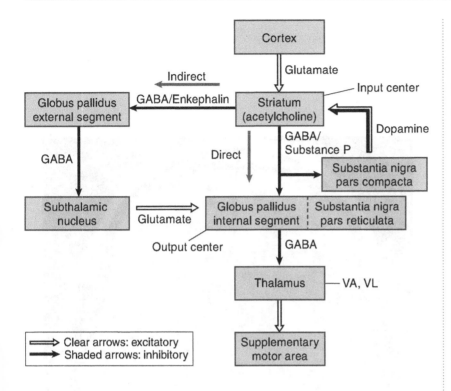

Note

Both basal ganglia pathways utilize 2 GABA neurons in series, and a "disinhibition."

Note

Dopamine drives the direct pathway; acetylcholine (ACh) drives the indirect pathway.

VA/VL: ventral anterior/ventral lateral thalamic nuclei

Figure III-7-2.

Dopamine and cholinergic effects

In addition to the GABA neurons, 2 other sources of chemically significant neurons enhance the effects of the direct or indirect pathways.

Dopaminergic neurons in the substantia nigra in the midbrain project to the striatum. The effect of dopamine excites or drives the direct pathway, increasing cortical excitation. Dopamine excites the direct pathway through D_1 receptors and inhibits the indirect pathway through D_2 receptors.

Cholinergic neurons found within the striatum have the opposite effect. Acetylcholine (Ach) drives the indirect pathway, decreasing cortical excitation.

Note

All basal ganglia connections are with ipsilateral cortex.

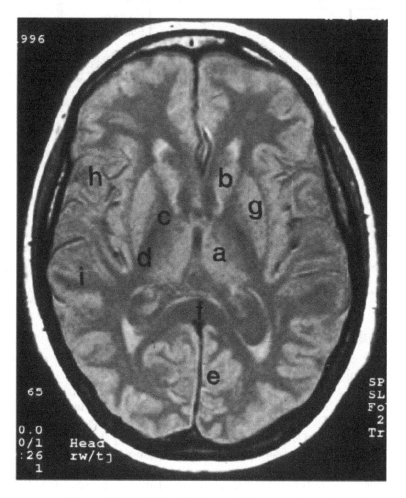

Figure III-7-3. MRI of Horizontal Section through Diencephalon, Basal Ganglia, and Cortex.

(a) Thalamus (b) Head of Caudate Nucleus (c) Genu of Internal Capsule Containing Corticobulbar Axons (d) Posterior Limb of Internal Capsule (e) Primary Visual Cortex (f) Splenium of Corpus Callosum (g) Putamen (h) Broca's Motor Speech Area (i) Wernicke's Oral Comprehension Area

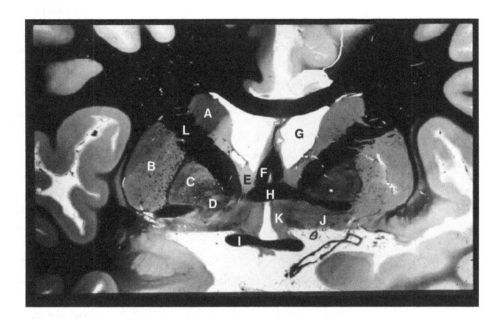

Figure III-7-4. Coronal Section through Basal Ganglia and Other Subcortical Structures

(A) caudate nucleus (B) putamen (C) globus pallidus external segment
(D) globus pallidus internal segment (E) septal nuclei (F) fornix (G) lateral
ventricle (H) anterior commissure (I) optic chiasm (J) basal nucleus of
Meynert (K) preoptic hypothalamus (L) internal capsule, anterior limb

Table III-7-1. Diseases of the Basal Ganglia

Disease	Clinical Manifestations	Notes
Parkinson disease	Bradykinesia, cogwheel rigidity, pill- rolling (resting) tremor, shuffling gate, stooped posture, masked face, depression, dementia	**Loss of pigmented dopaminergic neurons from substantia nigra** **Lewy bodies:** intracytoplasmic eosinophilic inclusions, contain α-synuclein Known causes of parkinsonism: infections, vascular, and toxic insults (e.g., **MPTP**)
Huntington disease	Chorea (multiple, rapid, random movements), athetosis (slow, writhing movements), personality changes, dementia Onset: 20–40 years	**Degeneration** of GABAergic neurons in **neostriatum**, causing atrophy of head of caudate nucleus (and ventricular dilatation) **Autosomal dominant** **Unstable nucleotide repeat** on gene in chromosome 4, which codes for huntingtin protein Disease shows **anticipation** and **genomic imprinting** **Treatment:** antipsychotic agents, benzodiazepines, anticonvulsants
Wilson disease (hepatolenticular degeneration)	Tremor, asterixis, parkinsonian symptoms, chorea, neuropsychiatric symptoms; fatty change, hepatitis, or cirrhosis of liver, tremor may be "wing beating"	**Autosomal recessive defect in copper transport** Accumulation of copper in liver, brain, and eye (Descemet membrane, producing **Kayser-Fleischer ring**) Lesions in basal ganglia (especially putamen) **Treatment: penicillamine** (a chelator), zinc acetate (blocks absorption)
Hemiballism	Wild, flinging movements of limbs	Hemorrhagic destruction of **contralateral subthalamic nucleus** Hypertensive patients
Tourette syndrome	Motor tics and vocal tics (e.g., snorting, sniffing, uncontrolled and often obscene vocalizations), commonly associated with OCD and ADHD	**Treatment:** Antipsychotic agents

Abbreviations: ADHD, attention deficit hyperactivity disorder; MPTP, 1-methyl-4-phenyl-1,2,3, 6-tetrahydropyridine; OCD, obsessive-compulsive disorder

Clinical Correlate

Lesions or Diseases of the Basal Ganglia

Lesions or diseases of the basal ganglia generally present with movement disorders, known as dyskinesias, and an involuntary tremor, or tremor at rest.

Most basal ganglia disorders seem to preferentially affect either the direct or the indirect pathways, altering the balance between the two.

Lesions of the direct pathway

Lesions of the direct pathway result in an underactive cortex and hypokinetic disturbances in which there is a slowing or absence of spontaneous movements. The best-known disorder of the direct pathway is caused by the degeneration of dopaminergic neurons of the substantia nigra in Parkinson disease. Because the cortex is underactive, Parkinson patients have problems initiating movements, combined with a reduction in the velocity and amplitude of the movements. The tremor at rest is the classic pill-rolling tremor seen in the fingers. Skeletal muscles in the upper limbs exhibit a cogwheel rigidity because of increased muscle tone. Patients also present with a stooped posture, an expressionless face, and a festinating or accelerating gait during which individuals seem to chase their center of gravity. One strategy for Parkinson patients is to give them L-dopa, a dopamine precursor that crosses the blood–brain barrier. Another strategy is to give anticholinergic drugs to inhibit the effects of acetylcholine on the indirect pathway.

Lesions of the indirect pathway

Other common disorders of the basal ganglia (chorea, athetosis, dystonia, tics) result from lesions to parts of the indirect pathway, which result in an overactive motor cortex. An overactive cortex produces hyperkinetic disturbances, expressed in numerous spontaneous movements. The involuntary tremors seen in these diseases range from being dancelike in chorea to ballistic with lesions to the subthalamic nucleus.

Chorea produces involuntary movements that are purposeless, quick jerks that may be superimposed on voluntary movements. Huntington chorea exhibits autosomal dominant inheritance (chromosome 4) and is characterized by severe degeneration of GABA neurons in the striatum. In addition to chorea, these patients frequently suffer from athetoid movements, progressive dementia, and behavioral disorders. Sydenham chorea is a transient complication in some children with rheumatic fever.

Athetosis refers to slow, wormlike, involuntary movements that are most noticeable in the fingers and hands but may involve any muscle group. It is present in Huntington disease and may be observed in many diseases that involve the basal ganglia.

Dystonia refers to a slow, prolonged movement involving predominantly the truncal musculature. Dystonia often occurs with athetosis. Blepharospasm (contraction of the orbicularis oculi causing the eyelids to close), spasmodic torticollis (in which the head is pulled toward the shoulder), and writer's cramp (contraction of arm and hand muscles on attempting to write) are all examples of dystonic movements.

(Continued)

Clinical Correlate (*Continued*)

Hemiballismus results from a lesion of the subthalamic nucleus usually seen in hypertensive patients. Hemiballismus refers to a violent projectile movement of a limb and is typically observed in the upper limb contralateral to the involved subthalamic nucleus.

Tourette syndrome involves facial and vocal tics that progress to jerking movements of the limbs. It is frequently associated with explosive, vulgar speech.

Wilson disease results from an abnormality of copper metabolism, causing the accumulation of copper in the liver and basal ganglia. Personality changes, tremor, dystonia, and athetoid movements develop. Untreated patients usually succumb because of hepatic cirrhosis. A thin brown ring around the outer cornea, the Kayser-Fleischer ring, may be present and aid in the diagnosis.

Chapter Summary

- The basal ganglia play important motor functions in starting and stopping voluntary motor functions and inhibiting unwanted movements. The basal ganglia consists of 3 nuclei masses deep in the cerebrum (caudate nucleus, putamen, and globus pallidus), one nucleus in the midbrain (substantia nigra), and the subthalamic nucleus of the diencephalon. The striatum combines the caudate nucleus and the putamen while the corpus striatum consists of these 2 nuclei plus the globus pallidus.

- There are 2 parallel circuits (direct and indirect) through the basal ganglia. These circuits receive extensive input from the cerebral cortex that project back to the motor cortex after a relay in the ventrolateral (VL) nucleus of the thalamus. Both of these pathways demonstrate disinhibition. The direct pathway increases the level of cortical excitation and promotes movement. The indirect pathway decreases the level of cortical excitation and suppresses unwanted movement.

- The striatum is the major input center and the globus pallidus is the major output center for the pathways through the basal ganglia. Critical to proper function of the striatum is dopamine production by the substantia nigra. Dopamine excites the direct pathway and inhibits the indirect pathway.

- Lesions of the direct pathway result in an underactive cortex, which produces hypokinetic motor disturbances. The classic disorder caused by degeneration of dopaminergic neurons of the substantia nigra is Parkinson disease. These patients are characterized by tremor at rest (pill-rolling), increased muscle tone, mask face, and hypokinetic movement.

- Hyperkinetic disorders result from lesions of the indirect pathway and cause an overactive motor cortex. These movements occur spontaneously at rest and cannot be controlled by the patient. Examples of these disorders include chorea (multiple quick movements), athetosis (slow serpentine movements), and hemiballismus (violent flinging movements). Hemiballismus results from hemorrhagic destruction of the contralateral subthalamic nucleus.

Visual Pathways

8

Learning Objectives

❏ Use knowledge of eyeball and optic nerve

❏ Solve problems concerning visual reflexes

❏ Answer questions about lesions of the visual pathways

EYEBALL AND OPTIC NERVE

Light must pass through the cornea, aqueous humor, pupil, lens, and vitreous humor before reaching the retina (Figure III-8-1). It must then pass through the layers of the retina to reach the photoreceptive layer of rods and cones. The outer segments of rods and cones transduce light energy from photons into membrane potentials. Photopigments in rods and cones absorb photons, and this causes a conformational change in the molecular structure of these pigments. This molecular alteration causes sodium channels to close, a hyperpolarization of the membranes of the rods and cones, and a reduction in the amount of neurotransmitter released. Thus, rods and cones release less neurotransmitter in the light and more neurotransmitter in the dark.

Rods and cones have synaptic contacts on bipolar cells that project to ganglion cells (Figure III-8-2). Axons from the ganglion cells converge at the optic disc to form the optic nerve, which enters the cranial cavity through the optic foramen. At the optic disc, these axons acquire a myelin sheath from the oligodendrocytes of the central nervous system (CNS).

Clinical Correlate

Vitamin A, necessary for retinal transduction, cannot be synthesized by humans. Dietary deficiency of vitamin A causes visual impairment resulting in night blindness.

Clinicate Correlate

Decreased drainage into the canal of Schlemm is the most common cause of open-angle glaucoma.

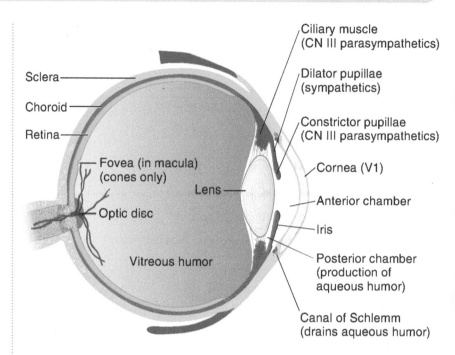

Figure III-8-1. The Eyeball

Labels (clockwise from top):
Ciliary muscle (CN III parasympathetics)
Dilator pupillae (sympathetics)
Constrictor pupillae (CN III parasympathetics)
Cornea (V1)
Anterior chamber
Iris
Posterior chamber (production of aqueous humor)
Canal of Schlemm (drains aqueous humor)
Lens
Vitreous humor
Optic disc
Fovea (in macula) (cones only)
Retina
Choroid
Sclera

Open-Angle Glaucoma

A chronic condition (often with increased intraocular pressure [IOP]) due to decreased reabsorption of aqueous humor, leading to progressive (painless) visual loss and, if left untreated, blindness. IOP is a balance between fluid formation and its drainage from the globe.

Narrow-Angle Glaucoma

An acute (painful) or chronic (genetic) condition with increased IOP due to blockade of the canal of Schlemm. Emergency treatment prior to surgery often involves cholinomimetics, carbonic anhydrase inhibitors, and/or mannitol.

VISUAL REFLEXES

Pupillary Light Reflex

When light is directed into an eye, it stimulates retinal photoreceptors and results in impulses carried in the optic nerve to the pretectal area. Cells in the pretectal area send axons to the Edinger-Westphal nuclei on both sides.

The Edinger-Westphal nucleus is the parasympathetic nucleus of the oculomotor nerve and gives rise to preganglionic parasympathetic fibers that pass in the third cranial nerve to the ciliary ganglion. Because cells in the pretectal area supply both Edinger-Westphal nuclei, shining light into one eye results in constriction of both the ipsilateral pupil (direct light reflex) and contralateral pupil (consensual light reflex).

Accommodation-Convergence Reaction

This reaction occurs when an individual attempts to focus on a nearby object after looking at a distant object. The oculomotor nerve carries the efferent fibers from the accommodation–convergence reaction, which consists of 3 components: accommodation, convergence, and pupillary constriction.

Accommodation refers to the reflex that increases the curvature of the lens needed for near vision. Preganglionic parasympathetic fibers arise in the Edinger-Westphal nucleus and pass via the oculomotor nerve to the ciliary ganglion. Postganglionic parasympathetic fibers from the ciliary ganglion supply the ciliary muscle. Contraction of this muscle relaxes the suspensory ligaments and allows the lens to increase its convexity (become more round). This increases the refractive index of the lens, permitting the image of a nearby object to focus on the retina.

Convergence results from contraction of both medial rectus muscles, which pull the eyes to look toward the nose. This allows the image of the near object to focus on the same part of the retina in each eye.

Pupillary constriction (miosis) results from contraction of the constrictor muscle of the iris. A smaller aperture gives the optic apparatus a greater depth of field. With Argyll Robertson pupils, both direct and consensual light reflexes are lost, but the accommodation–convergence reaction remains intact. This type of pupil is often seen in cases of neurosyphilis; however, it is sometimes seen in patients with multiple sclerosis, pineal tumors, or tabes dorsalis. The lesion site is believed to occur near the pretectal nuclei just rostral to the superior colliculi.

Table III-8-1. Pupillary Light Reflex Pathway

	Afferent Limb: CN II
Pretectal area Edinger-Westphal nucleus II III III II Pupil	Light stimulates ganglion retinal cells → impulses travel up **CNII**, which projects **bilaterally** to the **pretectal nuclei** (midbrain) The pretectal nucleus projects **bilaterally** → **Edinger-Westphal nuclei (CN III)**
	Efferent Limb: CN III
	Edinger-Westphal nucleus (preganglionic parasympathetic) → **ciliary ganglion** (postganglionic parasympathetic) → **pupillary sphincter muscle** → **miosis**

This is a simplified diagram; the ciliary ganglion is not shown.

Because cells in the pretectal area supply the Edinger-Westphal nuclei bilaterally, shining light in one eye → constriction in the ipsilateral pupil (direct light reflex) and the contralateral pupil (consensual light reflex).

Because this reflex does not involve the visual cortex, a person who is cortically blind can still have this reflex.

The eye is predominantly innervated by the parasympathetic nervous system. Therefore, application of muscarinic antagonists or ganglionic blockers has a large effect by blocking the parasympathetic nervous system.

Table III-8-2. Pharmacology of the Eye

Structure	Predominant Receptor	Receptor Stimulation	Receptor Blockade
Pupillary sphincter ms. (iris)	M_3 receptor (PANS)	Contraction → miosis	Relaxation → mydriasis
Radial dilator ms. (iris)	α receptor (SANS)	Contraction → mydriasis	Relaxation → miosis
Ciliary ms.	M_3 receptor (PANS)	Contraction → accommodation for near vision	Relaxation → focus for far vision
Ciliary body epithelium	β receptor (SANS)	Secretion of aqueous humor	Decreased aqueous humor production

Abbreviations: ms., muscle; PANS, parasympathetic nervous system; SANS, sympathetic nervous system

Table III-8-3. Accommodation–Convergence Reaction

When an individual focuses on a nearby object after looking at a distant object, 3 events occur:

1. Accommodation
2. Convergence
3. Pupillary constriction (miosis)

In general, stimuli from light → visual cortex → superior colliculus and pretectal nucleus → Edinger-Westphal nucleus (1, 3) and oculomotor nucleus (2).

Accommodation: Parasympathetic fibers contract the ciliary muscle, which relaxes suspensory ligaments, allowing the lens to increase its convexity (become more round). This increases the refractive index of the lens, thereby focusing a nearby object on the retina.

Convergence: Both medial rectus muscles contract, adducting both eyes.

Pupillary constriction: Parasympathetic fibers contract the pupillary sphincter muscle → miosis.

Table III-8-4. Clinical Correlates

Pupillary Abnormalities	
Argyll Robertson pupil (pupillary light-near dissociation)	• No direct or consensual light reflex; accommodation–convergence intact • Seen in **neurosyphilis**, diabetes
Relative afferent (Marcus Gunn) pupil	• Lesion of afferent limb of pupillary light reflex; diagnosis made with swinging flashlight • Shine light in Marcus Gunn pupil → pupils do not constrict fully • Shine light in normal eye → pupils constrict fully • Shine light immediately again in affected eye → apparent dilation of both pupils because stimulus carried through that CN II is weaker; seen in multiple sclerosis
Horner syndrome	• Caused by a lesion of the oculosympathetic pathway; syndrome consists of miosis, ptosis, apparent enophthalmos, and hemianhidrosis
Adie pupil	• Dilated pupil that reacts sluggishly to light, but better to accommodation; often seen in women and often associated with loss of knee jerks. Ciliary ganglion lesion
Transtentorial (uncal) herniation	• Increased intracranial pressure → leads to uncal herniation → CN III compression → fixed and dilated pupil, "down-and-out" eye, ptosis

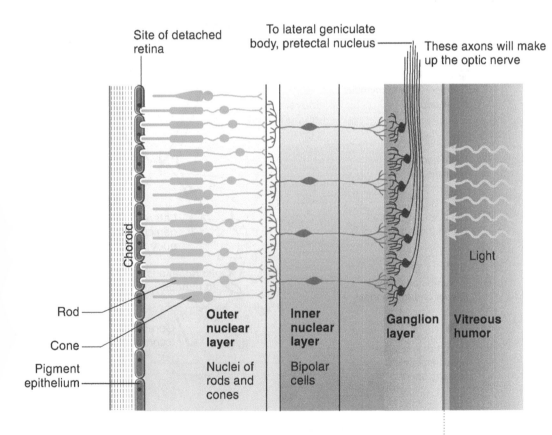

Figure III-8-2. Retina

Note:

Photoreceptor Rods: one kind

- Achromatic
- Low-light sensitive
- Night vision, motion

Cones: 3 kinds

- Red, green, blue
- Chromatic
- Bright light
- Sensitive
- Object recognition

Note

Visual information from **lower** retina courses in **lateral** fibers forming Meyer's **loop,** which projects to the lingual gyrus.

Clinical Correlate

Unilateral optic nerve lesions are seen in MS, where there is an immune-related inflammatory demyelination of the nerve. The lesion typically presents with a central scotoma due to involvement of the deep fibers in the nerve from the macula.

Note

Lesions to the visual radiations are more common than lesions to the optic tract.

At the optic chiasm, 60% of the optic nerve fibers from the nasal half of each retina cross and project into the contralateral optic tract (Figure III-8-3). Fibers from the temporal retina do not cross at the chiasm and instead pass into the ipsilateral optic tract. The optic tract contains remixed optic nerve fibers from the temporal part of the ipsilateral retina and fibers from the nasal part of the contralateral retina. Because the eye inverts images like a camera, in reality each nasal retina receives information from a temporal hemifield, and each temporal retina receives information from a nasal hemifield. Most fibers in the optic tract project to the lateral geniculate nucleus. Optic tract fibers also project to the superior colliculi for reflex gaze, to the pretectal area for the light reflex, and to the suprachiasmatic nucleus of the hypothalamus for circadian rhythms.

Visual Field Defects

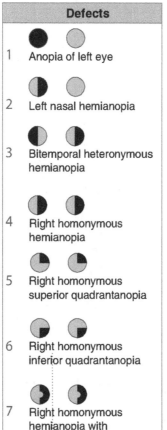

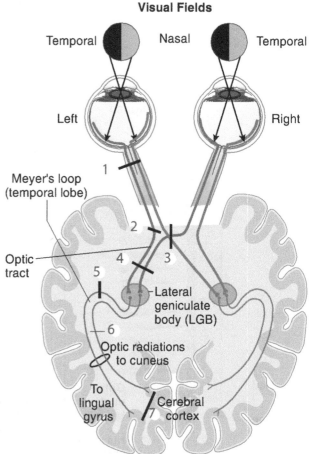

Figure III-8-3. Visual Pathways

1, 2 Optic nerve, 3 Chiasm, 4 Tract

Clinical Correlate

Some Causes of Lesions

1. Optic neuritis, central retinal artery occlusion
2. Internal carotid artery aneurysm
3. Pituitary adenoma (begins as superior quadrantanopia)
   Craniopharyngioma (begins as inferior quadrantanopia)
4. Vascular
5. Middle cerebral artery (MCA) occlusion
6, 7. Posterior cerebral artery occlusion
   Macula is spared in 7 due to collateral blood supply from MCA.

Notes

Like a camera, the lens inverts the image of the visual field, so the nasal retina receives information from the temporal visual field, and the temporal retina receives information from the nasal visual field.

At the **optic chiasm,** optic nerve fibers from the nasal half of each retina cross and project to the contralateral optic tract.

Most fibers from the **optic tract** project to the **lateral geniculate body (LGB)**; some also project to the pretectal area (light reflex), the superior colliculi (reflex gaze), and the suprachiasmatic nuclei (circadian rhythm). The LGB projects to the **primary visual cortex** (striate cortex, Brodmann area 17) of the occipital lobe via the optic radiations.

- Visual information from the lower retina (upper contralateral visual field) → temporal lobe (**Meyer loop**) → **lingual gyrus**
- Visual information from the upper retina (lower contralateral visual field) → parietal lobe → **cuneus gyrus**

The lateral geniculate body (LGB) is a laminated structure that receives input from the optic tract and gives rise to axons that terminate on cells in the primary visual cortex (striate cortex, Brodmann area 17) of the occipital lobe. The LGB laminae maintain a segregation of inputs from the ipsilateral and contralateral retina.

The axons from the LGB that project to the striate cortex are known as optic radiations, visual radiations, or the geniculocalcarine tract. The calcarine sulcus divides the striate cortex (primary visual cortex or Brodmann area 17) into the cuneus and the lingual gyri. The cuneus gyrus, which lies on the superior bank of the calcarine cortex, receives the medial fibers of the visual radiations. The lingual gyrus, which lies on the inferior bank of the calcarine cortex, receives the lateral fibers of the visual radiation. The medial fibers coursing in the visual radiations, which carry input from the upper retina (i.e., the lower contralateral visual field), pass from the LGB directly through the parietal lobe to reach the cuneus gyrus. Significantly, the lateral fibers coursing in the visual radiations, which carry input from the lower retina (i.e., the upper contralateral visual field), take a circuitous route from the LGB through Meyer loop anteriorly into the temporal lobe. The fibers of Meyer loop then turn posteriorly and course through the parietal lobe to reach the lingual gyrus in the striate cortex.

LESIONS OF THE VISUAL PATHWAYS

Lesions of the retina that include destruction of the macula produce a central scotoma. The macula is quite sensitive to intense light, trauma, aging, and neurotoxins.

Lesions of an optic nerve produce blindness (anopsia) in that eye and a loss of the sensory limb of the light reflex. The pupil of the affected eye constricts when light is shined into the opposite eye (consensual light reflex) but not when light is shined into the blinded eye (absence of direct light reflex).

Compression of the optic chiasm, often the result of a pituitary tumor or meningioma, results in a loss of peripheral vision in both temporal fields because the crossing fibers from each nasal retina are damaged. The resulting visual field defect is called a bitemporal heteronymous hemianopia.

All lesions past the chiasm produce contralateral defects. Lesions of the optic tract result in a loss of visual input from the contralateral visual field. For example, a lesion of the right optic tract results in a loss of input from the left visual field. This is called a homonymous hemianopia; in this example, a left homonymous hemianopia.

Lesions of the visual radiations are more common than lesions to the optic tract or lateral geniculate body and produce visual field defects (a contralateral homonymous hemianopia) similar to those of the optic tract if all fibers are involved.

Lesions restricted to the lateral fibers in Meyer loop, usually in the temporal lobe, result in a loss of visual input from the contralateral upper quarter of the visual field. For example, a lesion of the temporal fibers in the **right** visual radiation results in loss of visual input from the upper left quarter of the field (a **left** superior quadrantanopia).

Lesions restricted to the medial fibers in the visual radiation in the parietal lobe result in a loss of visual input from the contralateral lower quarter of the field (an inferior quadrantanopia).

Lesions inside the primary visual cortex are equivalent to those of the visual radiations, resulting in a contralateral homonymous hemianopsia, except that macular (central) vision is spared.

Lesions of the cuneus gyrus are equivalent to lesions restricted to the parietal fibers of the visual radiation, with macular sparing.

Lesions of the lingula are similar to lesions of the Meyer's loop fibers except for the presence of macular sparing. The pupillary light reflex is spared in lesions of the radiations or inside visual cortex because fibers of the pupillary light reflex leave the optic tracts to terminate in the pretectal area. The combination of blindness with intact pupillary reflexes is termed cortical blindness.

Chapter Summary

- The eyeball is formed by 3 layers: the sclera, choroid, and retina. The shape of the lens is modified for near and far vision by the ciliary muscle during the accommodation reflex. The sclera is the external layer and continues anteriorly as the cornea, which is transparent and allows light to enter the eye. The intermediate choroid layer is highly vascularized and pigmented. Anteriorly, the choroid layer forms the ciliary body and iris. The retina contains the photoreceptive layer of rods (for night vision and dim light) and cones (for color vision and high visual acuity).

- The axons of the ganglionic cells of the retina form the optic nerve at the optic disc.

- The visual pathway is a 3-neuron pathway with the first neuron (bipolar neurons) and the second neuron (ganglionic neurons) located in the retina. The ganglionic axons project from the retina through the optic nerve, optic chiasm, and optic tract to synapse with the third neuron located in the lateral geniculate body of the thalamus. These thalamic axons then project via the optic radiations (geniculocalcarine tract) in the parietal lobe to reach the primary visual (striate) cortex at the posterior pole of the occipital lobe. Because the lens inverts images like a camera, each nasal retina receives information from the temporal visual fields, and each temporal retina receives information from the nasal visual field. At the optic chiasm, the fibers from the nasal half of each retina decussate while the optic fibers from the temporal half of each retina pass through the chiasm without decussating. Thus, central to the chiasm ipsilateral visual fields project through the contralateral visual pathways. Lesions at the lateral aspect of the optic chiasm produce ipsilateral nasal hemianopsia, whereas midline lesions at the chiasm produce bitemporal heteronymous hemianopsia. Any lesion central to the chiasm results in contralateral homonymous hemianopsia.

- In addition, visual pathways carry optic fibers from the superior and inferior quadrants of the visual fields through the retina to the lateral geniculate body. The projections of the superior quadrants to the lower retina reach the lateral geniculate body laterally, synapse, and leave through the lateral course of Meyer loop in the temporal lobe before rejoining the optic radiation to reach the lower (lingual) gyrus of the striate cortex. Thus, lesions of the temporal lobe affecting Meyer loop result in contralateral homonymous superior quadrantanopia. Inferior quadrants of the visual fields project to the upper retina and then to the medial aspect of the lateral geniculate body. After synapsing in the geniculate body, the axons project completely through the optic radiations to reach the upper (cuneus) gyrus of the striate cortex. Lesions of these more medial fibers produce contralateral homonymous inferior quadrantanopia. Vascular lesions of the striate cortex due to occlusion of the posterior cerebral artery result in contralateral homonymous hemianopia with macular sparing.

Diencephalon 9

Learning Objectives

❑ Interpret scenarios on thalamus

❑ Demonstrate understanding of hypothalamus

❑ Use knowledge of epithalamus

The diencephalon can be divided into 4 parts: the thalamus, the hypothalamus, the epithalamus, and the subthalamus.

Diencephalon

Table III-9-1. Thala cerebellum mus

Thalamus—serves as a major sensory relay for information that ultimately reaches the neocortex. Motor control areas (basal ganglia, cerebellum) also synapse in the thalamus before reaching the cortex. Other nuclei regulate states of consciousness.

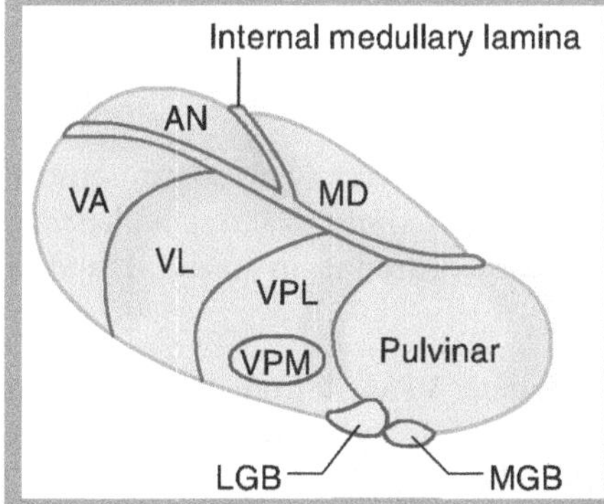

	Thalamic Nuclei	Input	Output
	VPL	Sensory from **body and limbs**	Somatosensory cortex
	VPM	Sensory from **face, taste**	Somatosensory cortex
	VA/VL	**Motor** info from BG, cerebellum	Motor cortices
	LGB	**Visual** from optic tract	First-degree visual cortex
	MGB	**Auditory** from inferior colliculus	First-degree auditory cortex
	AN	Mamillary nucleus (via mamillothalamic tract)	Cingulate gyrus (part of **Papez** circuit)
	MD	(Dorsomedial nucleus). Involved in **memory** Damaged in **Wernicke-Korsakoff** syndrome	
	Pulvinar	Helps integrate somesthetic, visual, and auditory input	
	Midline/intralaminar	Involved in **arousal**	

Diagram labels: Internal medullary lamina, AN, VA, MD, VL, VPL, VPM, Pulvinar, LGB, MGB

Abbreviations: AN, anterior nuclear group; BG, basal ganglia; LGB, lateral geniculate body; MD, mediodorsal nucleus; MGB, medial geniculate body; VA, ventral anterior nucleus; VL, ventral lateral nucleus; VPL, ventroposterolateral nucleus; VPM, ventroposteromedial nucleus

Clinical Correlate

Thiamine deficiency in alcoholics results in degeneration of the dorsomedial nucleus of thalamus and the mammillary bodies, hippocampus, and vermis of the cerebellum (see Chapter III-10).

Clinical Correlate

Thalamic pain syndrome affects the ventral nuclear group. Patients present with burning, aching pain in contralateral limbs or body. Involvement of the dorsal column-medial lemniscal part of VPL increases the sensitivity to pain and presents as contralateral loss of vibratory sense and gait ataxia. Thalamic pain syndrome is resistent to analgesic medications.

THALAMUS

The thalamus serves as the major sensory relay for the ascending tactile, visual, auditory, and gustatory information that ultimately reaches the neocortex. Motor control areas such as the basal ganglia and cerebellum also synapse in thalamic nuclei before they reach their cortical destinations. Other nuclei participate in the regulation of states of consciousness.

Major Thalamic Nuclei and Their Inputs and Outputs

Anterior nuclear group (part of the Papez circuit of limbic system)

Input is from the mammillary bodies via the mammillothalamic tract and from the cingulate gyrus; output is to the cingulate gyrus via the anterior limb of the internal capsule.

Medial nuclear group (part of limbic system)

Input is from the amygdala, prefrontal cortex, and temporal lobe; output is to the prefrontal cortex and cingulate gyrus. The most important nucleus is the dorso-medial nucleus.

Ventral nuclear group

Motor Nuclei

Ventral anterior nucleus (VA): Input to VA is from the globus pallidus, substantia nigra. Output is to the premotor and primary motor cortex.

Ventral lateral nucleus (VL): Input to VL is mainly from the globus pallidus and the dentate nucleus of the cerebellum. Output is to the primary motor cortex (Brodmann area 4).

Sensory Nuclei

Ventral posterolateral (VPL) nucleus: Input to VPL conveying somatosensory and nociceptive information ascends in the medial lemniscus and spinothalamic tract. Output is to primary somatosensory cortex (Brodmann areas 3, 1, and 2) of the parietal lobe.

Ventral posteromedial (VPM) nucleus: Input to VPM is from the ascending trigeminal and taste pathways. Output is to primary somatosensory cortex (Brodmann areas 3, 1, and 2) of the parietal lobe.

Medial geniculate body (nucleus): Input is from auditory information that ascends from the inferior colliculus. Output is to primary auditory cortex.

Lateral geniculate body (nucleus): Input is from the optic tract. Output is in the form of the geniculocalcarine or visual radiations that project to the primary visual (striate) cortex in the occipital lobe.

Midline and Intralaminar Nuclei

Midline and intralaminar nuclei receive input from the brain-stem reticular formation, and from the spinothalamic tract. Intralaminar nuclei send pain information to the cingulate gyrus.

These nuclei appear to be important in mediating desynchronization of the electroencephalogram (EEG) during behavioral arousal.

HYPOTHALAMUS

The hypothalamus is composed of numerous nuclei that have afferent and efferent connections with widespread regions of the nervous system, including the pituitary gland, the autonomic system, and the limbic system (Figure III-9-1).

Table III-9-2. Hypothalamus, Epithalamus, Subthalamus

Hypothalamus—helps maintain homeostasis; has roles in the autonomic, endocrine, and limbic systems	
Hypothalamic Nuclei	Functions and Lesions
Lateral hypothalamic	**Feeding center;** lesion → starvation
Ventromedial	**Satiety center;** lesion → hyperphagia, obesity, savage behavior
Suprachiasmatic	Regulates circadian rhythms, receives direct retinal input
Supraoptic and paraventricular	Synthesizes **ADH** and **oxytocin; regulates water balance** Lesion → **diabetes insipidus,** characterized by polydipsia and polyuria
Mamillary body	Input from hippocampus; damaged in Wernicke encephalopathy
Arcuate	Produces hypothalamic releasing and inhibiting factors and gives rise to tuberohypophysial tract Has neurons that produce dopamine (prolactin-inhibiting factor)
Anterior region	**Temperature regulation;** lesion → hyperthermia Stimulates the parasympathetic nervous system
Posterior region	**Temperature regulation;** lesion → poikilothermia (inability to thermoregulate) Stimulates sympathetic nervous system
Preoptic area	Regulates release of gonotrophic hormones; contains sexually dimorphic nucleus Lesion before puberty → arrested sexual development; lesion after puberty → amenorrhea or impotence
Dorsomedial	Stimulation → savage behavior
Epithalamus—Consists of pineal body and habenular nuclei. The **pineal body** secretes melatonin with a **circadian rhythm.**	
Subthalamus—The **subthalamic nucleus** is involved in **basal ganglia** circuitry. Lesion → **hemiballismus** (contralateral flinging movements of one or both extremities)	

Abbreviation: ADH, antidiuretic hormone

Major Hypothalamic Regions or Zones, and Their Nuclei

Clinical Correlate

Dopaminergic projections from the arcuate nuclei inhibit prolactin secretion from the anterior pituitary. Lesions result in galactorrhea (milk discharge) and amenorrhea.

Clinical Correlate

Korsakoff Syndrome

Lesions of the mammillary bodies occur in Korsakoff syndrome and are usually associated with thiamine deficiency associated with chronic alcoholism. Korsakoff syndrome results in both anterograde and retrograde amnesia with confabulations.

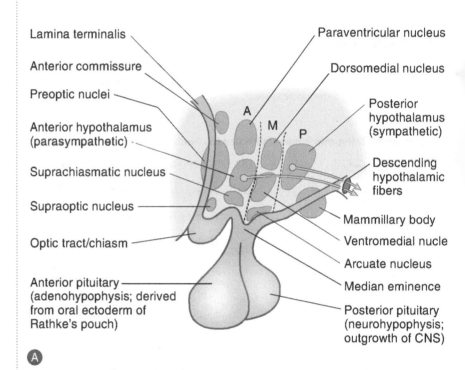

Lamina terminalis
Anterior commissure
Preoptic nuclei
Anterior hypothalamus (parasympathetic)
Suprachiasmatic nucleus
Supraoptic nucleus
Optic tract/chiasm
Anterior pituitary (adenohypophysis; derived from oral ectoderm of Rathke's pouch)

Paraventricular nucleus
Dorsomedial nucleus
Posterior hypothalamus (sympathetic)
Descending hypothalamic fibers
Mammillary body
Ventromedial nucle
Arcuate nucleus
Median eminence
Posterior pituitary (neurohypophysis; outgrowth of CNS)

A

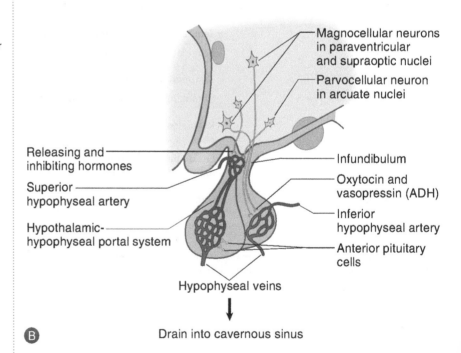

Releasing and inhibiting hormones
Superior hypophyseal artery
Hypothalamic-hypophyseal portal system

Magnocellular neurons in paraventricular and supraoptic nuclei
Parvocellular neuron in arcuate nuclei
Infundibulum
Oxytocin and vasopressin (ADH)
Inferior hypophyseal artery
Anterior pituitary cells

Hypophyseal veins
↓
Drain into cavernous sinus

B

Figure III-9-1. (A) Organization of the Hypothalamus (Sagittal Section) (B) Secretory Mechanisms of the Adeno- and Neuro-Hypophysis

Anterior region

Paraventricular and Supraoptic Nuclei

These nuclei synthesize the neuropeptides antidiuretic hormone (ADH) and oxytocin. Axons arising from these nuclei leave the hypothalamus and course in the supraopticohypophysial tract, which carries neurosecretory granules to the posterior pituitary gland, where they are released into capillaries. Lesions of the supraoptic nuclei lead to diabetes insipidus, which is characterized by polydipsia (excess water consumption) and polyuria (excess urination).

Suprachiasmatic Nucleus

Visual input from the retina by way of the optic tract terminates in the suprachiasmatic nucleus. This information helps set certain body rhythms to the 24-hour light-dark cycle (circadian rhythms).

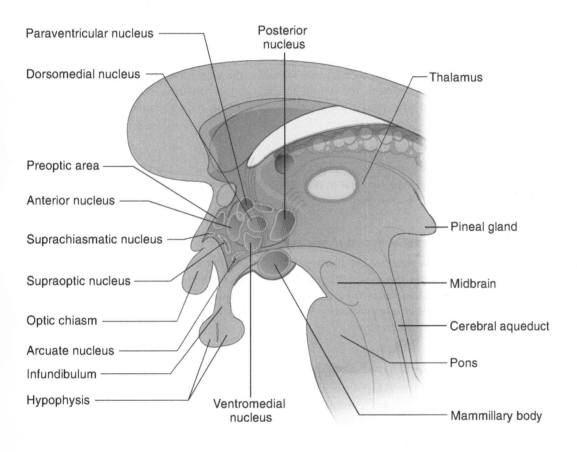

Figure III-9-2. The Hypothalamic Nuclei

Tuberal region

Arcuate Nucleus

Cells in the arcuate nucleus produce releasing hormones and inhibitory factors, which enter capillaries in the tuberoinfundibular tract and pass through the hypophyseal-portal veins to reach the secondary capillary plexus in the anterior pituitary gland. Releasing hormones and inhibitory factors influence the secretory activity of the acidophils and basophils in the anterior pituitary. (See Histology section.)

Ventromedial Nucleus

The ventromedial hypothalamus is a satiety center and regulates food intake. Lesions of the ventromedial hypothalamus result in obesity.

Posterior region

Mammillary Bodies

The mammillary nuclei are located in the mammillary bodies and are part of the limbic system. The mammillothalamic tract originates in the mammillary nuclei and terminates in the anterior nuclear group of the thalamus.

Anterior hypothalamic zone

The anterior hypothalamic zone senses an elevation of body temperature and mediates the response to dissipate heat. Lesions of the anterior hypothalamus lead to hyperthermia.

Posterior hypothalamic zone

The posterior hypothalamic zone senses a decrease of body temperature and mediates the conservation of heat. Lesions of the posterior hypothalamus lead to poikilothermy (i.e., cold-blooded organisms). An individual with a lesion of the posterior hypothalamus has a body temperature that varies with the environmental temperature.

Lateral hypothalamic zone

The lateral hypothalamic zone is a feeding center; lesions of the lateral hypothalamus produce severe aphagia.

Preoptic area

The preoptic area is sensitive to androgens and estrogens, whereas other areas influence the production of sex hormones through their regulation of the anterior pituitary. Before puberty, hypothalamic lesions here may arrest sexual development.

After puberty, hypothalamic lesions in this area may result in amenorrhea or impotence.

EPITHALAMUS

The epithalamus is the part of the diencephalon located in the region of the posterior commissure that consists of the pineal body and the habenular nuclei.

The pineal body is a small, highly vascularized structure situated above the posterior commissure and attached by a stalk to the roof of the third ventricle.

The pineal body contains pinealocytes and glial cells but no neurons. Pinealocytes synthesize melatonin, serotonin, and cholecystokinin.

The pineal gland plays a role in growth, development, and the regulation of circadian rhythms.

Environmental light regulates the activity of the pineal gland through a retinal–suprachiasmatic– pineal pathway.

The subthalamus is reviewed with the basal ganglia.

Clinical Correlate

Precocious Puberty

In young males, pineal lesions may cause precocious puberty.

Pineal Tumors

Pineal tumors may cause obstruction of CSF flow and increased intracranial pressure. Compression of the upper midbrain and pretectal area by a pineal tumor results in Parinaud syndrome, in which there is impairment of conjugate vertical gaze and pupillary reflex abnormalities.

Chapter Summary

- The diencephalon is divided into 4 parts: thalamus, hypothalamus, epithalamus, and subthalamus.

- The thalamus is the major sensory relay for many sensory systems. The long tracks of spinal cord and the trigeminal system synapse in the ventral posterolateral (VPL) and ventral posteromedial (VPM) nuclei, respectively. Auditory input is to the medial geniculate body, and the visual input is to the lateral geniculate body. Motor projections from the basal ganglia and cerebellum synapse in the ventral anterior and ventral lateral nuclei.

- The hypothalamus contains nuclei that have fiber connections with many areas of the nervous system, including the pituitary gland in the anterior and tuberal regions of the hypothalamus. Other areas control eating, drinking, body temperature, and provide connections with the limbic system.

- The epithalamus consists mainly of the pineal gland, which plays a major role in the regulation of circadian rhythms.

- The subthalamic projections are important circuits related to the basal ganglia.

Cerebral Cortex 10

Learning Objectives

❏ Answer questions about general features

❏ Solve problems concerning language and the dominant hemisphere

❏ Solve problems concerning blood supply

GENERAL FEATURES

The surface of the cerebral cortex is highly convoluted with the bulges or eminences, referred to as gyri; and the spaces separating the gyri, called sulci (Figures III-10-1 and III-10-2). Lobes of the cerebrum are divided according to prominent gyri and sulci that are fairly constant in humans.

Two prominent sulci on the lateral surface are key to understanding the divisions of the hemispheres. The lateral fissure (of Sylvius) separates the frontal and temporal lobes rostrally; further posteriorly, it partially separates the parietal and the temporal lobes. The central sulcus (of Rolando) is situated roughly perpendicular to the lateral fissure. The central sulcus separates the frontal and the parietal lobes. The occipital lobe extends posteriorly from the temporal and parietal lobes, but its boundaries on the lateral aspect of the hemisphere are indistinct. On the medial aspect of the hemisphere, the frontal and parietal lobes are separated by a cingulate sulcus from the cingulate gyrus. The cingulate is part of an artificial limbic lobe. Posteriorly, the parieto-occipital sulcus separates the parietal lobe from the occipital lobe. The calcarine sulcus divides the occipital lobe horizontally into a superior cuneus and an inferior lingual gyrus.

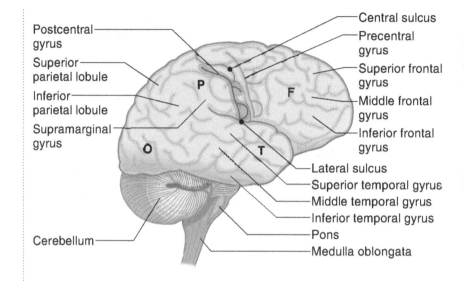

F: frontal lobe
P: parietal lobe
T: temporal lobe
O: occipital lobe

Postcentral gyrus
Superior parietal lobule
Inferior parietal lobule
Supramarginal gyrus
Cerebellum

Central sulcus
Precentral gyrus
Superior frontal gyrus
Middle frontal gyrus
Inferior frontal gyrus
Lateral sulcus
Superior temporal gyrus
Middle temporal gyrus
Inferior temporal gyrus
Pons
Medulla oblongata

Figure III-10-1. Lateral View of the Right Cerebral Hemisphere

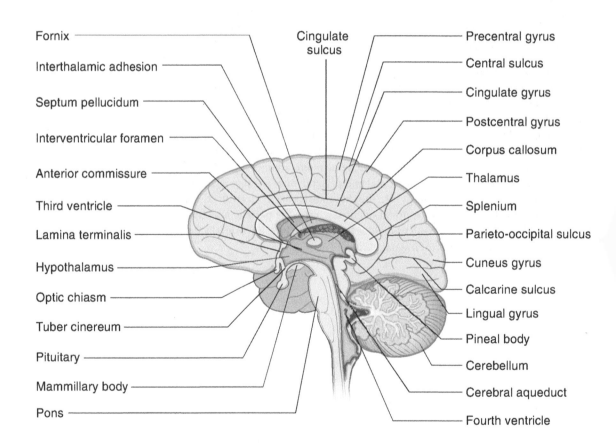

Fornix
Interthalamic adhesion
Septum pellucidum
Interventricular foramen
Anterior commissure
Third ventricle
Lamina terminalis
Hypothalamus
Optic chiasm
Tuber cinereum
Pituitary
Mammillary body
Pons

Cingulate sulcus

Precentral gyrus
Central sulcus
Cingulate gyrus
Postcentral gyrus
Corpus callosum
Thalamus
Splenium
Parieto-occipital sulcus
Cuneus gyrus
Calcarine sulcus
Lingual gyrus
Pineal body
Cerebellum
Cerebral aqueduct
Fourth ventricle

Figure III-10-2. Medial View of the Right Cerebral Hemisphere

About 90% of the cortex is composed of 6 layers, which form the neocortex (Figure III-10-5). The olfactory cortex and hippocampal formation are 3-layered structures and together comprise the allocortex. All of the neocortex contains a

6-layer cellular arrangement, but the actual structure varies considerably between different locations. On the basis of these variations in the cytoarchitecture, Brodmann divided the cortex into 47 areas, but only a few Brodmann numbers are used synonymously with functionally specific cortical areas.

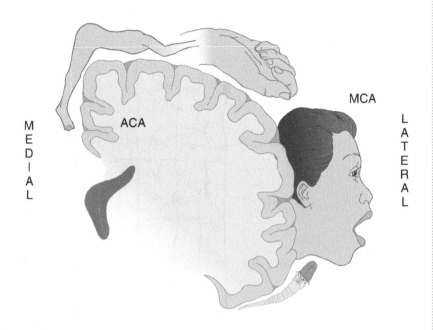

Figure III-10-3. Motor Homunculus in Precentral Gyrus (Area 4) Frontal Lobe (Coronal Section)

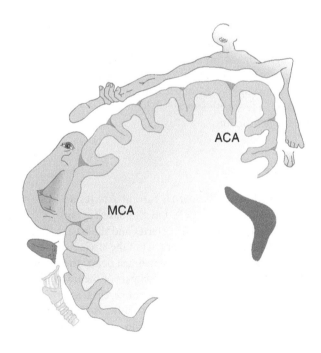

Figure III-10-4. Sensory Homunculus in Postcentral Gyrus (Areas 3, 1, 2) Parietal Lobe (Coronal Section)

Note

The internal granular layer is the site of termination of the thalamocortical projections. In primary visual cortex, these fibers form a distinct Line of Gennari. The internal pyramidal layer gives rise to axons that form the corticospinal and corticobulbar tracts.

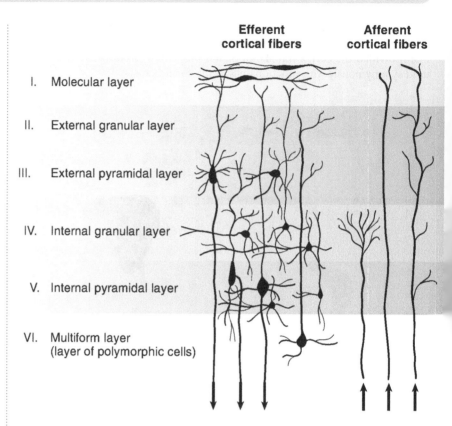

Figure III-10-5. The Six-Layered Neocortex

LANGUAGE AND THE DOMINANT HEMISPHERE

Most people (about 80%) are right-handed, which implies that the left side of the brain has more highly developed hand-controlling circuits. In the vast majority of right-handed people, speech and language functions are also predominantly organized in the left hemisphere. Most left-handed people show language functions bilaterally, although a few, with strong left-handed preferences, show right-sided speech and language functions.

BLOOD SUPPLY

The cortex is supplied by the 2 internal carotid arteries and the 2 vertebral arteries (Figures III-10-6 and III-10-7). On the base (or inferior surface) of the brain, branches of the internal carotid arteries and the basilar artery anastomose to form the circle of Willis. The anterior part of the circle lies in front of the optic chiasm, whereas the posterior part is situated just below the mammillary bodies. The circle of Willis is formed by the terminal part of the internal carotid arteries; the proximal parts of the anterior and posterior cerebral arteries and the anterior and posterior communicating arteries. The middle, anterior, and posterior cerebral arteries, which arise from the circle of Willis, supply all of the cerebral cortex, basal ganglia, and diencephalon.

The internal carotid artery arises from the bifurcation of the common carotid and enters the skull through the carotid canal. It enters the subarachnoid space and terminates by dividing into the anterior and middle cerebral arteries.

Just before splitting into the middle and anterior cerebral arteries, the internal carotid artery gives rise to the ophthalmic artery. The ophthalmic artery enters the orbit through the optic canal and supplies the eye, including the retina and optic nerve.

The middle cerebral artery is the larger terminal branch of the internal carotid artery. It supplies the bulk of the lateral surface of the hemisphere. Exceptions are the superior inch of the frontal and parietal lobes, which are supplied by the anterior cerebral artery, and the inferior part of the temporal lobe and the occipital pole, which are supplied by the posterior cerebral artery. The middle cerebral artery also supplies the genu and posterior limb of the internal capsule and the basal ganglia.

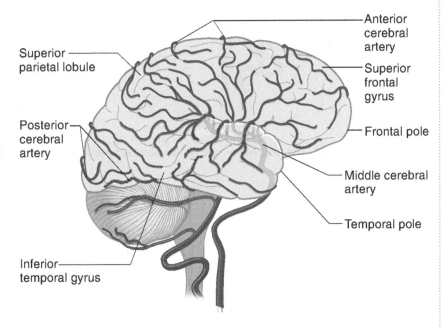

Figure III-10-6. The Distributions of the Cerebral Arteries: Part 1

The anterior cerebral artery is the smaller terminal branch of the internal carotid artery. It is connected to the opposite anterior cerebral artery by the anterior communicating artery, completing the anterior part of the circle of Willis. The anterior cerebral artery supplies the medial surface of the frontal and parietal lobes, which include motor and sensory cortical areas for the pelvis and lower limbs. The anterior cerebral artery also supplies the anterior four-fifths of the corpus callosum and approximately 1 inch of the frontal and parietal cortex on the superior aspect of the lateral aspect of the hemisphere.

Occlusion of the anterior cerebral artery results in spastic paresis of the contralateral lower limb and anesthesia of the contralateral lower limb. Urinary incontinence may be present, but this usually occurs only with bilateral damage. A transcortical apraxia of the left limbs may result from involvement of the anterior portion of the corpus callosum. A transcortical apraxia occurs because the left hemisphere (language dominant) has been disconnected from the motor cortex of the right hemisphere. The anterior cerebral artery also supplies the anterior limb of the internal capsule.

Clinical Correlate

Occlusion of the middle cerebral artery results in spastic paresis of the contralateral lower face and upper limb and anesthesia of the contralateral face and upper limb.

An aphasia (e.g., Broca, Wernicke, or conduction) may result when branches of the left middle cerebral artery are affected, and left-sided neglect may be seen with a blockage of branches of the right middle cerebral artery to the right parietal lobe.

The middle cerebral artery also supplies the proximal parts of the visual radiations as they emerge from the lateral geniculate nucleus of the thalamus and course in Meyer's loop. These fibers course into the temporal lobe before looping posteriorly to rejoin the rest of the visual radiation fibers.

Occlusion of the branches that supply Meyer's loop fibers in the temporal lobe results in a contralateral superior quadrantanopsia.

Note

The middle cerebral artery (MCA) supplies:

- the lateral surface of the frontal, parietal, and upper temporal lobes
- the posterior limb and genu of the internal capsule
- most of the basal ganglia

Note

The anterior cerebral artery (ACA) Supplies:

1. Medial surface of frontal and parietal lobes

2. Anterior four-fifths of corpus callosum

3. Anterior limb of internal capsule

The posterior cerebral artery (PCA) Supplies:

1. Occipital lobe

2. Lower temporal lobe

3. Splenium

4. Midbrain

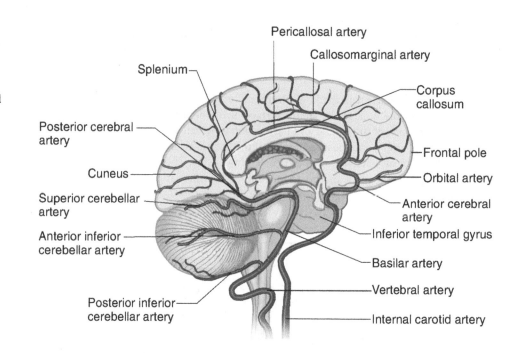

Figure III-10-7. The Distributions of the Cerebral Arteries: Part 2

Clinical Correlate

The most common aneurysm site in the circle of Willis is where the anterior communicating artery joins an anterior cerebral artery.

Circle of Willis
Anterior communicating
Anterior cerebral
Internal carotid
Posterior communicating
Posterior cerebral (medial midbrain)

Middle cerebral

Superior cerebellar (lateral pons)

Basilar

Vertebral

Anterior spinal (medial medulla)

Paramedian (medial pons)

Anterior inferior cerebellar (lateral pons)

Posterior inferior cerebellar (lateral medulla)

Figure III-10-8. Arterial Supply of the Brain

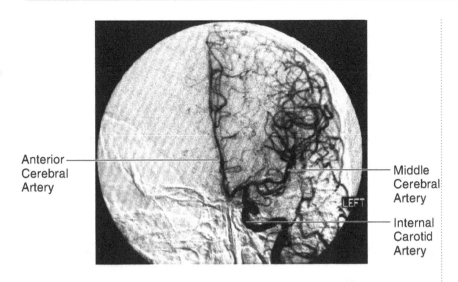

Figure III-10-9. Anteroposterior View of Left Internal Carotid

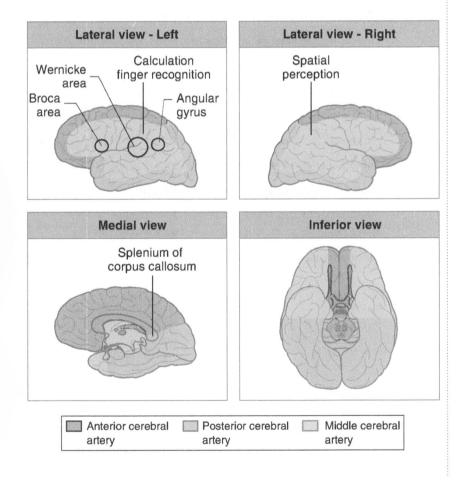

Figure III-10-10. Territories Supplied by the Cerebral Arteries

The posterior cerebral artery is formed by the terminal bifurcation of the basilar artery. The posterior communicating artery arises near the termination of the internal carotid artery and passes posteriorly to join the posterior cerebral artery. The posterior communicating arteries complete the circle of Willis by joining the vertebrobasilar and carotid circulations. The posterior cerebral artery supplies the occipital and temporal cortex on the inferior and lateral surfaces of the hemisphere, the occipital lobe and posterior 2/3 of the temporal lobe on the medial surface of the hemisphere, and the thalamus and subthalamic nucleus.

Occlusion of the posterior cerebral artery results in a homonymous hemianopia of the contralateral visual field with macular sparing.

Table III-10-1. Cerebrovascular Disorders

Disorder	Types	Key Concepts
Cerebral infarcts	Thrombotic	**Anemic/pale** infarct; usually atherosclerotic complication
	Embolic	**Hemorrhagic/red** infarct; from heart or atherosclerotic plaques; **middle cerebral artery** most vulnerable to emboli
	Hypotension	**"Watershed"** areas and **deep cortical layers** most affected
	Hypertension	**Lacunar** infarcts; **basal ganglia**, internal capsule, and pons most affected
Hemorrhages	Epidural hematoma	Almost always traumatic Rupture of **middle meningeal artery** after skull fracture Lucid interval before loss of consciousness ("talk and die" syndrome)
	Subdural hematoma	Usually caused by trauma Rupture of **bridging veins** (drain brain to dural sinuses)
	Subarachnoid hemorrhage	**Ruptured berry aneurysm** is most frequent cause Predisposing factors: Marfan syndrome, Ehlers-Danlos type 4, adult polycystic kidney disease, hypertension, smoking
	Intracerebral hemorrhage	Common causes: hypertension, trauma, infarction

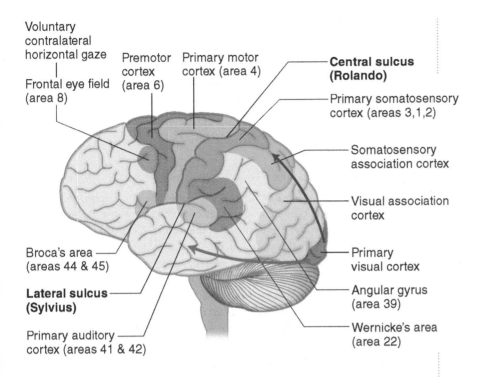

Figure III-10-11. Cerebral Cortex: Functional Areas of
Left (Dominant) Hemisphere

Frontal Lobe

A large part of the frontal cortex rostral to the central sulcus is related to the control of movements, primarily on the opposite side of the body. These areas include primary motor cortex (Brodmann area 4), premotor cortex (area 6), the frontal eye field (area 8), and the motor speech areas of Broca (area 44 and 45). Traditionally, area 4 is considered the primary motor cortex. It is in the precentral gyrus, immediately anterior to the central sulcus, and contains an orderly skeletal motor map of the contralateral side of the body.

The muscles of the head are represented most ventrally closest to the lateral fissure; then, proceeding dorsally, are the regions for the neck, upper limb, and trunk on the lateral aspect of the hemisphere. On the medial aspect of the hemisphere is the motor representation for the pelvis and lower limb.

Premotor cortex

Just anterior to area 4 is the premotor cortex (area 6). Neurons here are particularly active prior to the activation of area 4 neurons, so it is thought that the premotor cortex is involved in the planning of motor activities. Damage here results in an apraxia, a disruption of the patterning and execution of learned motor movements. Individual movements are intact, and there is no weakness, but the patient is unable to perform movements in the correct sequence.

Clinical Correlate

Lesion of the Frontal Eye Field

The frontal eye field lies in front of the motor cortex in Brodmann area 8. This cortical area is the center for contralateral horizontal gaze. A lesion here results in an inability to make voluntary eye movements toward the contralateral side. Because the activity of the intact frontal eye field in the opposite cortex would also be unopposed after such a lesion, the result is conjugate slow deviation of the eyes toward the side of the lesion.

If motor cortex is involved in the lesion, the patient may have a contralateral spastic paresis. The intact frontal eye field in the opposite hemisphere deviates the eyes **away** from the paralyzed limbs.

Prefrontal cortex

The prefrontal cortex is located in front of the premotor area and represents about a quarter of the entire cerebral cortex in the human brain. This area is involved in organizing and planning the intellectual and emotional aspects of behavior, much as the adjacent premotor cortex is involved in planning its motor aspects.

Clinical Correlate

Lesions in the Prefrontal Area

Lesions in the prefrontal area produce what is called the frontal lobe syndrome. The patient cannot concentrate and is easily distracted; there is a general lack of initiative, foresight, and perspective. Another common aspect is apathy (i.e., severe emotional indifference). Apathy is usually associated with abulia, a slowing of intellectual faculties, slow speech, and decreased participation in social interactions. Prefrontal lesions also result in the emergence of infantile suckling or grasp reflexes that are suppressed in adults. In the suckling reflex, touching the cheek causes the head to turn toward the side of the stimulus as the mouth searches for a nipple to suckle. In the grasp reflex, touching the palm of the hand results in a reflex closing of the fingers, which allows an infant to grasp anything that touches the hand.

Clinical Correlate

Expressive Aphasia

Broca area is just anterior to the motor cortex region that provides upper motoneuron innervation of cranial nerve motor nuclei. This area in the left or dominant hemisphere is the center for motor speech and corresponds to Brodmann areas 44 and 45. Damage to Broca area produces a motor, nonfluent, or expressive aphasia that reflects a difficulty in piecing together words to produce expressive speech. Patients with this lesion can understand written and spoken language but normally say almost nothing. When pressed on a question such as "What did you do today?" they might reply "Went town." The ability to write is usually also affected in a similar way (agraphia) in all aphasias, although the hand used for writing can be used normally in all other tasks. Patients are keenly aware of and frustrated by an expressive aphasia, because of their lack of the ability to verbalize their thoughts orally or in writing.

Broca area damage often extends posteriorly into the primary motor cortex and might be combined with a contralateral paralysis of the muscles of the lower face, resulting in a drooping of the corner of the mouth. If the lesion is larger, the patient might have a spastic hemiparesis of the contralateral upper limb.

Parietal Lobe

Primary somatosensory cortex

The parietal lobe begins just posterior to the central sulcus with the postcentral gyrus. The postcentral gyrus corresponds to Brodmann areas 3, 1, and 2 and contains primary somatosensory cortex. Like primary motor cortex, there is a similar somatotopic representation of the body here, with head, neck, upper limb, and trunk represented on the lateral aspect of the hemisphere, and pelvis and lower limb represented medially. These areas are concerned with discriminative touch, vibration, position sense, pain, and temperature. Lesions in somatosensory cortex result in impairment of all somatic sensations on the opposite side of the body, including the face and scalp.

Posterior parietal association cortex

Just posterior and ventral to the somatosensory areas is the posterior parietal association cortex, including Brodmann areas 5 and 7.

Clinical Correlate

Lesions, usually in the dominant hemisphere and which include areas 5 and 7 of the posterior parietal association areas, often result in apraxia (also seen with lesions to the premotor cortex). Apraxia is a disruption of the patterning and execution of learned motor movements. This deficit seems to reflect a lack of understanding how to organize the performance of a pattern of movements (i.e., what should be done first, then next, etc.). The patient may be unable, for example, to draw a simple diagram (constructional apraxia) or describe how to get from his home to his work.

Another deficit, with lesions of areas 5 and 7 is astereognosia (inability to recognize objects by touch). There is no loss of tactile or proprioceptive sensation; rather, it is the integration of visual and somatosensory information that is impaired. Both apraxia and astereognosia are more common after left hemisphere damage than in right hemisphere damage. The astereognosia is usually confined to the contralateral side of the body; in contrast, apraxia is usually bilateral. Apraxia is probably a result of the loss of input to the premotor cortex (area 6), which is involved in the actual organization of motor movements into a goal-directed pattern.

Wernicke area

The inferior part of the parietal lobe and adjacent part of the temporal lobe in the dominant (left) hemisphere, known as Wernicke area, are cortical regions that function in language comprehension. At a minimum, Wernicke area consists of area 22 in the temporal lobe but may also include areas 39 and 40 in the parietal lobe. Areas 39 (the angular gyrus) and 40 (the supramarginal gyrus) are regions of convergence of visual, auditory, and somatosensory information.

Note

Any blockage of the left middle cerebral artery that results in an aphasia (Broca Wernicke, conduction) or Gerstmann syndrome will also result in **agraphia**.

Clinical Correlate

Receptive Aphasia

Lesions in area 22 in the temporal lobe and area 39 or 40 in the parietal lobe produce a fluent, receptive, or Wernicke aphasia. The patient with Wernicke aphasia cannot comprehend spoken language and may or may not be able to read (alexia) depending on the extent of the lesion. The deficit is characterized by fluent verbalization but lacks meaning. Patients are paraphasic, often misusing words as if speaking using a "word salad."

Patients with Wernicke aphasia are generally unaware of their deficit and show no distress as a result of their condition.

Gerstmann Syndrome

If the lesion is confined to just the angular gyrus (area 39), the result is a loss of ability to comprehend written language (alexia) and to write it (agraphia), but spoken language may be understood. Alexia with agraphia in pure angular gyrus lesions is often seen with 3 other unique symptoms: acalculia (loss of the ability to perform simple arithmetic problems), finger agnosia (inability to recognize one's fingers), and right–left disorientation. This constellation of deficits constitutes Gerstmann syndrome and underscores the role of this cortical area in the integration of how children begin to count, add, and subtract using their fingers.

Conduction Aphasia

There is a large fiber bundle connecting areas 22, 39, and 40 with Broca area in the frontal lobe, known as the superior longitudinal fasciculus (or the arcuate fasciculus). A lesion affecting this fiber bundle results in a conduction aphasia. In this patient, verbal output is fluent, but there are many paraphrases and word-finding pauses. Both verbal and visual language comprehension are also normal, but if asked to, the patient cannot repeat words or execute verbal commands by an examiner (such as "Count backwards beginning at 100") and also demonstrates poor object naming. This is an example of a disconnect syndrome in which the deficit represents an inability to send information from one cortical area to another. As with an expressive aphasia, these patients are aware of the deficit and are frustrated by their inability to execute a verbal command that they fully understand.

Transcortical Apraxia

Lesions to the corpus callosum caused by an infarct of the anterior cerebral artery may result in another type of disconnect syndrome known as a transcortical apraxia. As in other cases of apraxia, there is no motor weakness, but the patient cannot execute a command to move the left arm. They understand the command, which is perceived in the Wernicke area of the left hemisphere, but the callosal lesion disconnects the Wernicke area from the right primary motor cortex so that the command cannot be executed. The patient is still able to execute a command to move the right arm because Wernicke area in the left hemisphere is able to communicate with the left primary motor cortex without using the corpus callosum.

(Continued)

Clinical Correlate (*Continued*)

Asomatognosia

The integration of visual and somatosensory information is important for the formation of the "body image" and awareness of the body and its position in space. Widespread lesions in areas 7, 39, and 40 in the nondominant right parietal lobe may result in unawareness or neglect of the contralateral half of the body, known as asomatognosia. Although somatic sensation is intact, the patients ignore half of their body and may fail to dress, undress, or wash the affected (left) side. Patients will have no visual field deficits, so they can see, but deny the existence of things in the left visual field. Asking them to bisect a horizontal line produces a point well to the right of true center. If asked to draw a clock face from memory, they will draw only the numbers on the right side, ignoring those on the left. Patients may deny that the left arm or leg belongs to them when the affected limb is passively brought into their field of vision. Patients may also deny their deficit, an anosognosia.

Occipital Lobe

The occipital lobe is essential for the reception and recognition of visual stimuli and contains primary visual and visual association cortex.

Visual cortex

The visual cortex is divided into striate (area 17) and extrastriate (areas 18 and 19). Area 17, also referred to as the primary visual cortex, lies on the medial portion of the occipital lobe on either side of the calcarine sulcus. Its major thalamic input is from the lateral geniculate nucleus. Some input fibers are gathered in a thick bundle that can be visible on the cut surface of the gross brain, called the line of Gennari. The retinal surface (and therefore the visual field) is represented in an orderly manner on the surface of area 17, such that damage to a discrete part of area 17 will produce a scotoma (i.e., a blind spot) in the corresponding portion of the visual field. A unilateral lesion inside area 17 results in a contralateral homonymous hemianopsia with macular sparing, usually caused by an infarct of a branch of the posterior cerebral artery. The area of the macula of the retina containing the fovea is spared because of a dual blood supply from both the posterior and middle cerebral arteries. The actual cortical area serving the macula is represented in the most posterior part of the occipital lobe. Blows to the back of the head or a blockage in occipital branches of the middle cerebral artery that supply this area may produce loss of macular representation of the visual fields. Bilateral visual cortex lesions result in cortical blindness; the patient cannot see, but pupillary reflexes are intact.

Visual association cortex

Anterior to the primary visual or striate cortex are extensive areas of visual association cortex. Visual association cortex is distributed throughout the entire occipital lobe and in the posterior parts of the parietal and temporal lobes. These regions receive fibers from the striate cortex and integrate complex visual input from both hemispheres. From the retina to the visual association cortex, information about form and color, versus motion, depth and spatial information are processed separately. Form and color information is processed by the parvocellular-blob system. This "cone stream" originates mainly in the central part of the retina, relays through separate layers of the lateral geniculate, and projects to blob zones of primary visual cortex. Blob zones project to the inferior part of the temporal lobe in areas 20 and 21. Unilateral lesions here result in achromatopsia, a complete loss of color vision in the contralateral hemifields. Patients see everything in shades of gray. Additionally, these patients may also present with prosopagnosia, an inability to recognize faces.

Motion and depth are processed by the magnocellular system. This "rod stream" originates in the peripheral part of the retina, relays through separate layers of the lateral geniculate, and projects to thick stripe zones of primary visual cortex. Striped areas project through the middle temporal lobe to the parietal lobe in areas 18 and 19. Lesions here result in a deficit in perceiving visual motion; visual fields, color vision, and reading are unaffected.

Clinical Correlate

Visual Agnosia

Damage to parts of the temporal lobes involving the cone stream produces a visual agnosia. Visual agnosia is the inability to recognize visual patterns (including objects) in the absence of a visual field deficit. For example, you might show a patient with an object agnosia a pair of glasses, and the patient would describe them as 2 circles and a bar. Lesions in areas 20 and 21 of the temporal lobe that also include some destruction of adjacent occipital lobe in either hemisphere result in prosopagnosia, a specific inability to recognize faces. The patient can usually read and name objects. The deficiency is an inability to form associations between faces and identities. On hearing the voice of the same person, the patient can immediately identify the person.

Alexia Without Agraphia

A principal "higher-order" deficit associated with occipital lobe damage is alexia without agraphia (or pure word blindness). The patients are unable to read at all and, curiously, often have a color anomia (inability to name colors). However, they are able to write. This is another example of a disconnect syndrome in which information from the occipital lobe is not available to the parietal or frontal lobes to either understand or express what has been seen.

(Recall that alexia *with* agraphia—inability to read or write—occurs with lesions encompassing the angular gyrus in the dominant parietal lobe.) The cause of the syndrome is usually an infarction of the left posterior cerebral artery that affects not only the anterior part of the occipital lobe but the splenium of the corpus callosum. Involvement of the left occipital cortex results in a right homonymous hemianopsia with macular sparing. Involvement of the splenium of the corpus callosum prevents visual information from the intact right occipital cortex from reaching language comprehension centers in the left hemisphere. Patients can see words in the left visual field but do not understand what the words mean.

Temporal Lobe

Primary auditory cortex

On its superior and lateral aspect, the temporal lobe contains the primary auditory cortex. Auditory cortex (areas 41 and 42) is located on the 2 transverse gyri of Heschl, which cross the superior temporal lobe deep within the lateral sulcus. Much of the remaining superior temporal gyrus is occupied by area 22 (auditory association cortex), which receives a considerable projection from both areas 41 and 42 and projects widely to both parietal and occipital cortices.

Patients with unilateral damage to the primary auditory cortex show little loss of auditory sensitivity but have some difficulty in localizing sounds in the contralateral sound field. Area 22 is a component of Wernicke area in the dominant hemisphere, and lesions here produce a Wernicke aphasia.

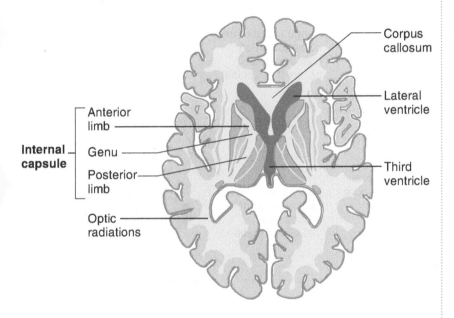

Figure III-10-12. Internal Capsule: Arterial Supply

Table III-10-2. Internal Capsule: Arterial Supply

Internal Capsule	Arterial Supply	Tracts
Anterior limb	Medial striate br. of ACA	Thalamocortical
Genu	Lenticulostriate br. of MCA	Corticobulbar
Posterior limb	Lenticulostriate br. of MCA	Corticospinal, all somatosensory thalamocortical projections

Note: The posterior cerebral artery also supplies the optic radiations.

Abbreviations: ACA, anterior cerebral artery; MCA, middle cerebral artery

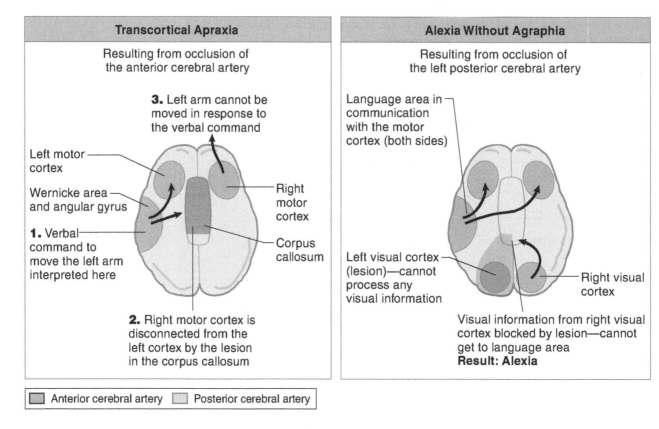

Transcortical Apraxia	Alexia Without Agraphia
Resulting from occlusion of the anterior cerebral artery	Resulting from occlusion of the left posterior cerebral artery

3. Left arm cannot be moved in response to the verbal command

Left motor cortex

Wernicke area and angular gyrus

1. Verbal command to move the left arm interpreted here

Right motor cortex

Corpus callosum

2. Right motor cortex is disconnected from the left cortex by the lesion in the corpus callosum

Language area in communication with the motor cortex (both sides)

Left visual cortex (lesion)—cannot process any visual information

Right visual cortex

Visual information from right visual cortex blocked by lesion—cannot get to language area
Result: Alexia

▢ Anterior cerebral artery   ▢ Posterior cerebral artery

Figure III-10-13. Disconnect Syndromes

Table III-10-3. CNS Blood Supply and Stroke-related Deficits

System	Primary Arteries	Branches	Supplies	Deficits after Stroke
Vertebrobasilar (posterior circulation)	**Vertebral arteries**	**Anterior spinal artery**	Anterior two-thirds of spinal cord	Dorsal columns spared; all else bilateral
		Posterior inferior cerebellar (PICA)	Dorsolateral medulla	See Brain-Stem Lesions in Chapter IV-5.
	Basilar artery	Pontine arteries	Base of pons	
		Anterior inferior cerebellar artery (AICA)	Inferior cerebellum, cerebellar nuclei	
		Superior cerebellar artery	Dorsal cerebellar hemispheres; superior cerebellar peduncle	
		Labyrinthine artery (sometimes arises from AICA)	Inner ear	
	Posterior cerebral arteries	—	Midbrain, thalamus, occipital lobe	**Contralateral hemianopia with macular sparing** Alexia without agraphia*
Internal carotid (anterior circulation)	Ophthalmic artery	Central artery of retina	Retina	Blindness
	Posterior communicating artery	—	—	Second most common **aneurysm** site (often with CN III palsy)
	Anterior cerebral artery	—	Primary motor and sensory cortex (leg/foot)	Contralateral spastic paralysis and anesthesia of **lower limb** Frontal lobe abnormalities
	Anterior communicating artery	—	—	Most common site of **aneurysm**
	Middle cerebral artery	Outer cortical	Lateral convexity of hemispheres	Contralateral spastic paralysis and anesthesia of **upper limb/face** **Gaze palsy** **Aphasia***
		Lenticulostriate	Internal capsule, caudate, putamen, globus pallidus	Gerstmann syndrome* Hemi inattention and neglect of contralateral body†

*If dominant hemisphere is affected (usually the left)

†Right parietal lobe lesion

Table III-10-4. Key Features of Lobes

Lobes	Important Regions	Deficit After Lesion
Frontal	Primary motor and premotor cortex	Contralateral spastic paresis (region depends on area of homunculus affected), premotor: apraxia
	Frontal eye fields	Eyes deviate to ipsilateral side
	Broca speech area* (Areas 44, 45)	**Broca aphasia (expressive, nonfluent aphasia):** patient can understand written and spoken language, but speech and writing are slow and effortful; patients are aware of their problem; often associated with right arm weakness and right lower face weakness.
	Prefrontal cortex	**Frontal lobe syndrome:** symptoms can include poor judgment, difficulty concentrating and problem solving, apathy, inappropriate social behavior
Parietal	Primary somatosensory cortex	Contralateral hemihypesthesia (region depends on area of homunculus affected)
	Superior parietal lobule	Contralateral astereognosis/apraxia
	Inferior parietal lobule (Angular gyrus; Area 39)	**Gerstmann syndrome** (if dominant hemisphere): right/left confusion, alexia, dyscalculia and dysgraphia, finger agnosia, contralateral hemianopia or lower quadrantanopia; unilateral neglect (nondominant)
Temporal	Primary auditory cortex	Bilateral damage → deafness Unilateral leads to slight hearing loss
	Wernicke area* (Area 22)	**Wernicke aphasia (receptive, fluent aphasia):** patient cannot understand any form of language; speech is fast and fluent, but not comprehensible
	Hippocampus	Bilateral lesions lead to inability to consolidate short-term to long-term memory
	Amygdala	**Klüver-Bucy syndrome:** hyperphagia, hypersexuality, visual agnosia
	Olfactory bulb, tract, primary cortex	Ipsilateral anosmia
	Meyer loop (visual radiations)	Contralateral upper quadrantanopia ("pie in the sky")
Occipital	Primary visual cortex	Cortical blindness if bilateral; macular sparing hemianopia

*In the dominant hemisphere. Eighty percent of people are left-hemisphere dominant.

Chapter Summary

- The external layer of the gray matter covering the surface of the cortex is characterized by numerous convolutions called gyri, separated by grooves called sulci. The cortex is divided into the frontal, parietal, occipital, and temporal lobes by several prominent sulci. Different areas of the cortex are concerned with sensory and motor functions. The frontal lobe contains the primary motor and premotor cortex, frontal eye field, and Broca speech area. The primary somatosensory and association cortex is found in the parietal lobe. The temporal lobe contains the primary auditory cortex and Wernicke area. The primary visual cortex is at the posterior pole of the occipital lobe.

- The blood supply of the cortex is supplied by branches of the 2 internal carotid arteries and 2 vertebral arteries. On the ventral surface of the brain, the anterior cerebral and middle cerebral branches of the internal carotid arteries connect with the posterior cerebral artery, derived from the basilar artery form the circle of Willis. This circle of vessels is completed by the anterior and posterior communicating arteries. The middle cerebral artery mainly supplies the lateral surface of the frontal, parietal, and upper aspect of the temporal lobe. Deep branches also supply part of the basal ganglia and internal capsule. The anterior cerebral artery supplies the medial aspect of the frontal and parietal lobes. The entire occipital lobe, lower aspect of temporal lobe, and the midbrain are supplied by the posterior cerebral artery.

- The homunculus of the motor and sensory cortex indicates that the upper limb and head are demonstrated on the lateral surface of the cortex. The pelvis and the lower limb are represented on the medial surface of the hemispheres. Therefore, the motor and sensory functions of the lower limb are supplied by the anterior cerebral artery while the motor and sensory functions of the upper limb and head are supplied by the middle cerebral artery.

- The primary language centers (Broca and Wernicke areas) are functionally located only in the dominant hemisphere, usually the left hemisphere. Both of these are supplied by the middle cerebral artery. Lesions of the Broca area result in motor or expressive aphasia (intact comprehension). Lesions of the Wernicke area produce receptive aphasia (lack of comprehension). Conduction aphasia results from a lesion of the arcuate fasciculus that connects the Broca and Wernicke areas.

- The internal capsule is a large mass of white matter that conducts almost all tracts to and from the cerebral cortex. It is divided into an anterior limb, genu, and posterior limb. The anterior limb is supplied by the anterior cerebral artery, and the genu and posterior limb are supplied by the middle cerebral artery. The primary motor and sensory systems course through the posterior limb and genu.

Limbic System 11

Learning Objectives

❑ Solve problems concerning general features

❑ Solve problems concerning olfactory system

❑ Demonstrate understanding of limbic system

GENERAL FEATURES

The limbic system is involved in emotion, memory, attention, feeding, and mating behaviors. It consists of a core of cortical and diencephalic structures found on the medial aspect of the hemisphere. A prominent structure in the limbic system is the hippocampal formation on the medial aspect of the temporal lobe. The hippocampal formation extends along the floor of the inferior horn of the lateral ventricle in the temporal lobe and includes the hippocampus, the dentate gyrus, the subiculum, and adjacent entorhinal cortex. The hippocampus is characterized by a 3-layered cerebral cortex. Other limbic-related structures include the amygdala, which is located deep in the medial part of the anterior temporal lobe rostral to the hippocampus, and the septal nuclei, located medially between the anterior horns of the lateral ventricle. The limbic system is interconnected with thalamic and hypothalamic structures, including the anterior and dorsomedial nuclei of the thalamus and the mammillary bodies of the hypothalamus. The cingulate gyrus is the main limbic cortical area. The cingulate gyrus is located on the medial surface of each hemisphere above the corpus callosum. Limbic-related structures also project to wide areas of the prefrontal cortex.

In A Nutshell

Functions of the Limbic System

- Visceral—smell

- Sex drive

- Memory/Learning

- Behavior and emotions

OLFACTORY SYSTEM

Central projections of olfactory structures reach parts of the temporal lobe without a thalamic relay and the amygdala. The olfactory nerve consists of numerous fascicles of the central processes of bipolar neurons, which reach the anterior cranial fossa from the nasal cavity through openings in the cribriform plate of the ethmoid bone. These primary olfactory neurons differ from other primary sensory neurons in 2 ways. First, the cell bodies of these neurons, which lie scattered in the olfactory mucosa, are not collected together in a sensory ganglion, and second, primary olfactory neurons are continuously replaced. The life span of these cells ranges from 30 to 120 days in mammals.

Within the mucosa of the nasal cavity, the peripheral process of the primary olfactory neuron ramifies to reach the surface of the mucous membrane. The central processes of primary olfactory neurons terminate by synapsing with neurons found in the olfactory bulb. The bulb is a 6-layered outgrowth of the brain that rests on the cribriform plate. Olfactory information entering the olfactory bulb undergoes a great deal of convergence before the olfactory tract carries axons from the bulb to parts of the temporal lobe and amygdala.

Clinical Correlate

Alzheimer disease results from neurons, beginning in the hippocampus, that exhibit neurofibrillary tangles and amyloid plaques. Other nuclei affected are the cholinergic neurons in the nucleus basalis of Meynert, noradrenergic neurons in the locus coeruleus, and serotonergic neurons in the raphe nuclei. Patients with Down syndrome commonly present with Alzheimer in middle age because chromosome 21 is one site of a defective gene.

Clinical Correlate

Olfactory deficits may be incomplete (hyposmia), distorted (dysosmia), or complete (anosmia). Olfactory deficits are caused by transport problems or by damage to the primary olfactory neurons or to neurons in the olfactory pathway to the central nervous system (CNS). Head injuries that fracture the cribriform plate can tear the central processes of olfactory nerve fibers as they pass through the plate to terminate in the olfactory bulb, or they may injure the bulb itself. Because the olfactory bulb is an outgrowth of the CNS covered by meninges, separation of the bulb from the plate may tear the meninges, resulting in cerebrospinal fluid (CSF) leaking through the cribriform plate into the nasal cavity.

LIMBIC SYSTEM

The limbic system is involved in emotion, memory, attention, feeding, and mating behaviors. It consists of a core of cortical and diencephalic structures found on the medial aspect of the hemisphere. The limbic system modulates feelings, such as fear, anxiety, sadness, happiness, sexual pleasure, and familiarity.

The Papez Circuit

A summary of the simplified connections of the limbic system is expressed by the Papez circuit (Figure III-11-1). The Papez circuit oversimplifies the role of the limbic system in modulating feelings, such as fear, anxiety, sadness, happiness, sexual pleasure, and familiarity; yet, it provides a useful starting point for understanding the system. Arbitrarily, the Papez circuit begins and ends in the hippocampus. Axons of hippocampal pyramidal cells converge to form the fimbria and, finally, the fornix. The fornix projects mainly to the mammillary bodies in the hypothalamus. The mammillary bodies, in turn, project to the anterior nucleus of the thalamus by way of the mammillothalamic tract. The anterior nuclei project to the cingulate gyrus through the anterior limb of the internal capsule, and the cingulate gyrus communicates with the hippocampus through the cingulum and entorhinal cortex.

The amygdala functions to attach an emotional significance to a stimulus and helps imprint the emotional response in memory.

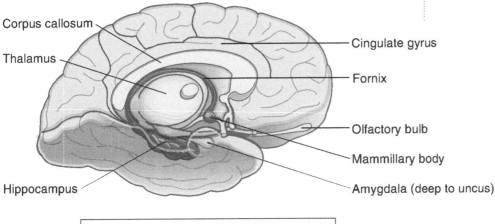

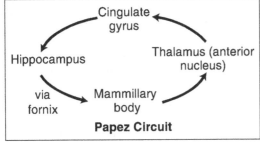

Figure III-11-1. The Limbic System and Papez Circuit

Limbic Structures and Function

- Hippocampal formation (hippocampus, dentate gyrus, the subiculum, and entorhinal cortex)
- Amygdala
- Septal nuclei
- The hippocampus is important in learning and memory. The amygdala attaches an emotional significance to a stimulus and helps imprint the emotional response in memory.

Limbic Connections

- The limbic system is interconnected with anterior and dorsomedial nuclei of the thalamus and the mammillary bodies.
- The cingulate gyrus is the main limbic cortical area.
- Limbic-related structures also project to wide areas of the prefrontal cortex.
- Central projections of olfactory structures reach parts of the temporal lobe and the amygdala.

Papez Circuit

Axons of hippocampal pyramidal cells converge to form the fimbria and, finally, the fornix. The fornix projects mainly to the mammillary bodies in the hypothalamus. The mammillary bodies project to the anterior nucleus of the thalamus (mammillo-thalamic tract). The anterior nuclei project to the cingulate gyrus, and the cingulate gyrus projects to the entorhinal cortex (via the cingulum). The entorhinal cortex projects to the hippocampus (via the perforant pathway).

Clinical Correlate

Anterograde Amnesia

Bilateral damage to the medial temporal lobes including the hippocampus results in a profound loss of the ability to acquire new information, known as anterograde amnesia.

Korsakoff Syndrome

Anterograde amnesia is also observed in patients with Korsakoff syndrome. Korsakoff syndrome is seen mainly in alcoholics who have a thiamine deficiency and often follows an acute presentation of Wernicke encephalopathy. Wernicke encephalopathy presents with ocular palsies, confusion, and gait ataxia and is also related to a thiamine deficiency. In Wernicke-Korsakoff syndrome, lesions are always found in the mammillary bodies and the dorsomedial nuclei of the thalamus.

In addition to exhibiting an anterograde amnesia, Korsakoff patients also present with retrograde amnesia. These patients confabulate, making up stories to replace past memories they can no longer retrieve.

Klüver-Bucy Syndrome

Klüver-Bucy syndrome results from bilateral lesions of the amygdala and hippocampus. These lesions result in:

- Placidity—there is marked decrease in aggressive behavior; the subjects become passive, exhibiting little emotional reaction to external stimuli.

- Psychic blindness—objects in the visual field are treated inappropriately. For example, monkeys may approach a snake or a human with inappropriate docility.

- Hypermetamorphosis—visual stimuli (even old ones) are repeatedly approached as though they were completely new.

- Increased oral exploratory behavior—monkeys put everything in their mouths, eating only appropriate objects.

- Hypersexuality and loss of sexual preference

- Anterograde amnesia

Alzheimer Disease

- Alzheimer disease accounts for 60% of all cases of dementia. The incidence increases with age.

- **Clinical:** insidious onset, progressive memory impairment, mood alterations, disorientation, aphasia, apraxia, and progression to a bedridden state with eventual death

- Five to 10% of Alzheimer cases are hereditary, early onset, and transmitted as an autosomal dominant trait.

Lesions involve the neocortex, hippocampus, and subcortical nuclei, including forebrain cholinergic nuclei (i.e., basal nucleus of Meynert). These areas show atrophy, as well as characteristic microscopic changes. The earliest and most severely affected areas are the hippocampus and temporal lobe, which are involved in learning and memory.

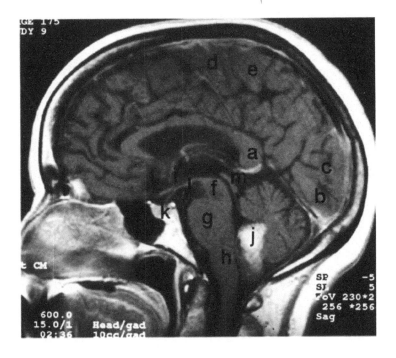

Figure III-11-2. MRI of Medial View of the Central Nervous System

(a) Corpus callosum (splenium) (b) Lingual gyrus (c) Cuneus gyrus (d) Primary motor cortex (e) Primary somatosensory cortex (f) Midbrain (g) Pons (h) Medulla (i) Hypothalamus in wall of third ventricle (j) Posterior vermis of cerebellum with intracerebral hemorrhage (k) Pituitary (l) Mammillary body (m) Pineal

Chapter Summary

- The limbic system is involved in emotion, attention, feeding, and mating behaviors. The major limbic system structures include the hippocampus, amygdala, mammillary body, cingulate gyrus, and the anterior nucleus of the thalamus. The Papez circuit represents possible connections of the limbic system between the diencephalon, temporal lobe, thalamus, and cortical areas.

- Clinical presentations of lesions related to the limbic system are Alzheimer disease, anterograde and retrograde amnesia, Korsakoff syndrome, and Klüver-Bucy syndrome.

Index

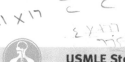